ORTHOPEDIC ASSISTANTS AND PLASTER TECHNICIANS

TEXTBOOK FOR
ORTHOPEDIC ASSISTANTS AND PLASTER TECHNICIANS

John Ebnezar

(A "Padma Shri Awardee"2016) ("Dr BC Roy National Awardee" 2015)
Honorary Doctorate in Medicine-Orthopedics (2016)
PhD(Yoga) MD(Ortho-Hons) MBBS D'Ortho DNB(Orthopedics) MNAMS Sports Medicine(Australia)
IOA-INOR Fellow(United Kingdom)

Consulting Orthopedic, Sports Specialist, Spine Surgeon and Holistic Orthopedic Expert
Geriatric Orthopedic Surgeon
Formerly, Vice-President, Indian Orthopedic Association
Founder President, Geriatric Orthopedic Society of India (GOSI)
Founder Director, Geriatric Orthopedic Association of India (GOAI)
Founder President, Orthopedic Author's Association, and All India Medical Author's Association (AIMAA)
President, Neuro-Spinal Surgeons Association of India (Karnataka)
Chairman, Swasthya Health Foundation (R); Chairman, Karnataka Orthopedic Academy®
President, Bangalore WHOlistic Academy; Chairman, Rakesh Cultural Academy
President, Vaidya Kala Ranga, Bengaluru, Karnataka, India
Former Medical Superintendent, CV Raman General Hospital, Bengaluru, Karnataka, India
Visiting Consultant, CSI Hospital, Bengaluru, Karnataka, India
CEO, Parimala Health Care Services (AN ISO 9001:2008 Hospital); India Chief Orthopedic and Spine Surgeon,
Dr John's Orthopedic Center; Chairman, Ebnezar Medical Institute, Bengaluru, Karnataka, India
Author of Over 200 Books in Orthopedics
Editor-in-Chief, Journal of the Geriatric Orthopedic Association of India Editor; Journal of Yoga and Physiotherapy
District Chairman for Health, Rotary District 3190
Guinness World Record Achiever in Book Writing—2010; 2nd World Record in Book Writing (103 Books)—2012
Guinness World Record Achiever in Social Service—2015; Guinness World Record in Social Service—2016
Two Guinness World Record Achiever in Health Awareness—2018
Winner of over 350 International, National and State Awards/Felicitations
A "Karnataka Rajyotsava Awardee—2010" (Highest Karnataka Civilian Award)

Co-author
Rakesh John

FRCS(Orthopedics) FRCS(International) MBBS MS(Orthopedics) DNB(Orthopedics) MNAMS MRCS(England) Diploma SICOT
Former Senior Resident Department of Orthopedics
Postgraduate Institute of Medical Education and Research, Chandigarh, India
Upper Limb Fellow, Wirral University Teaching Hospital, UK
Arthroscopy and Sports Medicine Fellow, QEII Hospital, Halifax, NS, Canada
Currently Consultant in Macclesfield, Cheshire, England, UK

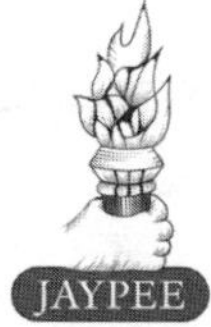

JAYPEE BROTHERS MEDICAL PUBLISHERS
The Health Sciences Publisher
New Delhi | London

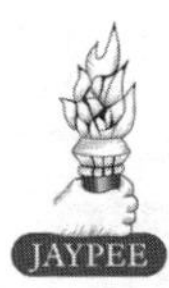 **Jaypee Brothers Medical Publishers (P) Ltd**

Headquarters
EMCA House
23/23-B, Ansari Road, Daryaganj
New Delhi 110 002, India
Landline: +91-11-23272143, +91-11-23272703
+91-11-23282021, +91-11-23245672
E-mail: jaypee@jaypeebrothers.com

Corporate Office	**Overseas Office**
Jaypee Brothers Medical Publishers (P) Ltd.	JP Medical Ltd.
4838/24, Ansari Road, Daryaganj	83, Victoria Street, London
New Delhi 110 002, India	SW1H 0HW (UK)
Phone: +91-11-43574357	Phone: +44-20 3170 8910
Fax: +91-11-43574314	Fax: +44(0)20 3008 6180
E-mail: jaypee@jaypeebrothers.com	E-mail: info@jpmedpub.com

Website: www.jaypeebrothers.com

Website: www.jaypeedigital.com

© 2025, Jaypee Brothers Medical Publishers

The views and opinions expressed in this book are solely those of the original contributor(s)/author(s) and do not necessarily represent those of editor(s) or publisher of the book.

All rights reserved. No part of this publication may be reproduced, stored or transmitted in any form or by any means, electronic, mechanical, photocopying, recording or otherwise, without the prior permission in writing of the publishers.

All brand names and product names used in this book are trade names, service marks, trademarks or registered trademarks of their respective owners. The publisher is not associated with any product or vendor mentioned in this book.

Medical knowledge and practice change constantly. This book is designed to provide accurate, authoritative information about the subject matter in question. However, readers are advised to check the most current information available on procedures included and check information from the manufacturer of each product to be administered, to verify the recommended dose, formula, method and duration of administration, adverse effects and contraindications. It is the responsibility of the practitioner to take all appropriate safety precautions. Neither the publisher nor the author(s)/editor(s) assume any liability for any injury and/or damage to persons or property arising from or related to use of material in this book.

This book is sold on the understanding that the publisher is not engaged in providing professional medical services. If such advice or services are required, the services of a competent medical professional should be sought.

Every effort has been made where necessary to contact holders of copyright to obtain permission to reproduce copyright material. If any have been inadvertently overlooked, the publisher will be pleased to make the necessary arrangements at the first opportunity.

Inquiries for bulk sales may be solicited at: jaypee@jaypeebrothers.com

Textbook for Orthopedic Assistants and Plaster Technicians / John Ebnezar, Rakesh John

First Edition: **2025**

ISBN: 978-93-5696-473-0

Printed at: Sterling Graphics Pvt. Ltd. India.

Dedicated to

My mother (Late) Sampath Kumari
Who taught me that life is more than self and
there is more joy in giving and sharing than taking.
My family and all my teachers
Who made me what I am today
and
All my students past and present

Preface

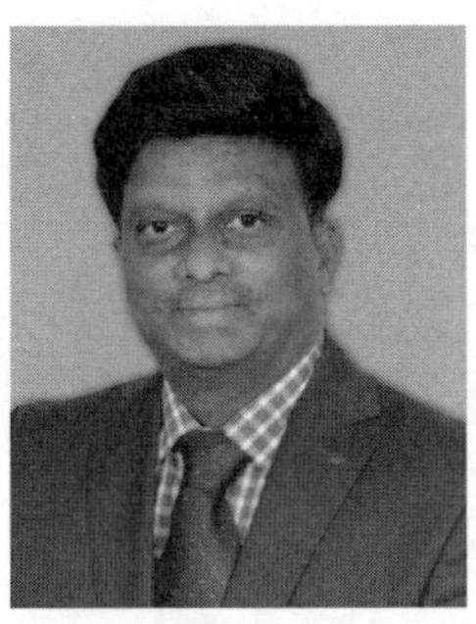

John Ebnezar
"Padma Shri Awardee",
"Dr BC Roy National
Awardee"

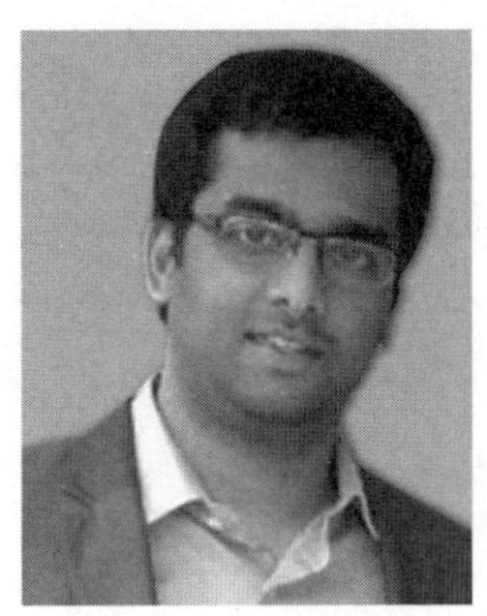

Rakesh John
Consultant
Macclesfield, Cheshire
England

I am delighted to bring this book to all those who are pursuing the plaster diploma course and are an integral part of the conservative treatment of fractures, when they either assist the orthopedic surgeons or apply the plasters themselves to the patients with fractured limbs. Plaster is very fascinating in orthopedics. In fact, while I was a young child, during a hospital round with my mother in the hospital, where she worked as a nursing tutor, I saw a plaster technician applying a plaster on a patient's forearm in the plaster room in the department of orthopedics. The white glistening plaster attracted me and I felt thrilled seeing it! I decided that I should be a part of the team that puts plasters. I desired to be a plaster boy one day and fulfill my dream of applying plaster but became a doctor. While I was a final-year MBBS student, I fell in love with orthopedics lock, stock, and barrel. The subject fascinated me so much that I was drawn toward it like a magnet. I always wanted to do something to the subject I loved most and wrote many books in the field of orthopedics. This book is a small effort on my part to train young students, who want to pursue the course of plaster technicians. Such a book is first of its kind.

Applying plaster is a skill that needs to be acquired with rigorous training and by understanding the basics of plasters and their application. This book will help the young graduates to know all about plasters and their indications, techniques, complications, and advantages. It will also help them train in the correct techniques of plaster application which is very important to avoid problems for optimum results. We hope that students will find this book very useful, and any constructive criticisms are always welcome to improve the book further.

Acknowledgments

Bringing out the first edition of the *"Textbook for Orthopedic Assistants and Plaster Technicians"* turned out to be an exciting effort. My belief that it would be a smooth sailing considering the experience of the previous book writing was proved right. Nevertheless, I ended working harder for this venture. A huge effort like this cannot be stage managed by a single person; hence, I would like to recall with gratitude the role played by these good Samaritans in making my dream a reality.

First and foremost, I would like to offer my reverence to my beloved Mother Late Smt Sampath Kumari, a disciplinarian and idealistic mother to the core. I owe my very existence and success to her. I thank my Son Rakesh John, for co-authoring this book with me. I thank all my family members for their constant support and encouragement.

I thank all my teachers who shaped my personality and career right from primary school to my postgraduation in orthopedics. I thank Ms Asfiya Sultana, my secretary, who helped me in compiling this book and I also thank all the staff of my hospital, for helping me at various stages of the writing of this book.

I thank Shri Jitendar P Vij (Group Chairman), Mr Ankit Vij (Managing Director), Dr Madhu Choudhary (Director—Publishing), and Dr Sangeeta Yadav (Development Editor). My special thanks go to M/s Jaypee Brothers Medical Publishers (P) Ltd, New Delhi, India, for kindly agreeing to publish this book and accomplishing the task in a splendid manner.

I thank all the teachers and students for patronizing and supporting my book. Finally, I thank the God Almighty, for all the blessings and the gift of life.

John Ebnezar

Contents

Section II: Practical Orthopedics

Upper Limbs

Lower Limbs

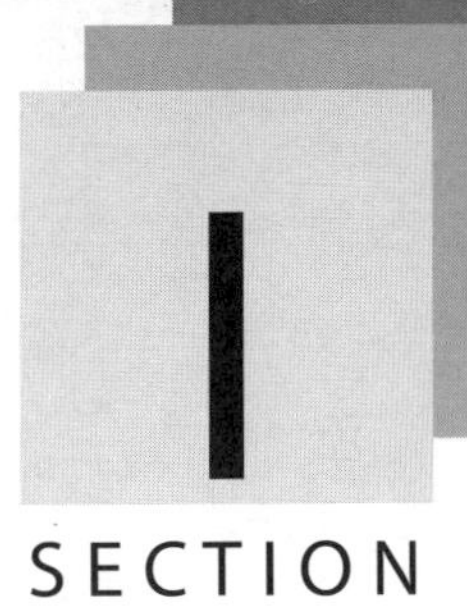

THEORY

SECTION OUTLINE

Traumatic

History Taking

History taking in medicine and in orthopedics is the most important aspect of making a diagnosis. It is not just form filling; it is an art which needs to be developed by students **(Fig. 1.1)**.

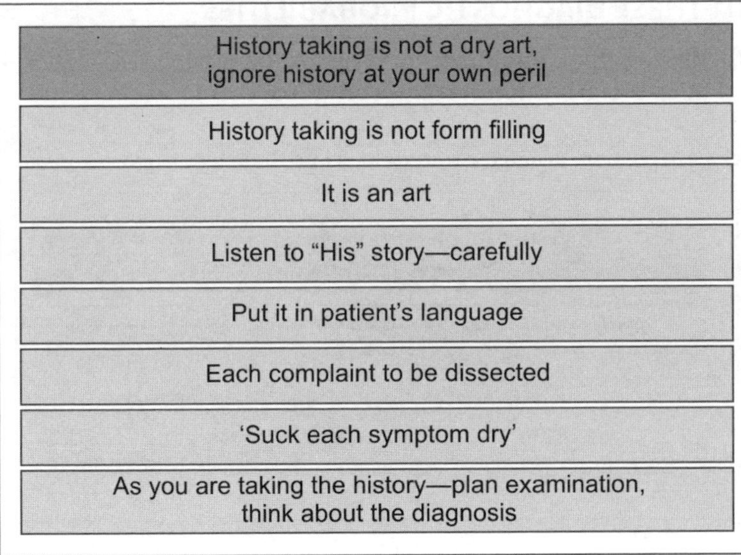

Fig. 1.1: History taking is an art.

COMPONENTS OF HISTORY TAKING

History taking has three components.
History triad: Present, past, others—family, socioeconomic, personal and occupational **(Fig. 1.2)**.

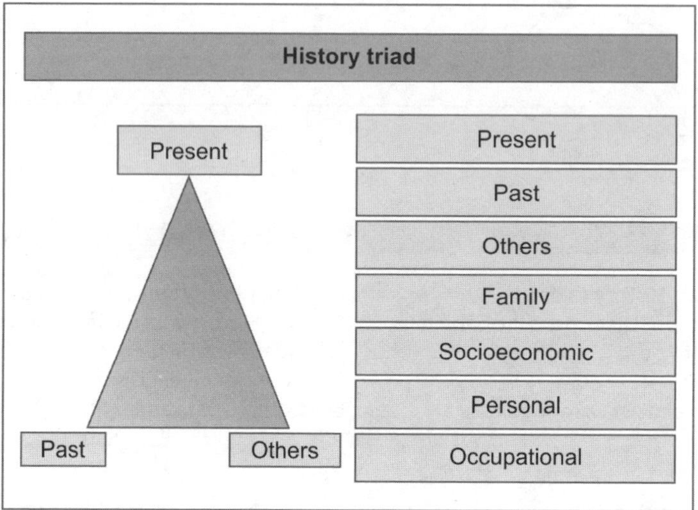

Fig. 1.2: History triad.

KNOW ABOUT THESE DIAGNOSTIC PROBABILITIES

Before taking the history, look into these for diagnostic possibilities—age, sex, occupation, nationality, education, social economic status **(Flowchart 1.1)**.

Flowchart 1.1: Before taking the history, look into these for diagnostic possibilities.

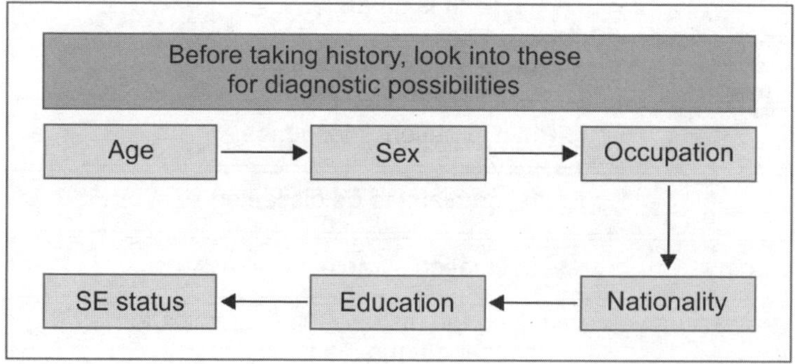

IMPORTANCE OF AGE

Age gives away vital diagnostic clues—looking at the age of the patient gives a bird's eye—view of the possible diagnosis, e.g., hip—in children, young adults (STAIIR) **(Fig. 1.3)**.

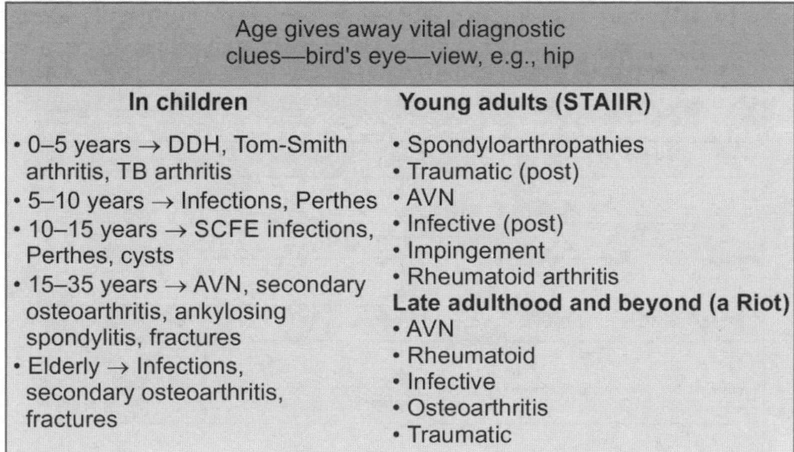

Fig. 1.3: Age gives away vital diagnostic clues—bird's eye—view, e.g., hip.

IMPORTANCE OF SEX

Sex predilection: Females—SLE, rheumatoid; males—spondyloarthropathy **(Fig. 1.4)**.

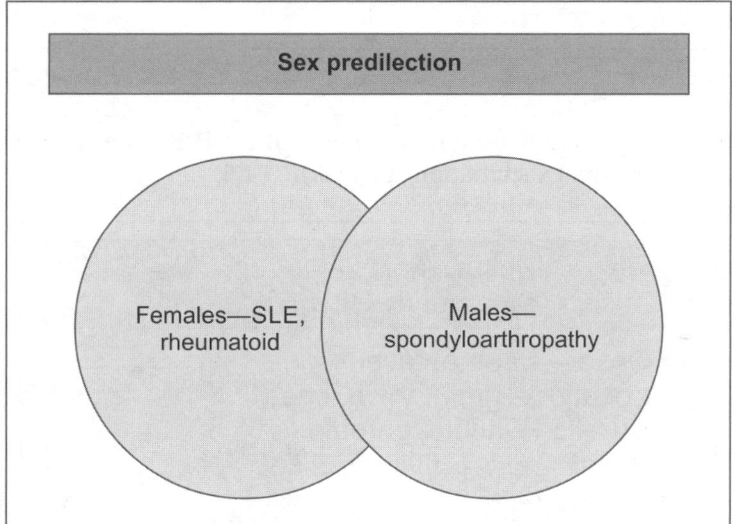

Fig.1. 4: Sex predilection.

TYPICAL COMPLAINTS IN ORTHOPEDICS

Complaints in order of importance—pain, early morning stiffness, limp, swelling, limb length discrepancy, deformity, inability to squat, inability to walk **(Flowchart 1.2)**.

Flowchart 1.2: Typical complaints in orthopedics—complaints in order of importance.

```
Typical complaints in orthopedics:
Compliants in order of importance
            ↓
           Pain
            ↓
   Early morning stiffness
            ↓
           Limp
            ↓
         Swelling
            ↓
  Limb length discrepancy
            ↓
         Deformity
            ↓
     Inability to squat
            ↓
     Inability to walk
```

Pain: What to look for? Remember the mnemonic—**OLD RIPE**—Onset, Location, Duration, Relief, Intensity, Progression, Exacerbation **(Fig. 1.5)**.

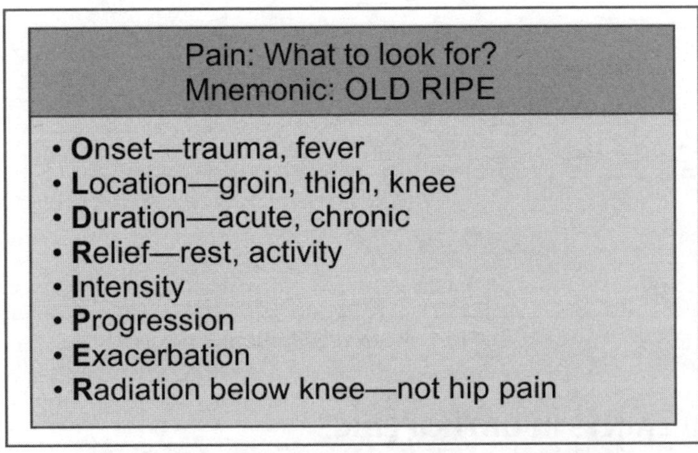

Fig. 1.5: Pain: What to look for? Mnemonic: OLD RIPE.

Morning stiffness: Duration gives you the clue—1 hour—RA, 1 hour—OA **(Fig. 1.6)**.

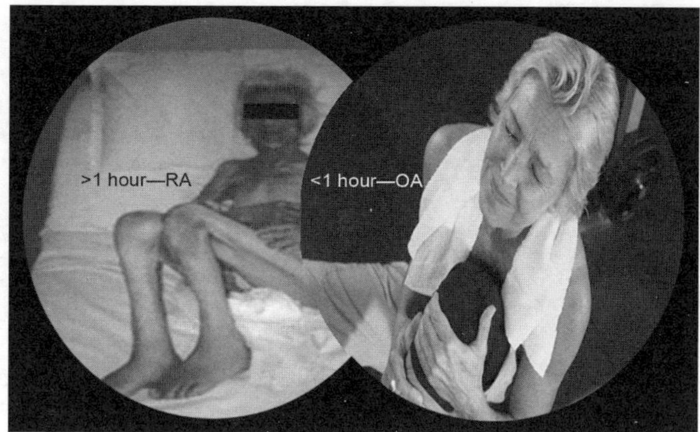

Fig. 1.6: Morning stiffness—duration gives you the clue.

Limp: Onset, duration, severity, progression, walking affected or not affected, associated or not associated with pain **(Flowchart 1.3)**.

Flowchart 1.3: Limp.

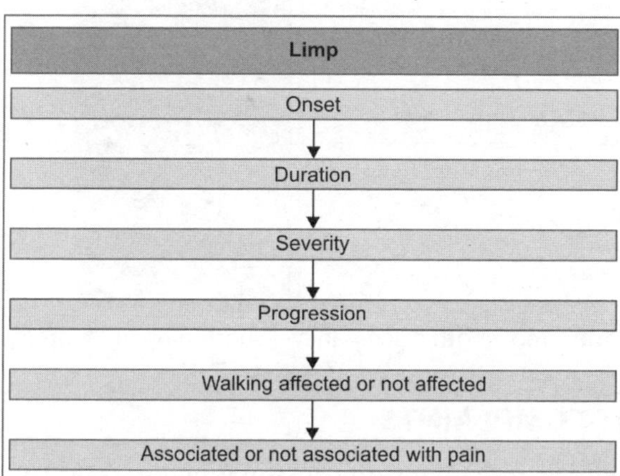

Hip Conditions

Hip conditions causing it—painful, painless **(Flowchart 1.4)**.

Flowchart 1.4: Limp—hip conditions.

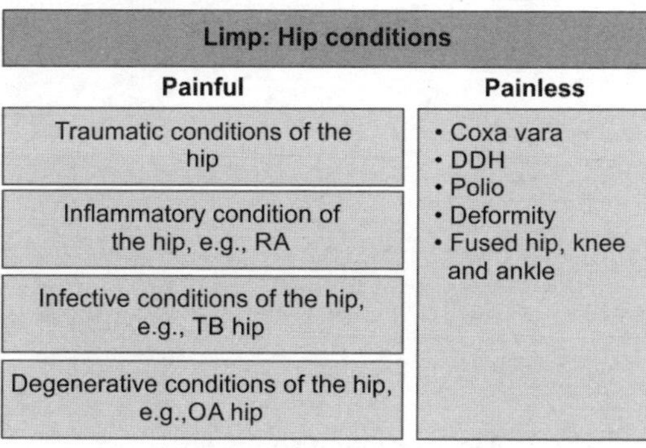

Swelling: Onset, progression, duration, pain, site **(Fig. 1.7)**.

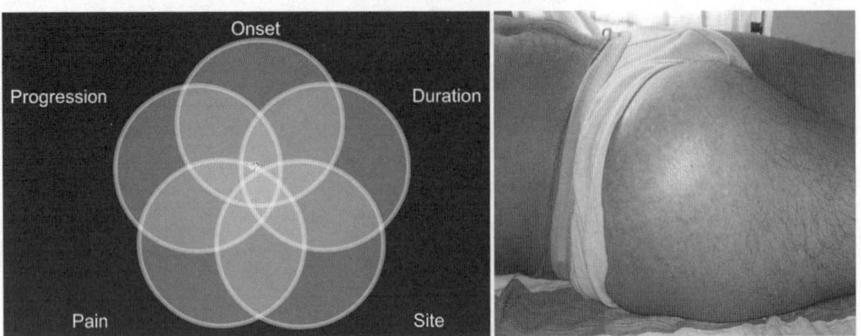

Fig. 1.7: Swelling.

Limb length discrepancy: Shortening or lengthening?—One side/both sides, duration, pain, progression, limp **(Fig. 1.8)**.

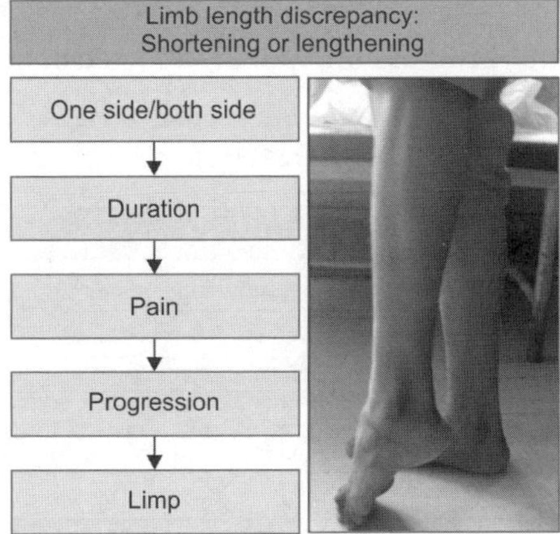

Fig. 1.8: Limb length discrepancy—shortening or lengthening?

OTHER IMPORTANT COMPLAINTS

Inability to squat, inability to walk, deformity, loss of function **(Fig. 1.9)**.

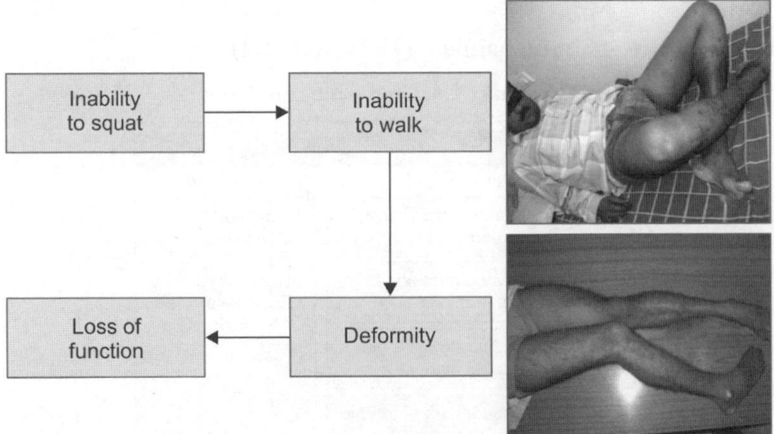

Fig. 1.9: Other complaints.

PAST HISTORY AND ITS IMPORTANCE

Past history: We are told not to brood into the past, but not here—TB, any systemic illness, bleeding diseases, surgery, trauma, drugs steroids—can lead to AVN, flare up of TB **(Fig. 1.10)**.

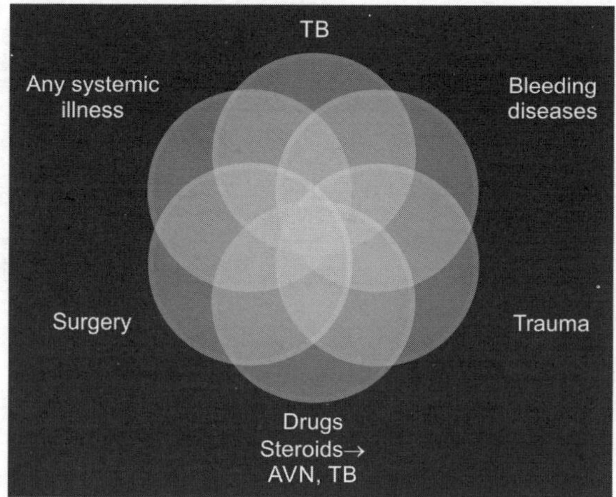

Fig. 1.10: Past history—we are told not to brood into the past, but not here.

Family History and Its Relevance

Family history has a relevance—tuberculosis, spondyloarthropathy, gout, RA, ankylosing spondylitis, etc. **(Fig. 1.11)**.

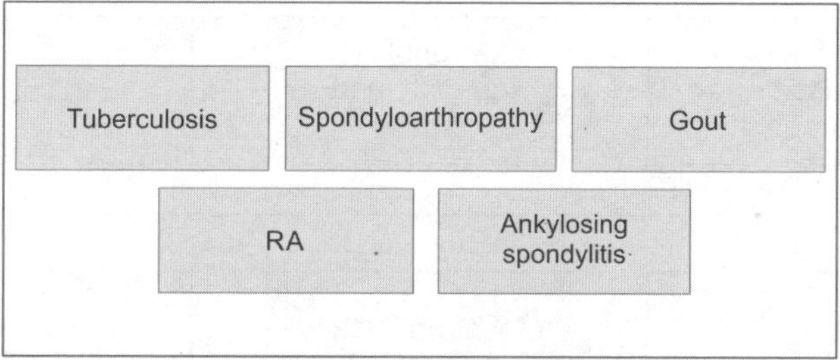

Fig. 1.11: Family history has a relevance.

Socioeconomic history: Rich, average, BPL, poor has diagnostic relevance **(Fig. 1.12)**.

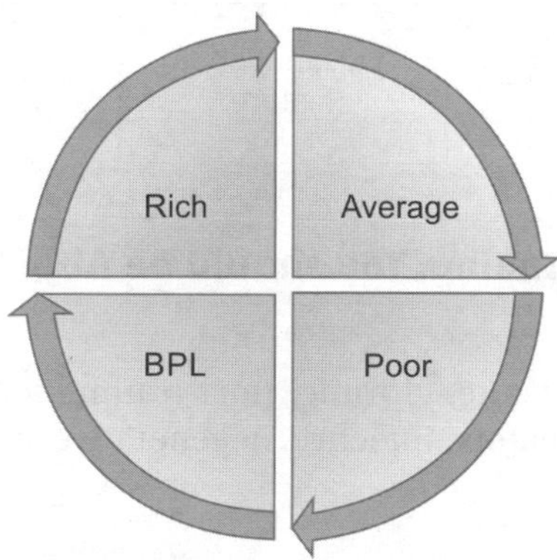

Fig. 1.12: Socioeconomic history.

TREATMENT HISTORY

For tuberculosis, for any chronic hip or spine conditions, regularity of treatment, duration of treatment, complications and side effects **(Flowchart 1.5)**.

Flowchart 1.5: Treatment history.

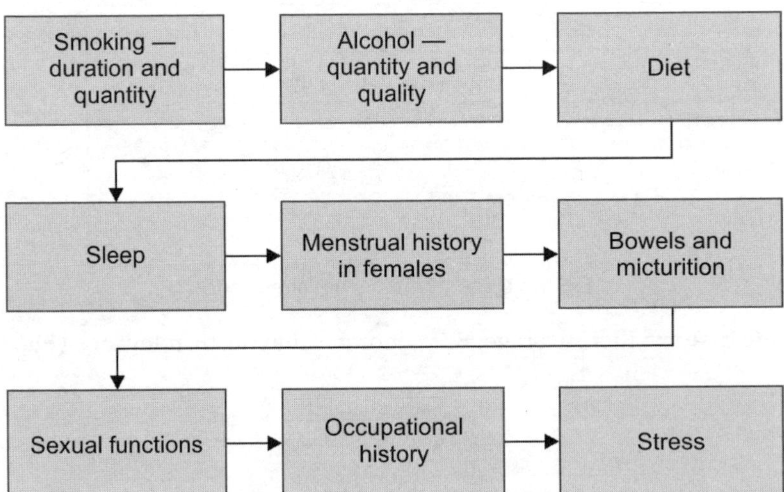

IMPORTANCE OF PERSONAL HISTORY

Smoking—duration and quantity, alcohol—quantity and quality, diet, sleep, menstrual history in females, bowels and micturition, sexual functions, occupational history, stress, etc. **(Flowchart 1.6)**.

Flowchart 1.6: Personal history.

At the End of the History Taking, You should be Able to Arrive at a Probable Diagnosis

Types of disease—acute, subacute, chronic, post-traumatic, non-traumatic. If chronic—congenital, metabolic, inflammatory, infective, degenerative, tumor **(Flowchart 1.7)**.

Flowchart 1.7: At the end of history taking, you need to make a likely diagnosis.

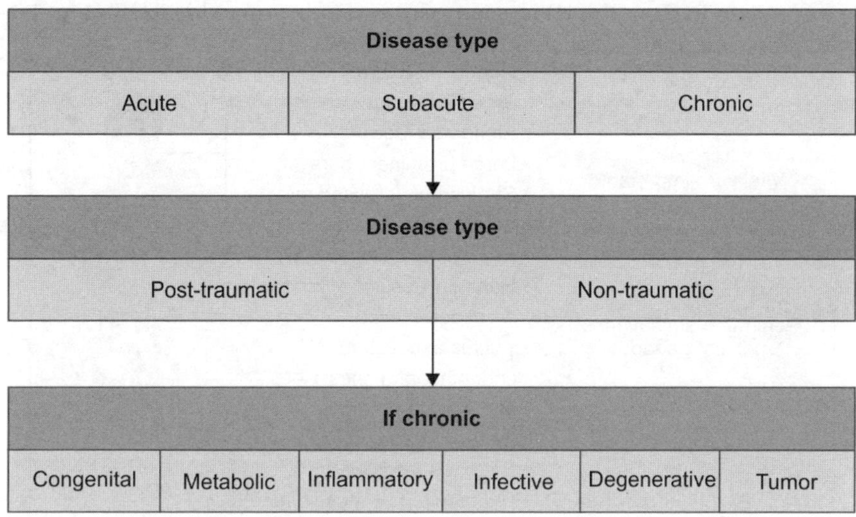

After History, it is Examination (Fig. 1.13)

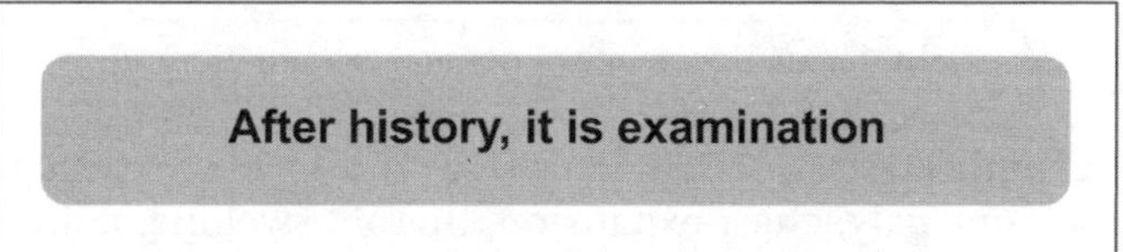

Fig. 1.13: After history, it is examination.

SCHEME OF EXAMINATION

Vitals, general examination, gait, look, feel, move **(Flowchart 1.8)**.

Flowchart 1.8: Scheme of examination.

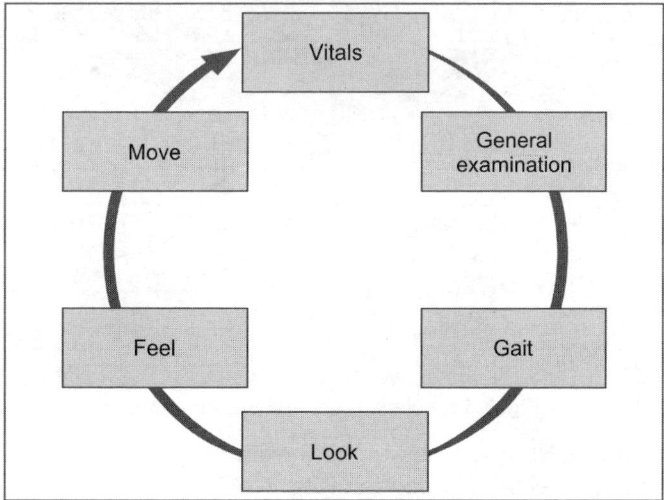

Importance of general examination: Vitals are important, general examination is not just general. It can lead on to something very concrete and help you to localize!! **(Fig. 1.14)**.

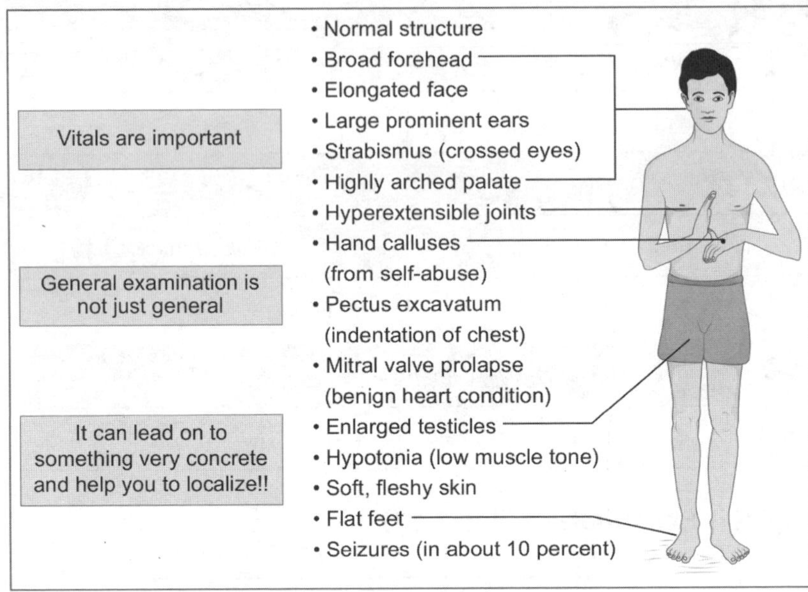

Fig. 1.14: Importance of general examination.

Relevant general examination: Anemia, icterus, cyanosis, blue sclera, lymphadenopathy, cachexia, hepatosplenomegaly, chest expansion, thyroid swelling, nails—clubbing/pitting, high arched palate, pectus excavatum **(Fig. 1.15)**.

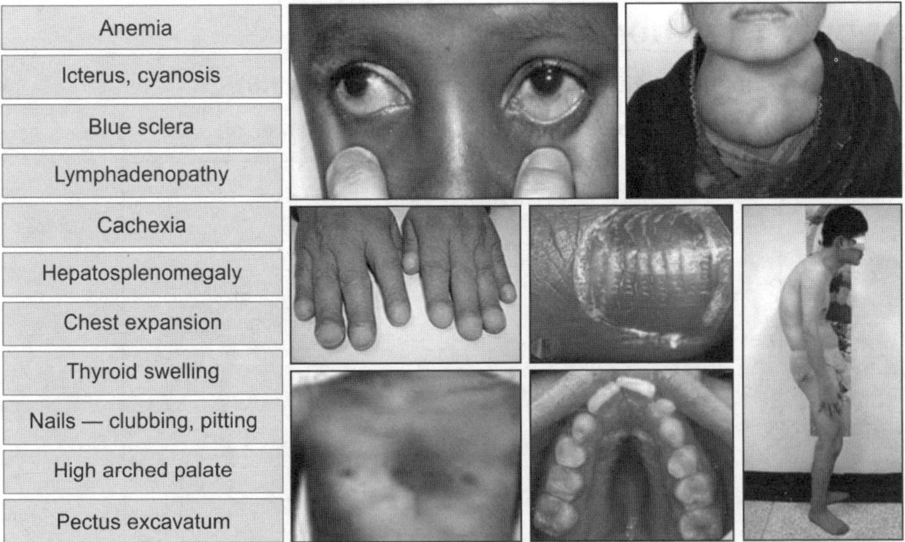

Fig. 1.15: Relevant general examination.

Systemic examination: CNS examination, CVS examination, per abdomen examination, genitourinary systems, per rectal examination **(Fig. 1.16)**.

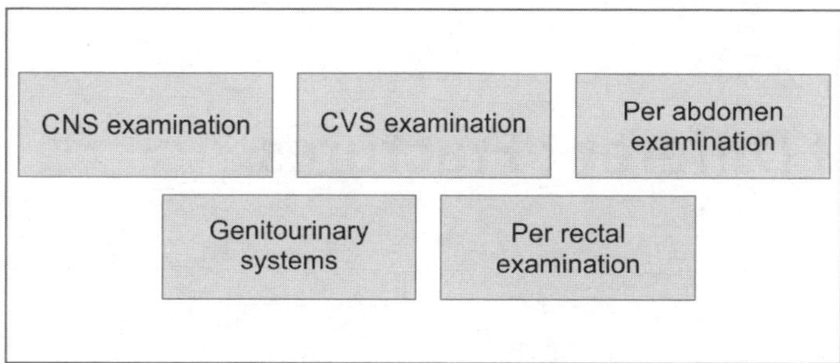

Fig. 1.16: Systemic examination.

Local Examination

After general examination it is time for local examination. Cardinal points—look, feel, move, measure **(Fig. 1.17)**.

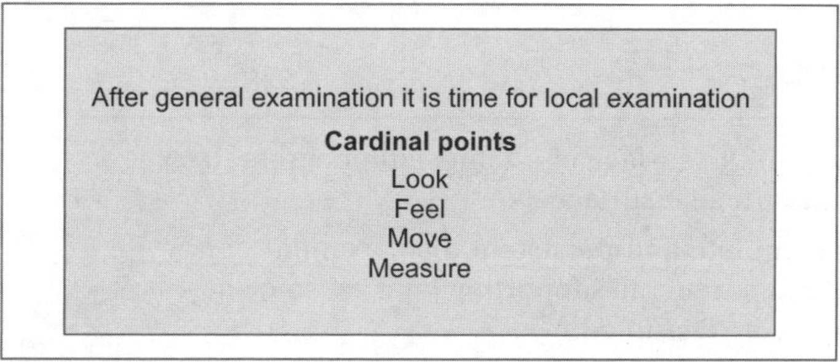

Fig. 1.17: After general examination it is time for local examination.

A careful history taking and systematic examination both general, systemic and local helps a student to arrive at a diagnosis. Unfortunately this art is lost in today's world of investigations. Students should learn to make a clinical diagnosis and not become slave of investigations.

Details of Different Fractures

DEFINITIONS

Fracture is a break in the surface of a bone, either across its cortex or through its articular surface.

Dislocation is a complete and persistent displacement of a joint in which at least part of the supporting joint capsule and some of its ligaments are disrupted.

Subluxation is a partial dislocation of a joint.

Sprain is the temporary subluxation of a joint and the articular surfaces return to normal alignment.

Strain is a tear in the muscle.

The bone can break within its soft tissue envelope and may not communicate to the exterior *(simple* or *closed fractures)* **(Fig. 2.1A)** or it may rip through its soft tissues or the soft tissue itself may be damaged by the external forces, exposing the bone to the external atmosphere *(compound* or *open fractures)* **(Fig. 2.1B)**.

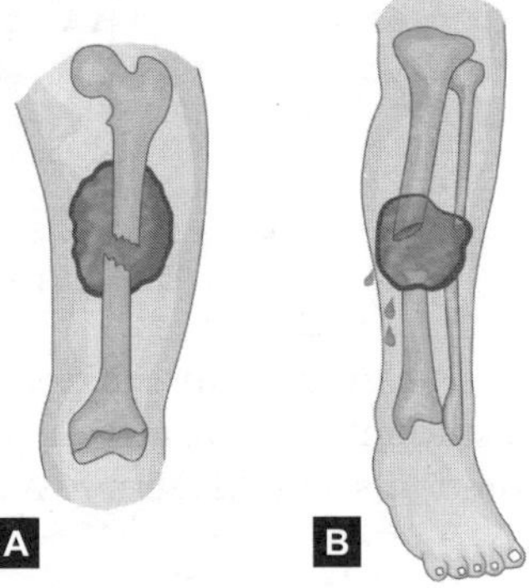

Figs. 2.1A and B: Simple and compound fractures.

Remember

Force required to break a bone could be:
- Large and sudden (e.g., RTA).
- Repetitive (e.g., a stress fracture).
- Trivial (e.g., pathological fractures).

TYPES OF FRACTURE

1. **Simple or compound (Figs. 2.2A and B)**—this has already been explained.
2. **Based on the extent of fracture line.**
   - *Incomplete fractures*—it involves only one surface or cortex of the bone.
   - *Complete fracture*—here the fracture involves the entire bone. A complete fracture could be *undisplaced* or *displaced*.

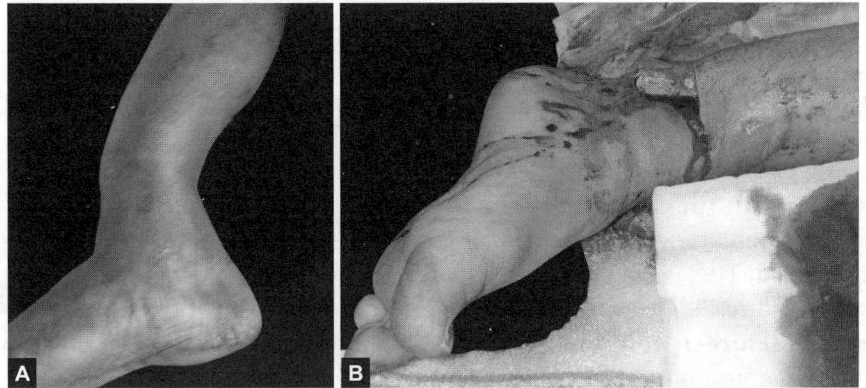

Figs. 2.2A and B: Clinical photograph showing: (A) Simple fracture; and (B) Compound fracture of the tibia.

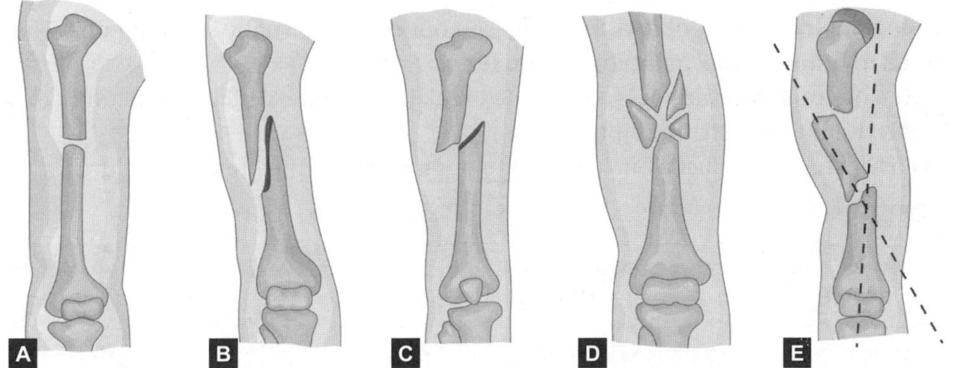

Figs. 2.3A to E: Types of fractures based on fracture patterns: (A) Transverse; (B) Spiral; (C) Oblique; (D) Comminuted; (E) Segmental fractures.

Causes for displacement

- Muscle forces.
- Gravity.
- Obliquity of the fracture line.
- Improper handling of the fracture.

3. **Based on fracture patterns [orthopedic trauma association classification (Figs. 2.3A to E)].**
   - *Linear fractures:* These could be *transverse, oblique or spiral.* Any fracture, which forms an angle less than 30° with the horizontal line, is called transverse. Angle equal to or more than 30° is termed oblique.
   - *Comminuted fractures:* Here the fracture fragments are more than two in number. They are further subclassified into *≤50% comminution* or more than *50% comminution. Butterfly-shaped fractures* are also included in this group.
   - *Segmental fractures:* A fracture can break into segments and the segment could be two levels, three levels, and a longitudinal split or comminuted.
   - *Bone loss:* This could be a <50% bone loss or >50% bone loss or a complete bone loss.

Atypical Fractures (Figs. 2.4A to D)

* **Greenstick fractures:** It is seen exclusively in children. Here the bone is elastic and usually bends due to buckling or breaking of one cortex when a force is applied. This is called a greenstick fracture.
* **Impacted fractures:** Here the fracture fragments are impacted into each other and are not separated and displaced.

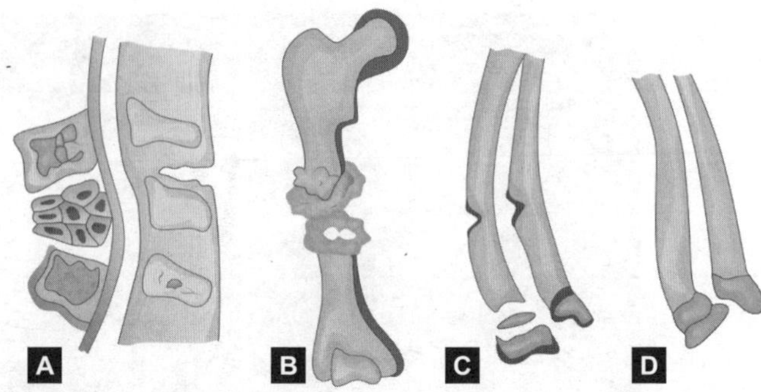

Figs. 2.4A to D: Showing atypical fractures: (A) Compression; (B) Pathological; (C) Greenstick; (D) Torus fractures.

* **Stress or fatigue fracture:** It is usually an incomplete fracture commonly seen in athletes and in bones subjected to chronic and repetitive stress (e.g., third metatarsal fracture, fracture tibia, etc.).
* **Pathological fracture:** It occurs in a diseased bone and is usually spontaneous. The force required to bring about a pathological fracture is trivial.
* **Hair line or crack fracture:** It is a very fine break in the bone, which is difficult to diagnose clinically. Radiology usually helps.
* **Torus fracture:** This is just a buckling of the outer cortex of the bones in children.

> **Remember**
> - Greenstick fracture—occurs in children.
> - Torus fracture—buckling of outer cortex in children.
> - Stress fracture—common in athletes.
> - Fatigue fractures—in occupations like police, nurse, etc.
> - Pathological fractures—usually seen in elderly people.
> - Hair line or crack fracture—is a special variety of incomplete fracture.

DISPLACEMENT OF FRACTURES

A complete fracture usually is displaced due to various factors already mentioned. Depending on the direction of force, mode of injury, pull of the muscles, a fracture can show any one of the following displacements or angulation **(Figs. 2.5A to D)**.

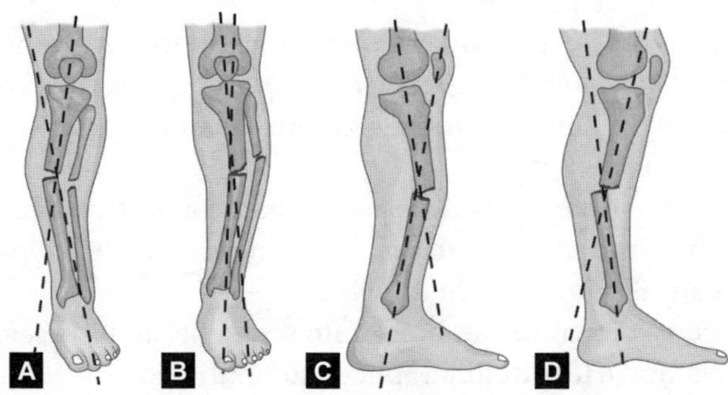

Figs. 2.5A to D: Showing types of angulation in fractures: (A) Medial; (B) Lateral; (C) Anterior; (D) Posterior.

❖ Anterior angulations or displacement.
❖ Posterior angulations or displacement.
❖ Varus or medial angulations or displacement.
❖ Valgus or lateral displacement or angulations.
❖ Shortening.
❖ Translational.

Note: Deformities following fractures are due to displacements of the bone fragments.

Fracture Healing and its Problems

"Fracture healing is as fascinating as fracture happening!"

GENERAL STRUCTURE OF A BONE

The general structure of a bone has an epiphysis and epiphyseal plate (which disappears with growth), metaphysis and diaphysis **(Fig. 3.1)**.

Epiphysis: This is an expanded portion at the end develops usually under pressure and forms a support for the joint surface. It is easily affected by developmental problems like epiphyseal dysplasias, trauma, overuse, degeneration and damaged blood supply. The end result is distorted joints due to avascular necrosis and degenerative changes.

Growth plate (physis) though mechanically weak it helps longitudinal growth. It responds to growth and sex hormones. It is affected by conditions like osteomyelitis, tumor, slipped epiphysis resulting in short stature or deformed growth or growth arrest.

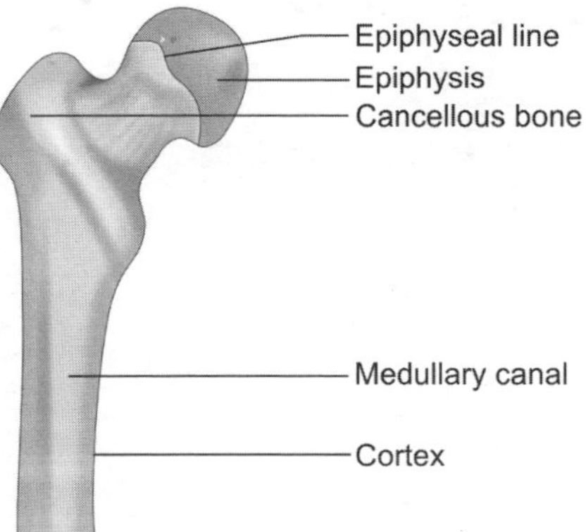

Fig. 3.1: General structure of a bone.

Metaphysis: This is concerned with remodeling of bone. It is the cancellous portion and heals readily. It gives attachment to ligament and tendons. It is vulnerable to develop osteomyelitis, dysplasias and tumors resulting in distorted growth and altered bone shapes.

Diaphysis: This is a significant compact cortical bone which is strong in compression and which gives origin to muscles. It forms the shafts of the bones. Healing is slow when compared to metaphysis. In remodeling it can remodel angulations but not rotation. It may develop fractures, dysplasias, infection and rarely tumors. The internal structure of the bone is depicted in **Figure 3.2**.

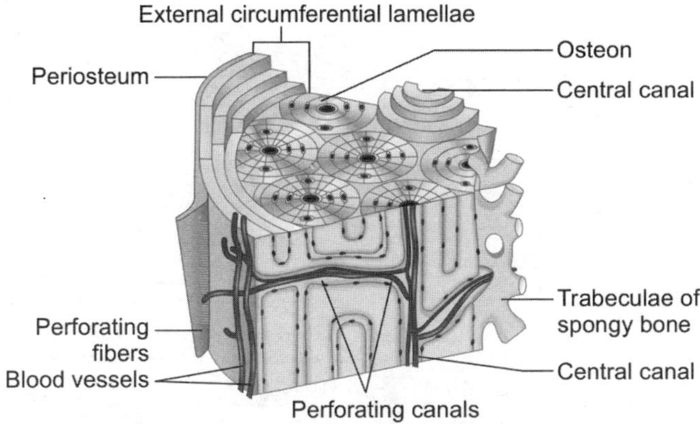

Fig. 3.2: Bone cross section showing its internal structure.

Organization of the bones: They are 206 in number and are grouped into two subdivisions namely:

1. Axial skeleton—80 bones.
2. Appendicular skeleton—126 bones

Axial skeleton forms the upright axis of the body and the *appendicular skeleton* forms the *appendages* and *girdles* that attach them to the axial skeleton **(Fig. 3.3)**.

Out of these 206, some of us are short and some are long. We have different shapes. The shape and size depend upon the functions attributed to us.

Blood supply to the bones: A typical long bone derives its blood supply from the following important sources:

1. **Peripheral:** This is through the periosteal vessels which penetrate the cortex in adults.
2. **Central:** This is through the nutrient artery which seeks entry into a long bone at the middle, divides into two and proceeds to either ends of the bones. They divide into many branches near the ends of the growth plates.
3. **Ends:** Here the blood supply is through two sources:
   a. *Epiphyseal vessels:* These vessels enter straight into the epiphysis.
   b. *Metaphyseal vessels:* From in and around the vascular anastomosis near the joints, some vessels pierce the metaphysis at their capsular attachments.

Thus bones have abundant and rich blood supply which gets disrupted during injuries **(Fig. 3.2)**.

A 'Quick Vascular Recap'—a long bone has four important blood supplies:	
1. Nutrient artery	3. Metaphyseal vessels
2. Periosteal vessels	4. Epiphyseal vessels

TYPES OF BONES (FIGS. 3.4A TO C)

Flat bones (Fig. 3.4A), e.g., scapula, skull, etc.

Irregular bones (Figs. 3.4B), e.g., pelvic bones.

Sesamoid bones: Their name is derived from their resemblance to "sesame seeds", e.g., patella (largest and most definitive of the sesamoid bones).

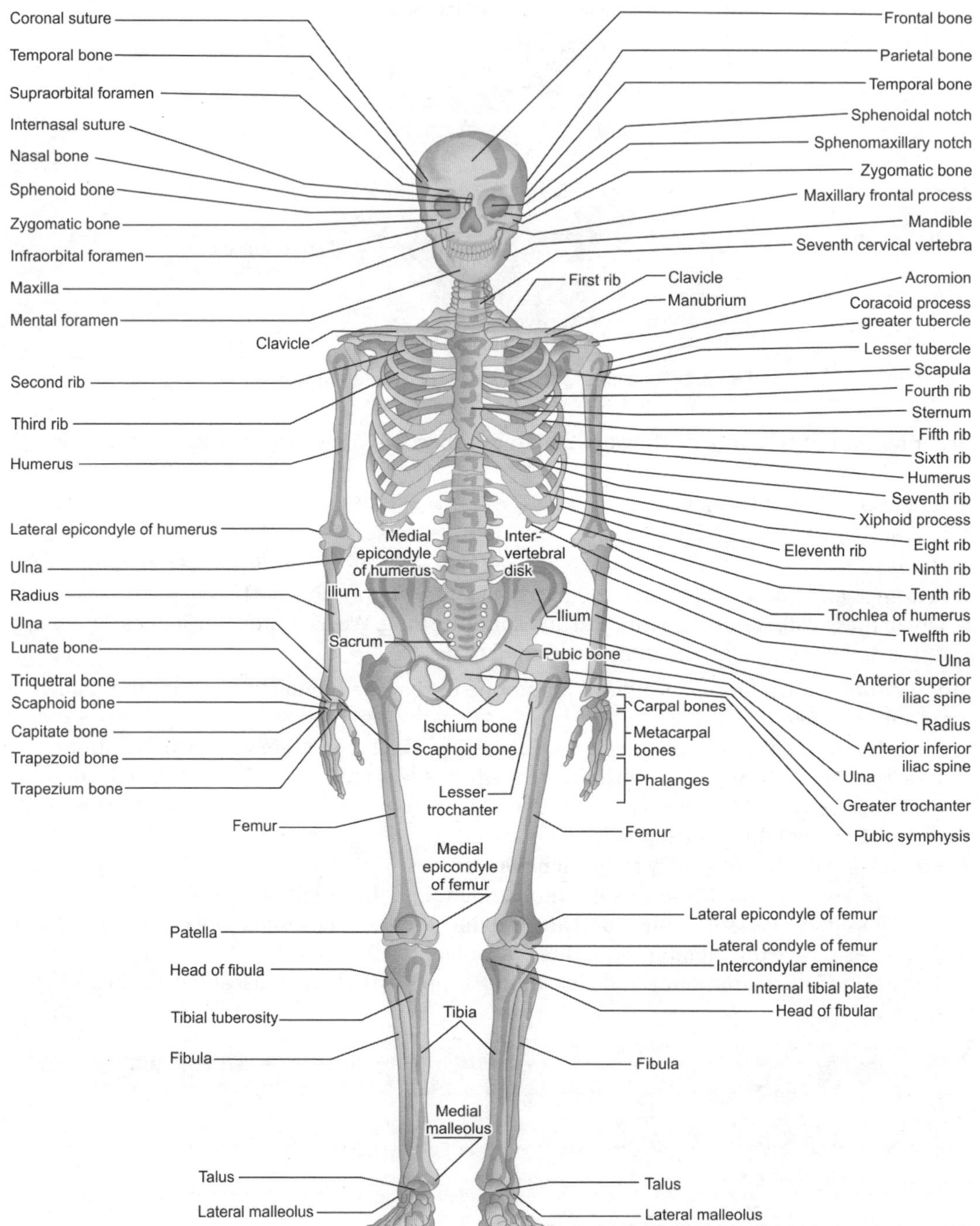

Fig. 3.3: Showing human skeletal framework (axial and appendicular).

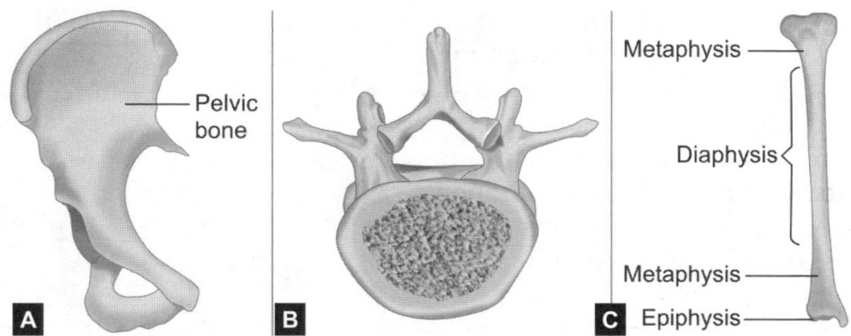

Figs. 3.4A to C: Types of bone: (A) Flat bone; (B) Irregular bone; (C) Long bone.

Long bones (Fig. 3.4C): These serve as levers for the muscle action, e.g., femur, tibia, etc.

Short bones: Their principle role is to provide strength **(Fig. 3.2)**.

FRACTURE HEALING

Bone is repaired by *callus* which is a new tissue that may develop externally or internally. An *external callus* envelops around the outer aspect of the opposing ends of bone fragments. An *internal callus* forms between the bone ends.

During the first two days at the fracture sites and away from the fracture site, in the deep layer of periosteum the *osteogenic cells* proliferate and lift the fibrous layer of the periosteum away from the bone. *Marrow cells* also proliferate but to a lesser degree. These osteogenic cells differentiate into *osteoblasts* which form the bone trabeculae resembling the embryonic tissue. The osteogenic cells lying away from the fracture site due to *inadequate vascularity* differentiate into chondroblasts and chondrocytes which form the cartilage. The cartilage is finally converted into bone by endochondral ossification.

The internal callus is formed by the mesenchymal cells which convert into pro-osteoblasts and later to osteoblasts laying down new bone. *Remodeling* is an activity of *osteoclasts* which slowly remove the necrotic bone and create cavities. Osteoblasts line these cavities and lay new bone.

Methods of Fracture Healing in a Cortical Bone

A fracture in a cortical bone heals by three ways, indirect, direct and distraction histogenesis as described by Ilizarov.

Indirect Fracture

This is the common method of fracture healing where both external and internal callus are formed. Fractures treated by conservative methods heal by this method **(Fig. 3.5)**. Hunter has described six stages in this method of healing **(Figs. 3.6A to F)**.

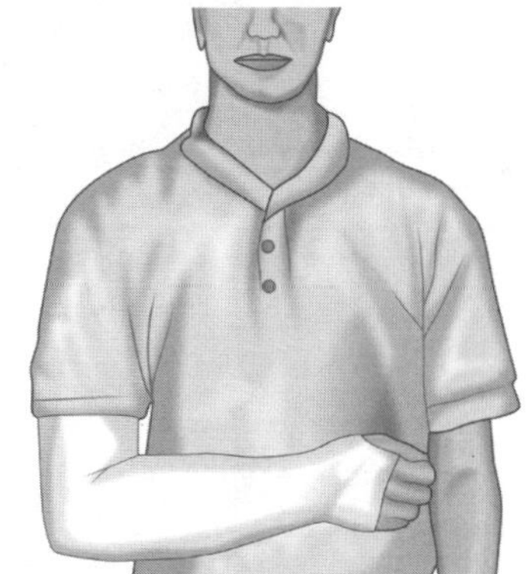

Fig. 3.5: This is an example of fracture healing by indirect method.

1. **Stage of impact:** This stage extends from the moment of impact till the complete dissipation of energy causing fractures.
2. **Stage of induction:** Following fractures cells possessing osteogenic potential are activated. Other inducing factors are BMP (bone morphogenic protein), fall in oxygen tension and bioelectric effects.
3. **Stage of inflammation:** In this stage the disruption of blood supply results in necrosis of the bone ends. There is hemorrhage, cellular proliferation and vascular ingrowths.

4. **Stage of soft callus:** Here the hematoma is organized with fibrous tissue, cartilage and woven bone. Fragments are united with fibrous or cartilaginous tissue or both.
5. **Stage of hard callus:** Bone fragments are firmly united with bone. If immobilization is complete, membranous bone healing takes place. If incomplete bone heals by endochondral ossification.
6. **Stage of remodeling:** Here fiber bone is converted to lamellar bone. Medullary canal is reconstituted and callus diameter begins to decrease in size which takes few months to several years. However, there will be no remodeling of rotational malalignment.

Primary Bone Healing (Direct Bone Healing, Healing by Primary Intention)

Figs. 3.6A to F: Hunter' stages of fracture healing: (A) Stage of induction; (B) Stage of inflammation; (C) Stage of soft callus; (D) Stage of hard callus; (E) Stage of remodeling; (F) Normal.

This type of bone repair is seen when bone fragments are anatomically reduced by open methods and rigidly fixed. This cannot be obtained by closed methods of fracture treatment but can be achieved by operative reduction and fixation with special techniques of plate and screws. Here ideally no external callus forms and there is no interposing fibrous tissue or cartilage tissue between the fracture sites. The fracture site is bridged by direct haversian remodeling which is almost a direct osteon to osteon hookup. The osteoclasts act as cutter heads to remove the bone and are in the forefront promptly followed by osteoblasts behind laying down new bone. This type of bone healing usually occurs in fractures treated by AO techniques developed by Swiss association for osteosynthesis **(Fig. 3.7)**.

Distraction Histogenesis (Fig. 3.8): Distraction histogenesis is a recent concept described by Ilizarov. Here bone repair is induced by gradual distraction of osteotomies and fracture

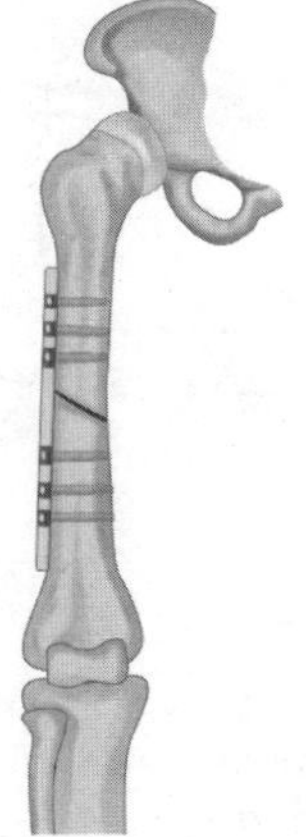

Fig. 3.7: This is an example of direct healing.

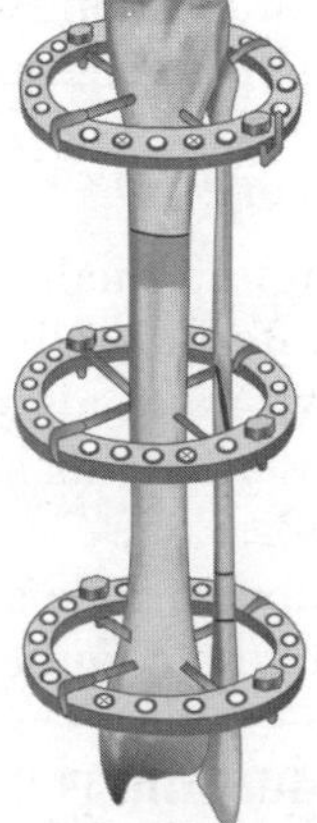

Fig. 3.8: Showing healing by distraction histogenesis.

after an interval of induction of say 5–7 days. For osteogenesis to occur the fracture or osteotomy must be stabilized and a slow distraction at the rate of 1 mm per day should be given.

Fracture Healing in Cancellous Bones

Mercifully fractures in cancellous bones generally unite well. In them the healing does not pass through the stage of callus and the bones unite readily. Unlike in the cortical bones, union in cancellous bones is direct and fast. The reasons being these bones have spongy constitution, have abundant blood supply and there is no medullary cavity. This increases the area of contact between the trabecular ends of the bones. The fracture hematoma is converted directly into bone by the mature osteoblasts.

Factors Influencing Healing is Features

Fracture healing is influenced by so many fractures some favorable and some unfavorable **(Box 3.1)**. Some of the important factors are:

- ❖ **Age:** In children the fractures unite readily. For reasons see chapters as fractures in children.
- ❖ **Type of fracture:** In terms of union, the incidence of good fractures union is as follows. Communited> segmented> oblige> transverse.
- ❖ **Type of bone:** Fracture in cancellous bones unite readily than cortical bones for other fracture.

<table>
<tr><td>Box 3.1: Factors affecting fracture repair.</td></tr>
</table>

Factors favoring union
- ◄◄ Adequate circulation
- ◄◄ Good reduction and fixations
- ◄◄ Hormones like growth hormone, parathormone, thyroxin, etc.
- ◄◄ Good nutrition and mineral supplements help passively
- ◄◄ Cancellous bone heal niece
- ◄◄ Bioelectric fixation

Factors detrimental to union
- ◄◄ Compound fractures
- ◄◄ Advanced age
- ◄◄ Poor circulation
- ◄◄ Infection
- ◄◄ Distraction
- ◄◄ Segmental fractures
- ◄◄ Comminution
- ◄◄ Osteoporosis
- ◄◄ Soft tissue interposition
- ◄◄ Inadequate and improper reduction and immobilization, etc.

Emergency Care of Fractures

FIRST AID

"First aid is the initial care of the injured at the scene of accident."

Anybody can give first aid, but to carry out cardiopulmonary resuscitation measures one should be trained in first aid and should possess a valid certificate issued by a competent body. First aid executed by a medical person is called a *medical aid.*

Goals of First Aid Treatment—is Aptly Described by Three Ps

❖ **P**reserve life by carrying out appropriate resuscitative measures.
❖ **P**revent further injuries by careful handling.
❖ **P**romote recovery.

To achieve these above goals, observe the following protocol in the emergency department of a hospital:

Initial Care of the Injured

At the Scene of Accident

❖ Remove the victim from the accident spot.
❖ Check his/her vital parameters quickly (pulse, consciousness, etc.).
❖ Seek the help of bystanders if trained in first aid.
❖ Ensure that police and ambulance have been informed.
❖ Remember to carry out the first aid as per the modus operandi described below.
❖ Ensure personal safety.
❖ Arrange to shift the injured to a hospital at the earliest.

MODUS OPERANDI IN FIRST AID

Airway

Human brain cannot survive look of oxygen for more than 3 minutes. Brain damage is irreversible. Hence, a quick effort should be made to ensure that as accident victim breathes normally for this clear airway is necessary. In the event of a blocked airway, proceed as follows:

❖ Clear the mouth of clots, dentures, loose teeth, etc.
❖ Extend the neck slightly as this opens up the pharynx.

Breathing

If the patient is not breathing, begin artificial respiration.

❖ First keep a thin cloth over the patient's mouth, blow into the patients mouth keeping his/her nostrils closed **(Fig. 4.1)**. Blow at the rate of 16/min and see for the chest raise.
❖ Mouth to nose respiration is carried out if there is extensive injury to the mouth.
❖ If the patient has suffered extensive facial injuries, put the patient prone, turn the face toward one side and apply pressure over the lower aspect of the chest (Holger-Nielsen's method).

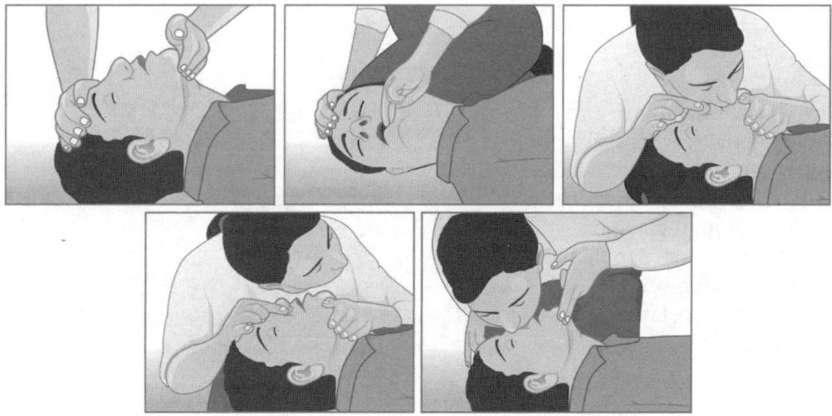

Fig. 4.1: Technique of mouth-to-mouth and mouth-to-nose respiration to resuscitate a victim.

Cardia

Examine the radial pulse at the wrist and the carotid pulse at the neck for the function of cardia. If the pulse is absent initiate cardiac resuscitative measures as follows:

❖ Ensure that patient is lying on a hard surface.
❖ Then pressure **(Fig. 4.2)** is applied with the heel of the palm at the lower end of sternum.
❖ Optimum pressure should be applied and the depth of each pressure should be 1¼ inch.
❖ Perform external cardiac massage at the rate of 72/min.
❖ It is preferable to carry out both external cardiac massage and artificial respiration

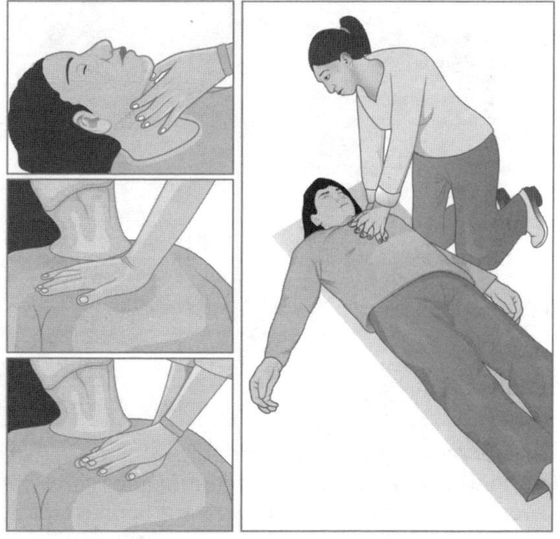

Fig. 4.2: Chest compression and technique of external cardiac massage.

simultaneously by two persons trained in first aid. But if there is no assistance available then cardiopulmonary resuscitation should be carried out by a single person as follows:

- First artificial respiration is given once and then the same person should quickly change position and carry out external cardiac massage 5 times. So, this 1:5 ratio should be maintained throughout.
- The cardiopulmonary resuscitation (CPR) should be carried out until the patient recovers or at least for half an hour.

Bleeding

It is advisable to arrest the bleeding by direct application of pressure over the bleeding points **(Fig. 4.3)**. *Tourniquet should be avoided and used only as a last resort.*

Now having ascertaining that the patient is breathing, has satisfactory heart function and with the arrest of any bleeding points, carry out the below mentioned examinations of the vital structures.

Remember

The ABC is first aid treatment:
A. Airway management is the first priority.
B. Breathing is very vital for the patient to survive.
   If the patient is not breathing, do the following:
   a. Mouth-to-mouth respiration
   b. Mouth-to-mouth nose reparation
   c. Holger-Nielsen method
C. Cardia and circulation: Ensure that the heart beats and the bleeding stops.

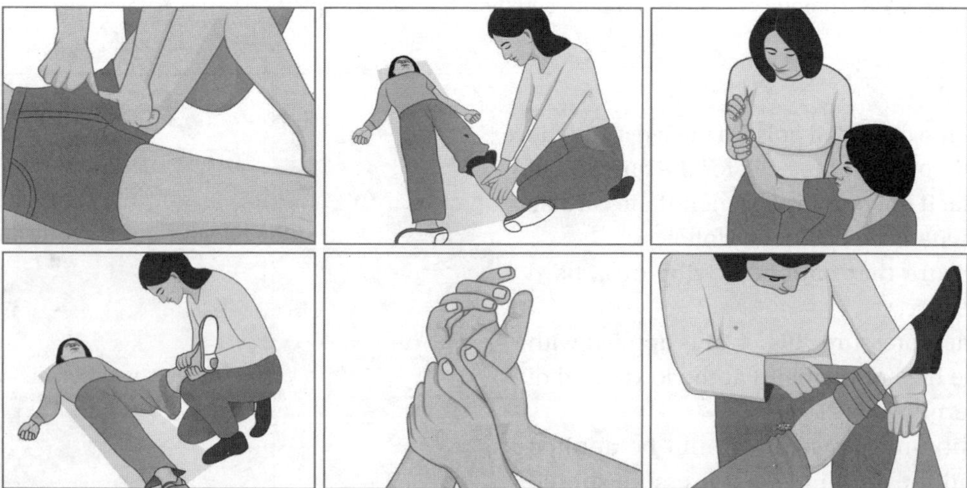

Fig. 4.3: Various measures to control bleeding—direct compression over the femoral artery in case of lower limb injuries, direct pressure over the injured site, elevation of the arm in upper limb injuries, elevation of the lower limb, direct compression over the injured area and application of compression bandage.

EXAMINATION OF THE VITAL STRUCTURES

Head injuries: Examine the patient for head injuries, cover the skull injuries with a clean cloth, and examine pupils and the level of consciousness. Look for neurological deficits.

Chest injuries: Open chest injuries are dangerous as they may cause tension pneumothorax. Application of a clean cloth with firm pressure over the open wounds is all that is required.

Abdominal injuries: All injured patients should be examined for intra-abdominal injuries as it is an emergency. Board-like rigid abdomen suggests blunt injury abdomen and there could be damage to the liver, spleen, colon, etc. Arrangement should be made to shift the patient immediately to a hospital. In open wounds of the abdomen, firm pressure should be applied by a clean cloth.

Pelvic fractures: Suspect pelvic fracture if the patient complains of pain during compression test or distraction test which is performed by applying pressure over the iliac bones. Tenderness over the symphysis pubis is also suggestive.

Injuries to the genitourinary system: Suprapubic swelling indicates bladder injury, injury to the scrotum or perineal hematoma indicates urethral rupture.

Spine injuries: Cervical spine injury should be suspected if the patient is lying still and loathes turning the neck. Injuries to the thoracic and lumbar spine should be suspected if the patient has developed paraplegia or complains of pain when individual spinous processes are palpated. *Extreme care should be exercised in managing and shifting a patient with spinal injuries.*

Fractures: Deformity, pain, swelling, loss of function of a limb are suggestive of fracture. Fracture needs to be splinted with whatever material is available at the scene of accident **(Fig. 4.4)**. The effective first aid measures during a bone and joint injuries are:

- Splinting the injuries limb with make shift or regular splints.
- Rest to the patient
- Limb elevation
- Firm compression bandage
- Cold sponging
- Folding pain killers
  They can be managed electively after shifting the patient to the hospital.

> **Remember**
> - Fracture is not an emergency.
> - Most of them can be managed electively at a later date.
> - In A to F management of injured fracture treatment comes last.
> - Prepare and improvise splints with available materials at the scene of accident.

MANAGEMENT AT THE HOSPITAL

Once as injured reaches, a hospital the role of the first aide's ends treatment at the hospital is not called first aid but is called medical aid. Trauma care at hospitals is given by various experts. Details of this treatment are outside the scope of this book. However, fracture management has been dealt at appropriate sections. Only as outline of the hospital, treatment is given below. Mac

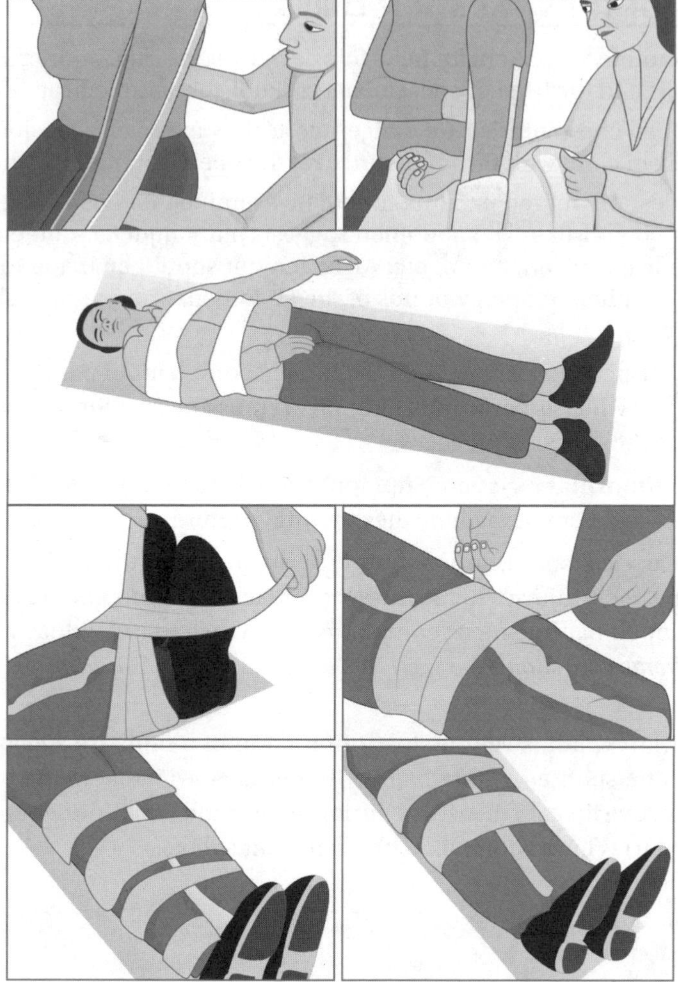

Fig. 4.4: Splinting of various injured sites—splinting of the elbow using news papers, using one's own body as a support, using ones own limb as a support.

Murthy has laid down the A to F management guidelines to be followed in the institutional care of the injured in the order of importance:

- ❖ **A**irway management
- ❖ **B**lood and fluid replacement
- ❖ **C**entral nervous system management
- ❖ **D**igestive system management
- ❖ **E**xcretory system management
- ❖ **F**racture management.

Other emergency measures like administration of antitoxin, antibiotics, antigas gangrene serum, and wound debridement should be carried out. Appropriate radiographs should be taken before treating the fractures. The treatment of bone and joint injuries are discussed in detail in the relevant chapters.

5
CHAPTER

Management of Fractures— Simple and Compound

Ironically, fractures pass through different levels of treatment, namely:

1. Treatment by unskilled people at the scene of accident.
2. Treatment by semiskilled people at the emergency department.
3. Treatment by skilled people, i.e., by the orthopedic surgeons.

So logically, fracture treatment commences from the scene of the accident, progresses through various methods of treatment, operative and non-operative and finally concludes with rehabilitation. Now let us analyze the treatment methodologies at the three important stages.

DIFFERENT LEVELS OF FRACTURE TREATMENT

Treatment by the Unskilled People

This happens at the scene of accident. From illiterate, to even a doctor could end up treating an accident victim. Nobody has any choice over the 'treating' persons in times of emergency. They are at the mercy of luck and God as to whom they end up being treated with. The principles of treatment at the accident site have to be:

1. **'Preserve life':** This takes precedence over the fracture management and consists of preserving life by ensuring proper respiration, circulation, heart functions and level of consciousness by various cardiopulmonary resuscitative measures.
2. **'Prevent' further damage:** By judicious handling of the vital organs and immobilizing the fractures by appropriate splinting with whatever material is available at your disposal on the roads (e.g. newspapers, umbrella, sticks, cardboards, rods, etc.). All these materials can be used to prepare a make-shift splint.

Remember

The principles of fracture treatment as emergency site: (4P's)
- **P**reserve life
- **P**revent further damage
- **P**romote recovery
- **P**atient to be shifted to the hospital at the earliest.

3. **Promote recovery:** By transporting the patient to the hospital at the earliest with utmost care, and entrusting, the patient to the trained personnel is at the hospital. Please refer chapter of First Aid for more details on emergency treatment of fractures.

> **Remember**
>
> The principle of fracture treatment at the scene of accident is splint, and splint the fractures with whatever material you could lay your hands on!

Treatment by Semiskilled People

Once the patient is transported to the hospital, semi-skilled professionals, at the causality, like the duty doctors, junior residents, postgraduate students, nurses and other paramedics now take up fracture treatment. Their job is to:

❖ Evaluate the whole body for injuries. Institute appropriate resuscitative measures to preserve and maintain life. Remove the tight bandages, tourniquets and make shift splints applied at the scene of the accidents.

After the general condition of the victim stabilizes:

1. Apply proper splints like, Thomas splints, BB splints, etc., to immobilize the fractures.
2. Subject the patient to appropriate investigations like laboratory tests, X-ray, MRI, CT scans, etc.
3. Transfer the patient to the care of a specialist like orthosurgeon, neurosurgeon, etc.

> **Remember**
>
> **The principles of treatment at the emergency department:**
> ◄◄ Evaluation
> ◄◄ Resuscitation
> ◄◄ Immobilization with proper splints
> ◄◄ Investigations
> ◄◄ Shifting the patient to the care of an orthopedic surgeon for the definitive treatment.

Treatment by Skilled Professionals (Definitive Treatment)

Now the role of an orthopedic surgeon in the fracture treatment begins. With the life preserved and saved, his job is to tackle the fractures with a vast armamentarium of choices of treatment methods available at his disposal, tailor making it to suit the needs of the individual patient. Fractures he needs to treat may range from simple, compound, complicated, fracture dislocations, and multiple fractures. There could be multisystem injuries for which he needs to summon the services of other specialists like neurosurgeons, faciomaxillary surgeons, thoracic surgeons, vascular surgeons, etc. Now he is part of a trauma team aiming to restore the individual back to his pre-injury status. His role can be discussed under the following subheadings:

❖ Appropriate investigations and decision making
❖ Management of simple fractures.
❖ Management of open fractures.
❖ Rehabilitation

Investigations in orthotrauma: For this he can rely on the investigations already ordered by the junior surgeons or get the below mentioned investigations done again to evaluate the spectrum of the fracture pathology to his satisfaction before deciding the most appropriate treatment methods.

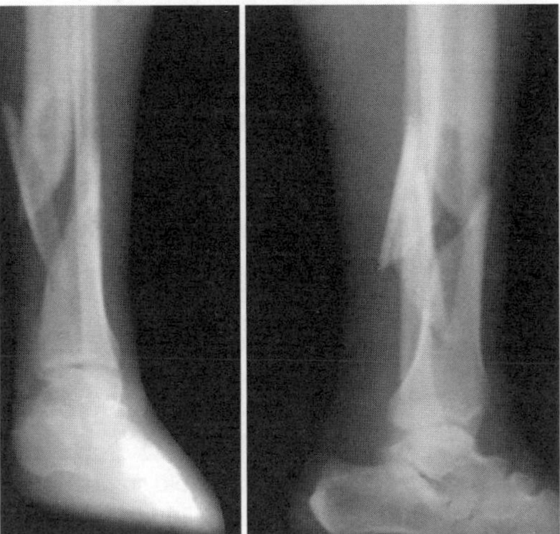

Fig. 5.1: Plain X-ray—anteroposterior and lateral views gold standard in limb fractures.

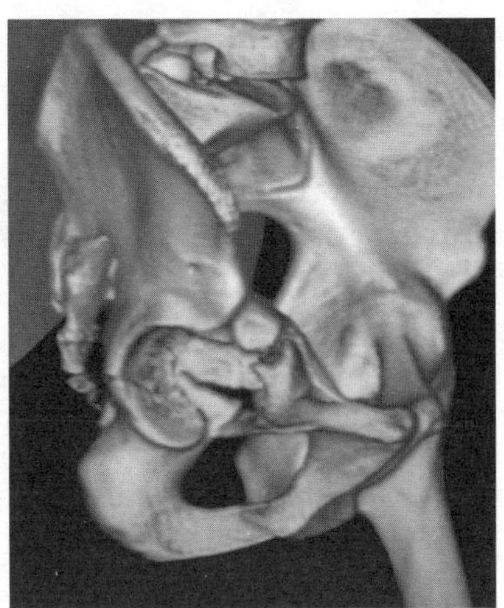

Fig. 5.2: CT scan is extremely valuable in the diagnosis of pelvic and acetabular injuries.

Radiography: It is an important diagnostic tool for fractures. Minimum two views, anteroposterior and lateral, are required as bone is a cylinder. Sometimes an oblique view and other special view are required depending upon the clinical situations and the bone under study **(Fig. 5.1)**.

CT scan and MRI: These are the most sophisticated investigative methods available now in orthopedics. Both are noninvasive and are extremely useful in evaluating both soft tissue and bony injuries. CT Scan is particularly useful in evaluating acetabular and pelvic injuries **(Fig. 5.2)** and MRI is of extreme value in assessing spine injuries **(Fig. 5.3)**.

Other Investigations

Include laboratory investigations, arthrography for joint injuries **(Fig. 5.4)**, arthroscopy especially for knee **(Fig. 5.5)**, shoulder, and ankle injuries, bone scans arteriogram, etc., except the first

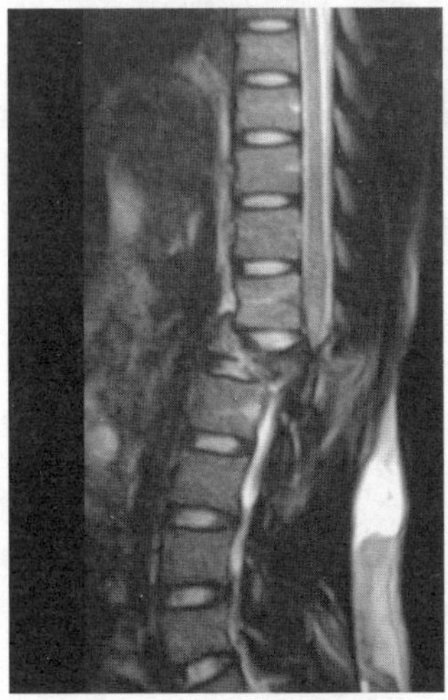

Fig. 5.3: MRI is extremely valuable in the diagnosis of spine injuries.

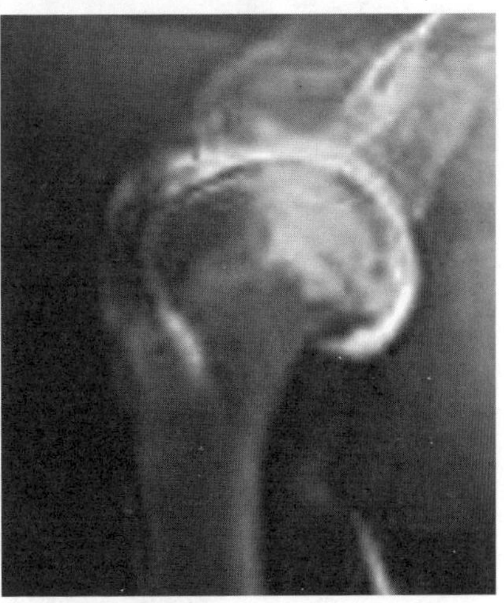

Fig. 5.4: Arthrography is useful in assessing knee ligament injuries.

the other investigations are required is special situations and is entirely the choice of the treating orthopedic surgeons.

Management of Fractures by the Orthosurgeon (Definitive Treatment)

The *goal* of an orthopedic surgeon in the fracture management is to restore the anatomy back to its normal or as near to normal as possible. The *responsibility* of an orthopedic surgeon is to ensure that there is no functional disability to the patient after the treatment of fractures. Management of fracture can be broadly classified and discussed under the following heads:

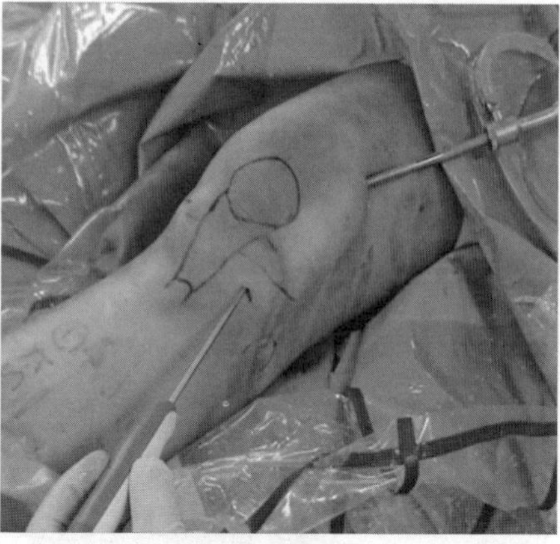

Fig. 5.5: Arthroscopy gold standard in assessing joint injuries.

MANAGEMENT OF SIMPLE/UNDISPLACED FRACTURES

Simple fractures are undisplaced or displaced and can be managed by conservative and operative methods. *Methods normally employed for* undisplaced fractures, incomplete fractures, impacted fractures, etc. Rest and just immobilization of the fractures seems to be enough in these cases and this can be achieved by:

* **Simple cuff and collar sling** for upper limb fractures **(Fig. 5.6A)**.
* **Strapping** for fracture clavicle, fracture ribs, etc. **(Figs. 5.6B to D)**.
* **Plaster casts and slabs:** Plaster of Paris slabs can be used to support the injured limb while the casts can be used for definitive treatment **(Figs. 5.7A to D)**.

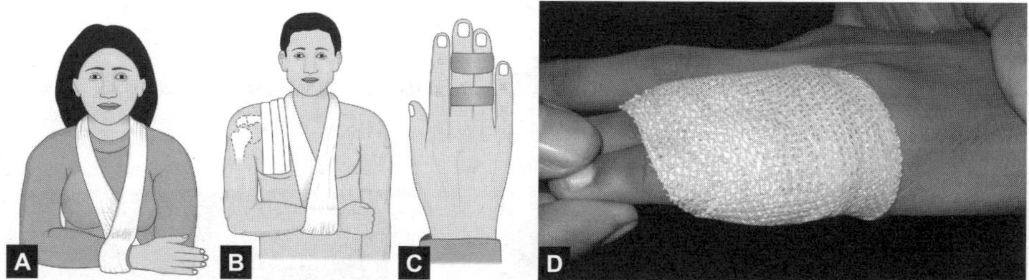

Figs. 5.6A to D: Various conservative treatment methods in orthopedics: (A) Simple cuff and collar sling; (B) Strapping; (C) Sling; (D) Buddy taping.

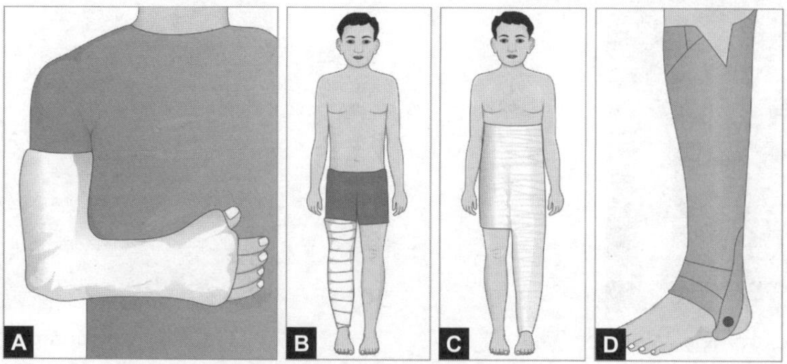

Figs. 5.7A to D: Various conservative treatment methods in orthopedics with plasters.

❖ **Rest and nonsteroidal anti-inflammatory drugs (NSAIDs)** for impacted fracture neck of femur, etc.
❖ **Splints:** Specialized splints like the Thomas splints **(Fig. 5.8)**, BB splints, pneumatic splints, etc., can be used for immobilization of the fractures.

MANAGEMENT OF DISPLACED FRACTURES

Here the aim is to restore back the normal anatomy of the bones by either closed or open reduction. This consists of resuscitation, reduction, retention and rehabilitation (4Rs).

1. **Resuscitation** is the top most priority if the patient is in shock following a fracture. A to F management proposed by Mac Murthy is to be followed in all situations of emergencies.
2. **Reduction** of the fracture fragments is mandatory if displaced. It is usually done under general anesthesia after adequate radiographic study. Reduction methods consist of:
   a. *Closed reduction:* The technique followed is traction (given by the orthosurgeon) and counter-traction (given by an assistant) methods **(Fig. 5.9)**.
   b. *Continuous traction:* Continuous traction used for reduction of fractures are Gallow's traction (for fracture shaft femur in children), balanced skeletal traction (for adult shaft femur fractures, etc.) **(Fig. 5.10)**. No longer used.
   c. *Open reduction:* It is done when the above methods fail or if there are specific indications.
3. **Retention:** Once the fracture fragments are reduced, it has to be retained in that position till the fracture unites, otherwise it tends to get displaced due to the action of muscles, gravity and inherent factors.

Retention methods after closed reduction are:
a. *By plaster of Paris splints:* This is the most common splint employed.
b. *By continuous traction:* To overcome the muscle forces after closed reduction. The traction could be skin or skeletal traction and is employed as fixed, balanced or combined types of tractions **(Figs. 5.11A to D)**. However, these are no longer followed due to the availability of newer and better techniques.

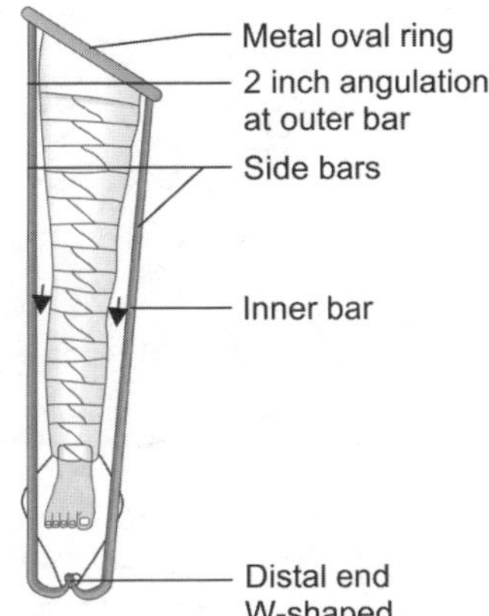

Fig. 5.8: Showing a Thomas splint.

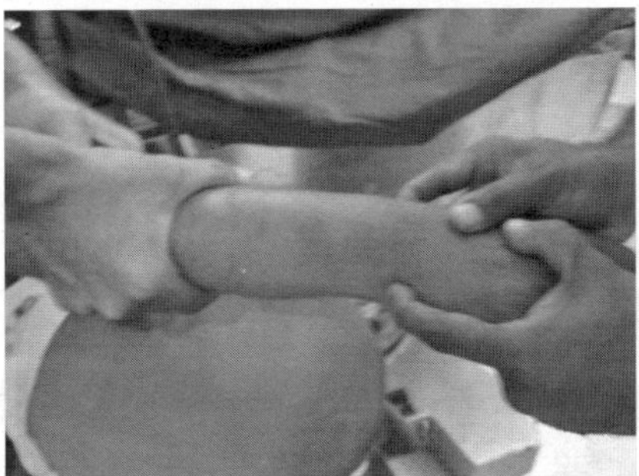

Fig. 5.9: Showing method of closed reduction by traction and countertraction methods for a Colles' fracture.

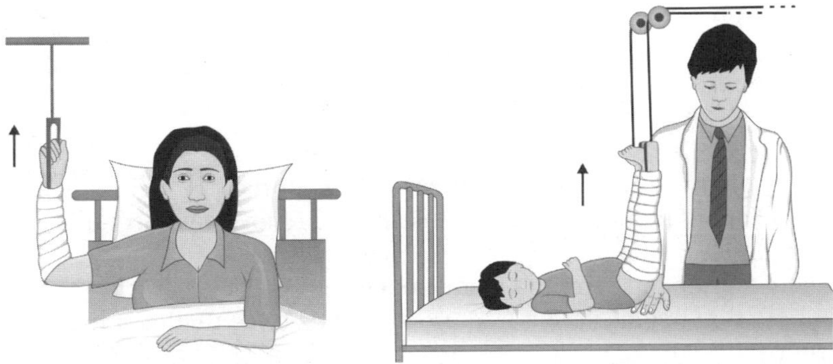

Fig. 5.10: Continuous traction in a child Dunlop's traction and Gallow's fractures.

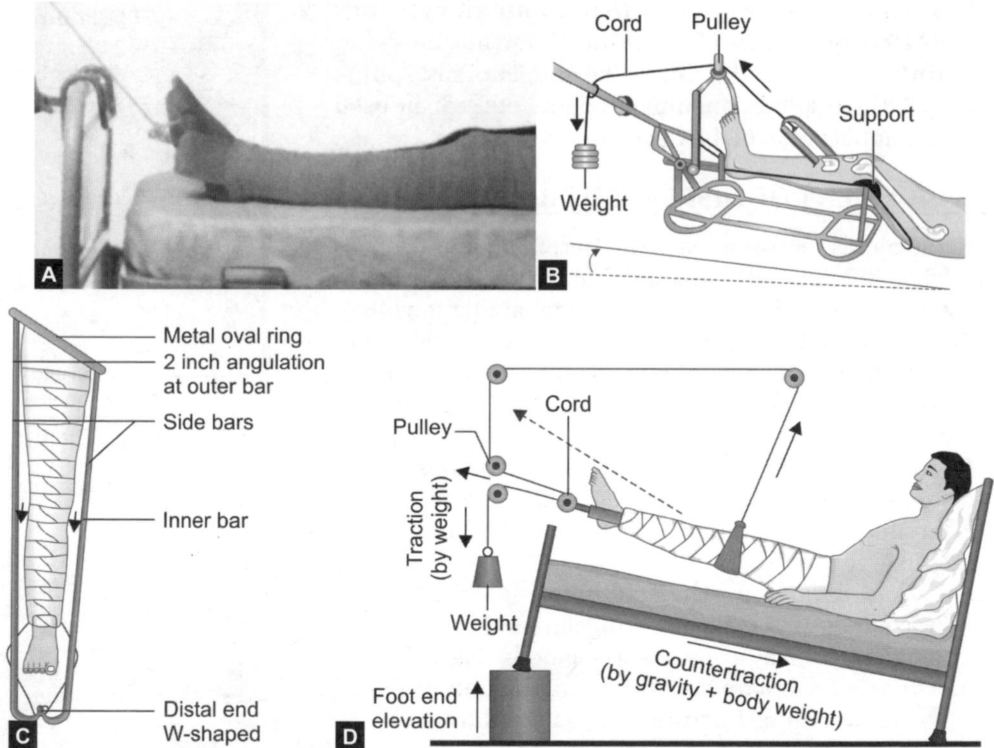

Figs. 5.11A to D: (A and B) Showing methods of skin traction and skeletal traction; (C and D) Showing methods of fixed traction and balanced traction.

  c. *Use of functional braces:* This can be used after 3 weeks, once the fracture becomes sticky **(Fig. 5.12)**. This enables the patient to mobilize his joints early and thus prevent joint stiffness.

4. **Rehabilitation (Figs. 5.13A to C):** Recourse to the following physiotherapeutic methods:
  a. Isotonic active exercises for the un-immobilized joints.
  b. Isometric exercises for the joints immobilized.
  c. Care of the plaster splints for loosening, breakage, tightness, skin excoriations, soiling, etc.
  d. Training to carry out the functional activities with the unaffected limb.
  e. Once the plaster is removed, mobilization of joints is done by appropriate active and passive exercises. Resistive exercises help to strengthen the muscles.
  f. Heat therapy to alleviate pain, swelling and spasm.
  g. Massaging of the joints after application of pain relieving gel or oils helps to relax the muscles and relieve pain. Isotonic exercises help to strength muscles.
  h. Counseling to keep the depression and anxiety away.

Thus, rehabilitation begins with a fracture and ends once the lost functions ore restored back completely.

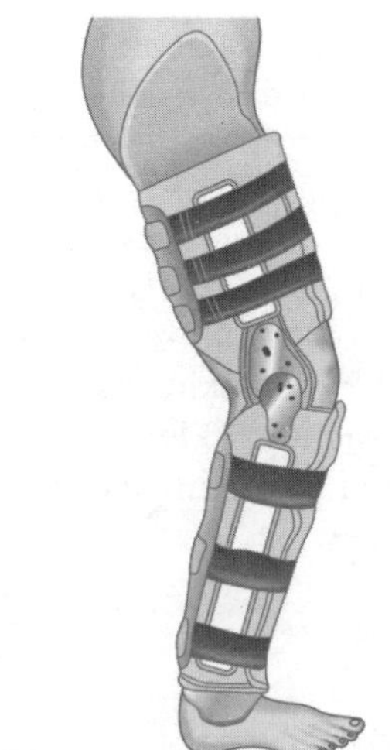

Fig. 5.12: Functional cast brace.

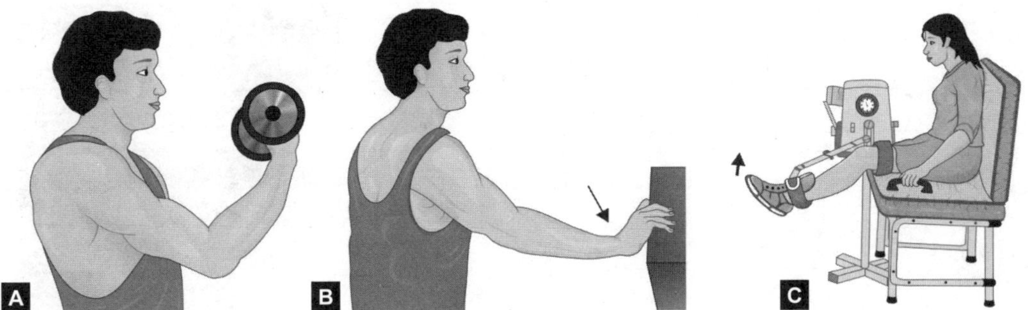

Figs. 5.13A to C: Rehabilitation is the most essential part of fracture management. Here are a few important methods: (A) Isotonic exercises; (B) Isometric exercises; (C) Continuous passive motion exercises.

Rehabilitation of Fractures after Open Reduction

This proceeds on the same lines as that of the fractures treated by closed reduction except that wound care has to be followed meticulously. In cases of internal fixations, the joints can be mobilized early by appropriate physiotherapy techniques.

> **Remember**
>
> **The 5R's in the management of closed fractures treated by closed reductions:**
> - **R**esuscitation if the patient is in shock
> - **R**eduction of the fracture if displaced
> - **R**etention of the fragment by plasters tractions, etc.
> - **R**ehabilitation
> - **R**eduction of lost anatomy and functions

Fracture Management by Open Reduction (Operative Management)

As mentioned earlier open method is indicated once the conservative methods fail and when there are specific indications. These indications could be absolute, relative or rare as mentioned below:

Indications

Absolute
- Failed closed reduction
- Displaced intra-articular fractures
- Types III and IV epiphyseal injuries
- Major avulsion fractures
- Nonunion
- Replantation of extremities

Relative
- Multiple fractures
- Delayed union
- Loss of reduction
- Pathological fractures
- For better nursing care
- To avoid prolonged bed rest
- Closed methods ineffective in Galeazzi fracture, Monteggia fracture, femoral neck fracture, etc.

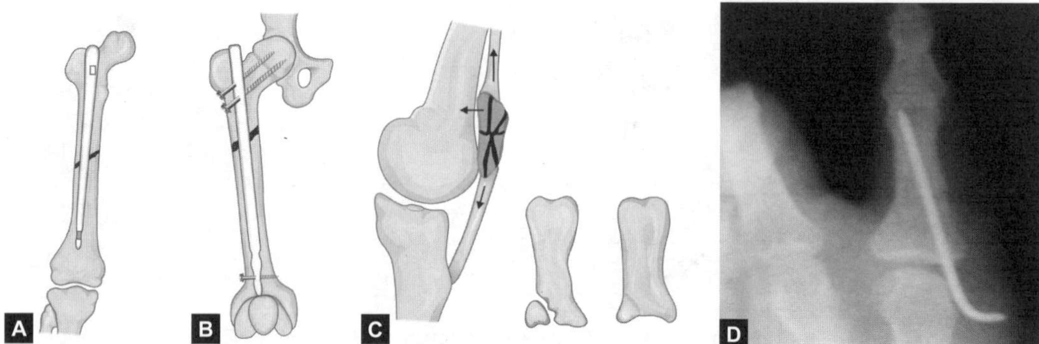

Figs. 5.14A to D: Various internal fixations methods in orthopedics: (A) IM nail; (B) Interlocking nail; (C) Tension bend wiring; (D) Fixations of small fractures with K-wires.

Questionable

- Neurovascular injury
- Open fractures
- Cosmetic reasons
- Economic consideration

Retention after open reduction: After open reduction the fracture fragment invariably needs to be fixed internally **(Figs. 5.14A to D)**.

The Choice of Implants

K-wire: For epiphyseal injuries and for small bones of hand and feet (diameter of the K-wires varies from 1 to 3 mm).

Screws: For avulsion fractures and butterfly fragments.

Intramedullary nails: For fracture through the narrowest portion of a medullary canal of a long bone **(Fig. 5.14A)**.

Interlocking nails: For segmental fractures comminuted fractures, etc., of long bones **(Fig. 5.14B)**.

Steel wires (No. 18–20 gauze): Useful for tension band wiring for fracture of patella, metacarpal and phalangeal fractures, etc. **(Figs. 5.14C and D)**.

Plate and screws: For proximal and distal third fractures of long bones **(Fig. 5.15)**.

Contraindications for Open Reduction

- Infection.
- Small fragments.
- Weak and porotic bone.
- Soft tissue damage.
- Undisplaced or impacted fractures.
- Poor general and medical condition.

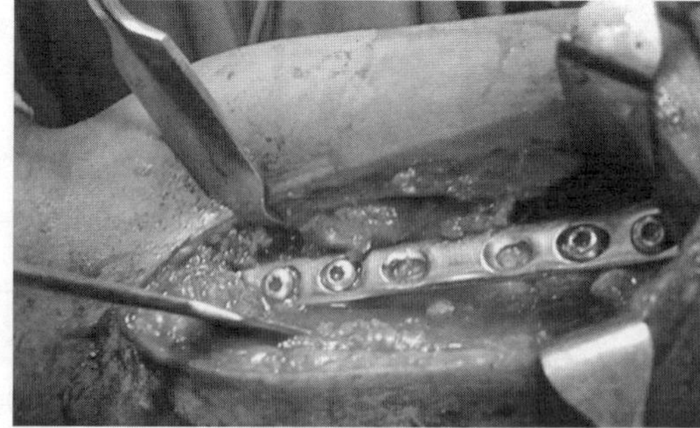

Fig. 5.15: Showing open reduction and internal fixation with DCP plate and screws in humerus fracture.

Disadvantages of Open Reduction

❖ Closed fracture converted into an open fracture.
❖ Fracture hematoma is disturbed.
❖ Scar tissue.
❖ Anesthetic problems.
❖ Foreign body reaction due to metals.

Important Splints in Orthopedics

"A splint lays the fracture to rest until an orthopedic surgeon mends it."

SPLINTS

The most dramatic discovery ever made in the treatment of fractures or orthopedic disorders is undoubtedly the "splints". Any substance used to immobilize a fracture or inflamed joint is called the splint. The credit of refining the splints from a crude variety to that of finesse and quality deservingly goes to the *Father of British Orthopedic Surgery, HO Thomas*. His epoch making discovery of a knee splint, named after him, as the Thomas splint has stood the test of time and still finds a pride place in the treatment armamentarium of orthopedics. Thus he richly deserves to be called "Father of Splints".

Uses

The splint has the following different uses:
* It can be used to immobilize the fractures.
* It can be used to transport the injured patient.
* It can be used to rest an inflamed joint.
* It can be used to correct or prevent deformities.
* It finds a place even in the definitive treatment of fractures.

Splints Used in Different Regions in Orthopedics

Neck

* Cervical collar **(Fig. 6.1A to C)**
* Four post-collar **(Fig. 6.2)**

Uses: To immobilized the neck in painful conditions.

Upper Limbs

* Aeroplanes splint —brachial plexus injury
* Carpal tunnel splint—for carpal tunnel syndrome **(Fig. 6.1)**

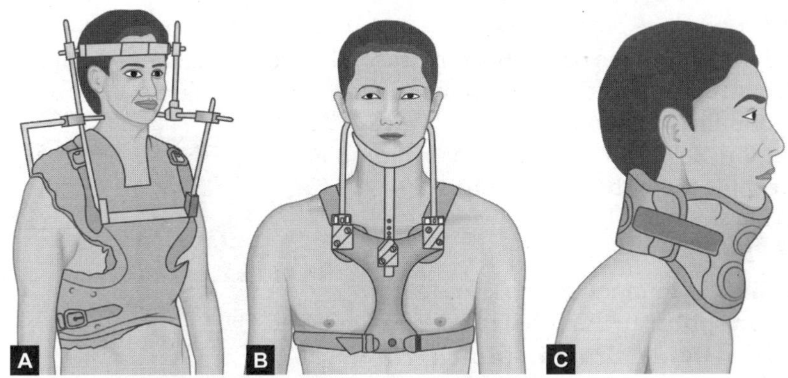

Figs. 6.1A to C: Methods of cervical immobilization: (A) Halo-vest traction; (B) Four post-cervical collar; (C) Cervical collar.

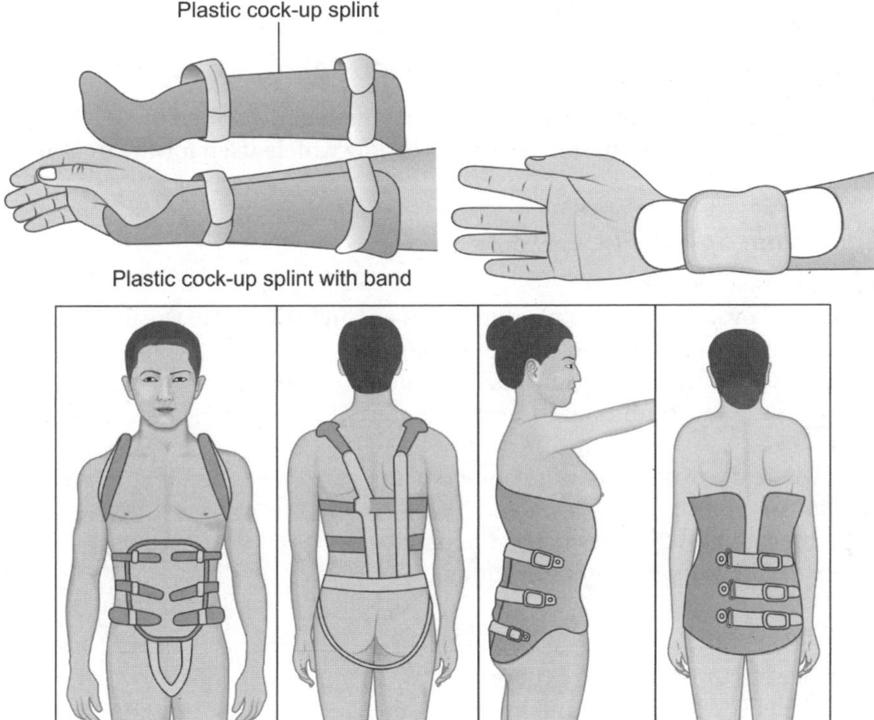

Fig. 6.2: Showing treatment of stable thoracolumbar fractures with brace.

- ❖ Cock-up splint—used in wrist drop **(Fig. 6.1)**
- ❖ Mallet splint—for Mallet injuries **(Fig. 6.2)**
- ❖ Finger splint—phalangeal fractures
- ❖ Knuckle benders splint—ulnar nerve palsy
- ❖ Volkmann's splint for VIC

Spine

- ❖ **Dorsal region:** Milwaukee brace, Boston Brace. Uses for correction of scoliosis.
- ❖ **Dorsolumbar region:** Anterior spinal hypertension brace **(Fig. 6.2)**, ASHE, Taylor's brace. Used to immobilize the thoracolumbar.
- ❖ **Lumbar region:** Belts and corsets. Used to immobilize the lumbar spine in low backache **(Fig. 6.2)**.

Lower Limb Splints

- ❖ **Thomas splint:** To immobilize the knee joint
- ❖ **Böhler-Braun splint:** To immobilize fracture femur
- ❖ **CTEV splint (Denis Brown splint):** For CTEV correction
- ❖ **Foot drop splint:** For foot drop condition **(Fig. 6.3)**
  Now let us focus our attention to some of the commonly used splints in orthopedics namely:

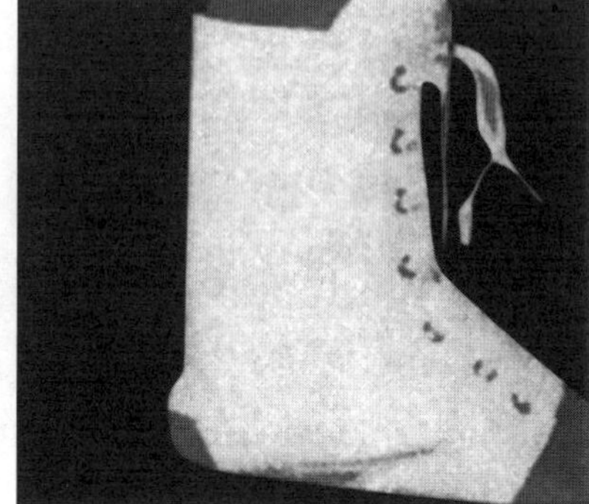

Fig. 6.3: Foot-drop splint (static type).

DIFFERENT TYPES OF SPLINTS

Thomas Splint (Also Called Thomas Knee-Bed Splint)

This is one of the very commonly used splints in orthopedics described by HO Thomas in 1876 to assist for ambulatory treatment of TB knee. It is now widely used for the treatment of shaft fractures of femur.

Parts of a Thomas Splint (Fig. 6.4)

A Thomas splint consists of four parts.
1. A padded metal oval ring with soft leather set at an angle of 120° to the inner bar.
2. Two side bars one inner and another outer bars of equal length. They bisect the oval ring. The outer bar has a curve to accommodate for the greater trochanter.
3. Distal end where the two side bars are joined in the form of a 'W'.
4. Outer side bar is angled 2 inches below the padded ring to clear the prominent greater trochanter.

Uses of Thomas Splint

- ❖ To immobilize fracture femur anywhere.
- ❖ As a first aid measure for lower limb injuries.
- ❖ For transportation of an injured patient.
- ❖ In the treatment of joint diseases like TB knee, septic arthritis, etc.

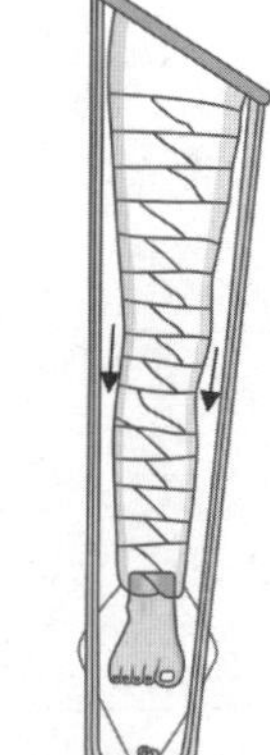

Fig. 6.4: Parts of a Thomas splint (the most famous splint in orthopedics).

Vital Thomas Splint Facts

- ❖ **How to choose the proper ring size:** Measure the thigh circumference at the highest point of the groin and add two inches.
- ❖ **How to choose the correct length:** Measure the highest point on the medial side of the groin to heel and then add six inches.

Böhler-Braun (BB) Splint (Fig. 6.5)

This is Böhler's modification of Braun splint. It consists of a heavy metallic frame with four pulleys:
1. Proximal pulley prevents foot drop.
2. Second pulley to apply traction in the line of femur.
3. Third pulley to apply traction in the line of supracondylar area of femur.
4. Fourth pulley to apply traction in line of the legs.

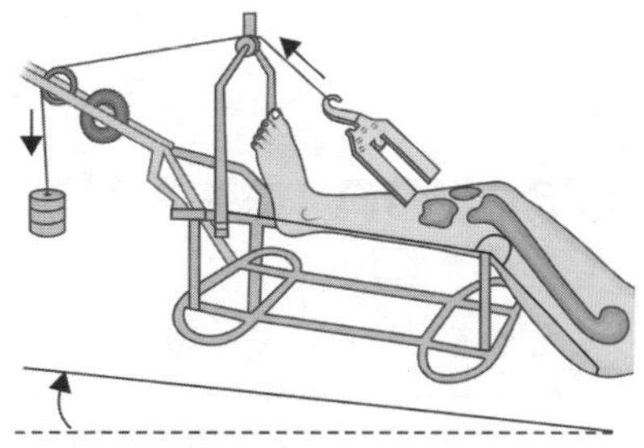

Fig. 6.5: Böhler-Braun splint.

Indications of BB Splint

Skeletal traction is applied through this frame for comminuted trochanteric fractures of the femur. It is also used for the treatment of fracture shaft femur and supracondylar fractures of the femur. Rarely can it be used for the fracture shaft of tibia and fibula.

One important precaution, which should be taken while using the BB splint, is to provide support at the fracture site and not at the knee joint to prevent angulations especially in supracondylar fractures of femur. This helps prevent troublesome knee stiffness.

Problems of BB Splint

❖ Makes nursing care difficult.
❖ It is a heavy and cumbersome frame.
❖ It is associated with recumbent problems like bed sores, hypostatic pneumonia, renal calculi, etc.

CARE OF THE SPLINTS

❖ **Padding:** The splint should be well padded at the bony prominences and at the injury sites.
❖ **Bandage:** This should be tied with optimum pressure.
❖ **Exercises:** Active exercises of the joints and muscles should be permitted within the splints.
❖ **Checking:** Daily checking and adjustments of the splints are recommended.
❖ **Neurovascular status:** Distal neurovascular status should be assessed daily.

Traction in Orthopedics

"Who says pulling can be distracting only it can be healing too!"

INTRODUCTION

Traction is a unique method of treatment in orthopedics. It plays multiple roles like providing stretching effect on the muscles, ligaments, other soft tissue structures including the bones and the discs. It helps in providing relaxation of the above structures. It also helps to keep the patient on the bed and thereby ensures total rest to the body which is otherwise not possible. It is mainly useful in the regional conditions like low backache, cervical spondylosis, etc. Traction also plays an important role in the management of fractures in orthopedics. Les us find out how?

USES OF TRACTION IN FRACTURES OR DISLOCATIONS

❖ To reduce a fracture or a dislocation.
❖ To retain the fracture after reduction.
❖ To overcome the muscle spasm.
❖ To control movement of an injured part of the body and to aid in healing.

METHODS OF TRACTION

There are four methods of applying traction, namely skin, skeletal, pelvic and spinal.

SKIN TRACTION (FIG. 7.1)

Here traction is applied over a large area of skin. Maximum weight that can be applied through skin traction is 15 lbs or 6.7 kg. If the weight used is more than this, the traction will slide down peeling off the skin. When used in fracture, skin traction is applied to the limb distal to the fracture site.

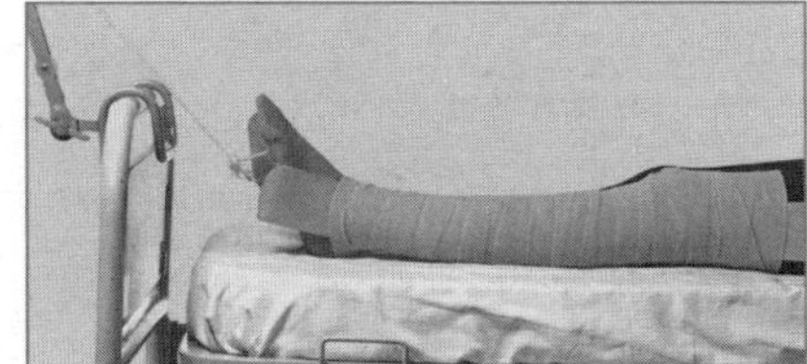

Fig. 7.1: Skin traction.

Types of Skin Traction

Adhesive Skin Traction

Here adhesive material is used for strapping which is applied anteromedial and posterolateral on either side of the lower limbs.

Nonadhesive Skin Traction

Useful in thin and atrophic skin and in patients sensitive to adhesive strap. It is less secure than the former.

Contraindications for Skin Traction

Abrasions, lacerations, impaired circulation, dermatitis, marked shortening, allergy to plaster are some of the important contraindications for skin tractions.

Complications

Allergy, excoriations, pressure sores around the malleoli, common peroneal nerve palsy, etc., are some of the known complications in skin tractions.

> **Remember**
>
> Rotation of the limb is difficult to control with skin tractions.

Important Skin Tractions

Bucks Extension Skin Traction

This is the most common type of traction employed for lower limbs. It is used for temporary treatment of fracture neck femur, undisplaced fractures of acetabulum, after reduction of hip dislocation, to correct minor fixed flexion deformity of hip and knee for low backache, etc.

Dunlop's Traction

Used in upper limbs and is indicated for supracondylar fractures, intercondylar fractures of humerus where elbow flexion causes circulatory embarrassment **(Fig. 7.2)**. No longer used, of historic importance.

Gallow's Traction (Fig. 7.3) or Bryant's Traction

Used for fracture shaft femur in children less than 2 years. If used in children above 2 years, it causes vascular complications. No longer used, of historic importance.

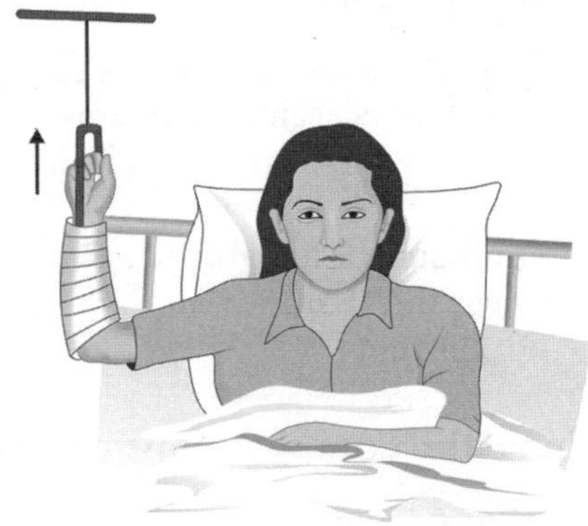

Fig. 7.2: Showing Dunlop's traction.

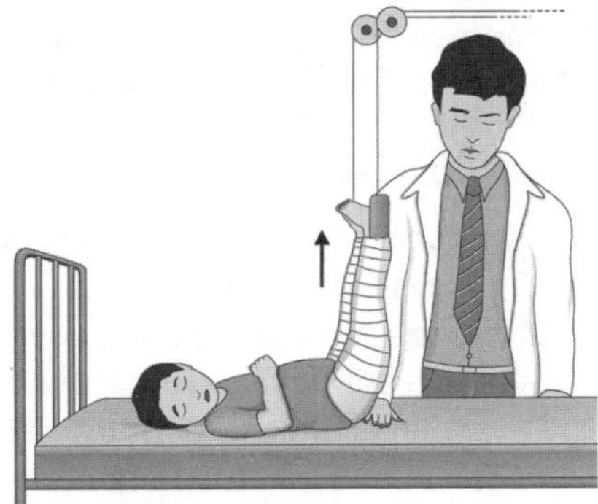

Fig. 7.3: Gallow's traction.

SKELETAL TRACTION

Here the traction is given through a metal or pin driven through the bone. It is seldom necessary for upper limb fractures but useful in lower limb fractures for reducing and maintaining the fracture reduction. It is reserved for those cases in which skin traction is contraindicated and where the need to be applied weight is more than 5 kg **(Fig. 7.4)**.

Know the Pins Used for Skeletal Traction

Steinmann Pin

It is a rigid stainless steel pin 4–6 mm in diameter. Böhler's stirrup allows the direction of the traction to be varied without turning the pin in the bone.

Denham Pin

This pin is threaded in the center and engages the bony cortex. It reduces the risk of pin sliding and is useful in cancellous bone like calcaneum and osteoporotic bones.

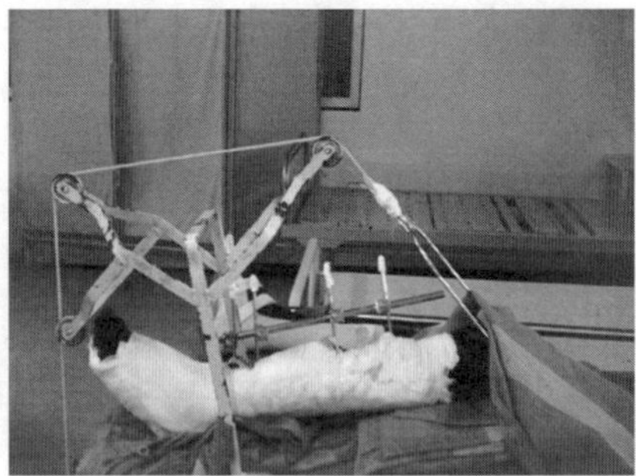

Fig. 7.4: Skeletal traction through Böhler-Braun frame.

K-wire

It is of small diameter and is often used in upper limbs for olecranon traction and through the metacarpal and metatarsal bones.

Know the Rules of Application

- Skeletal traction should be applied in a major OT under local anesthesia.
- Follow strict aseptic measures.
- Drive the pin from lateral to medial in case of upper tibial traction, to avoid injuring the lateral popliteal nerve.
- Pin should be at right angles to the limb and parallel to the ground.
- Cover the sharp tip on the medial side with a stopper bottle to prevent damage to the normal limb.

Know the Complications of Skeletal Traction

During Application

- Injury to the nerves (lateral popliteal nerve).
- Injury to the vessels.
- Injury to the muscles, ligaments and tendons.
- Injury to the epiphysis in children (upper tibial epiphysis).

When Pin is in Situ

- Infection—due to improper aseptic measures.
- Migration—due to loosening.
- Breakage—thin pin or more weight.
- Bending—same reasons as above.
- Loosening—due to osteoporosis, infection, etc.
- Distraction of fracture fragments—due to excessive weight.

Late Effects

- Pin tract infection.
- Chronic osteomyelitis with ring sequestra at the site.
- Genu recurvatum due to damage to the anterior epiphysis of tibia in children.
- Depressed scar.

PRECAUTIONS DURING TRACTION

- ❖ Carefully watch the pin tract sites everyday. Cleaning these sites with aseptic solutions should be a daily routine.
- ❖ Bed sores should be prevented at all costs. For this regular back care, use of waterbeds, turning the patient over for every 2 hours are some of the effective time tested methods to prevent bedsores.
- ❖ The feet should not be left touching the pulleys.
- ❖ The weight of the traction unit should not touch the ground.
- ❖ Ensure that the bandages are not too tight.
- ❖ Prevent chest complications by proper chest physiotherapy measures.
- ❖ To prevent stiffness, active exercises of the unimmobilized joints should be begun at the earliest.
- ❖ Proper bowel and bladder care is mandatory to prevent urinary tract infection and constipation.

Traction Points

Well-known traction in orthopedics	
Tractions	**Indications**
Head or cervical tractions	
Crutchfield or Garden wells	Cervical spine injuries
Head halter **(Fig. 12.9)**	Cervical spine injuries
Halo pelvic	Scoliosis
Upper limb tractions	
Dunlop's traction	Supracondylar fracture of humerus
Metacarpal traction	Compound forearm injuries
Lower limb tractions	
Gallow's or Bryant's	Fracture shaft femur (<2 years)
Russel's traction	Trochanteric fracture
Perkin's traction	Fracture shaft femur in adults
90–90° traction	Fracture shaft femur in children
Agnes Hunt traction	Correction of hip deformity
Well leg adduction deformity	To correct abduction and traction of hip
Calcaneal	Compound fractures of traction distal traction leg and ankle
Buck's traction	Low backache, etc.
Pelvic traction	Low backache, etc.

Countertraction force will overcome muscle spasm only if another force is acting in the opposite direction as countertraction.

Types

Fixed traction: Here countertraction is achieved through an appliance, which obtains a firm purchase on a part of the body. This can maintain but cannot obtain reduction, e.g., fixed traction on a Thomas splint for a fracture shaft femur **(Fig. 7.5)**.

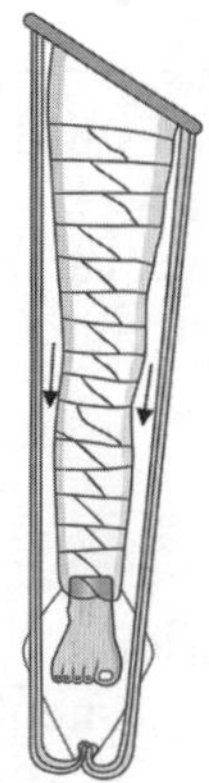

Fig. 7.5: Fixed traction through the Thomas splint.

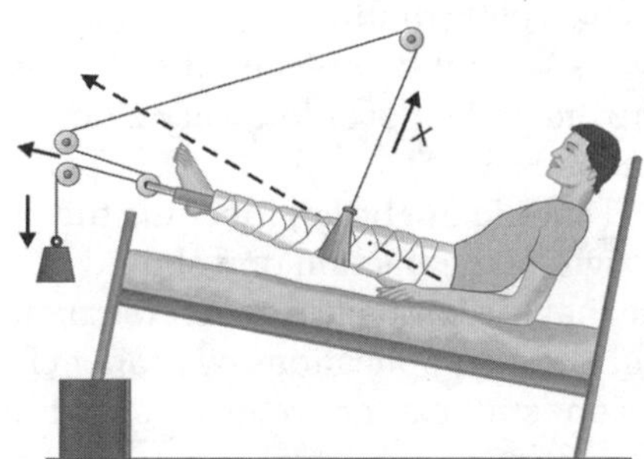

Fig. 7.6: Showing sliding or balanced traction.

Sliding or Balanced Traction

Here weight of all or part of the body acting under the influence of gravity is utilized to provide countertraction. This can be achieved by raising the foot end of the bed. *Unlike in a fixed traction, both reduction and maintenance of a fracture can be obtained* **(Fig. 7.6)**. This is of historic importance only. May be used only in very elderly patients who are unfit for surgery.

Pelvic Traction

Pelvic traction is mainly indicated in the conservative treatment of pelvic fractures. A detailed account of this is however available in the chapter on pelvic injuries.

Spinal Traction

Cervical Traction

This could a head halter or chin halter traction of skull traction through the Crutchfield tongs or Garden Wells tongs. The purpose of these tractions is to immobile the neck in fractures or dislocations of the cervical spine. It could be used as a first aid, reducing the fracture or dislocation, maintenance of the reduction, postoperative immobilization, etc. **(Fig. 7.7)**.

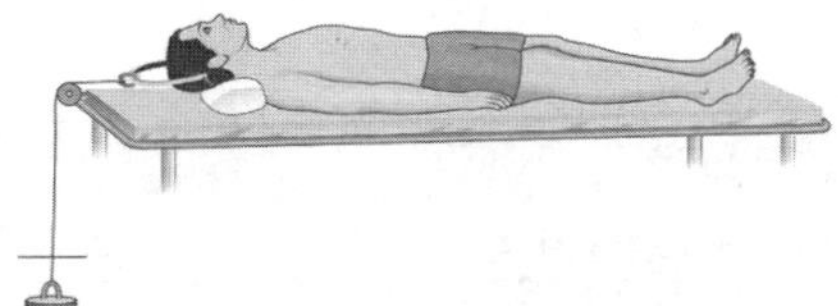

Fig. 7.7: Skull traction through Crutchfield tongs.

<table><tr><td>

Quick facts

Utility of a cervical traction in neck injuries:
- As a first aid measure for transport of the patient.
- For reduction of the fracture and dislocation and maintenance of the reduction.
- To relieve the neck muscle spasm.
- For postoperative immobilization.

</td></tr></table>

Nonskeletal cervical traction is used for common neck pains due to cervical spondylosis, etc. **(Fig. 7.8)**.

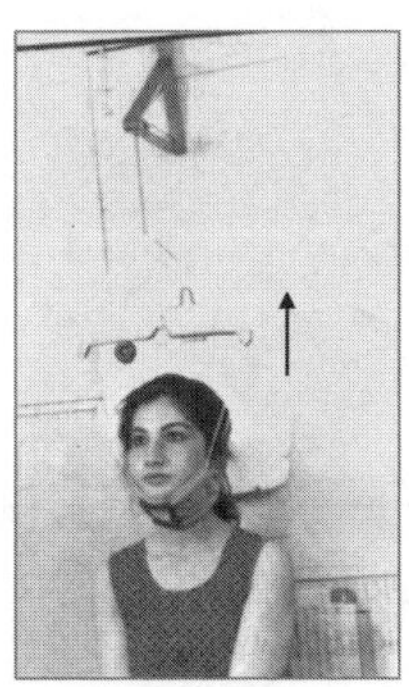

Fig. 7.8: Cervical traction in sitting position.

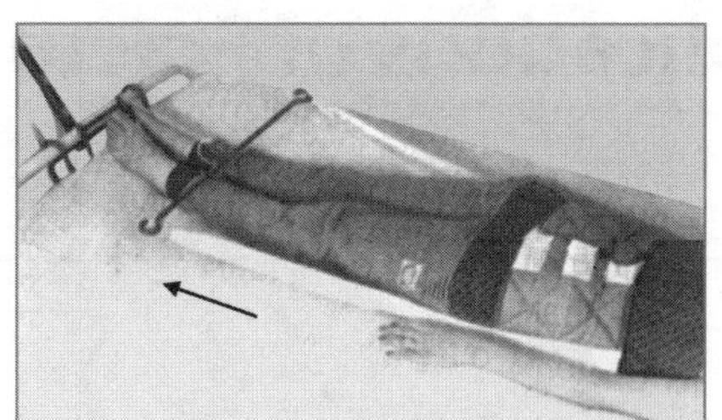

Fig. 7.9: Lumbar traction in low-backache.

Lumbar Traction

Traction to the lower back can be used in acute low backache situations like muscle strain or ligament sprain. It can also be used as a first aid measure to transport a patient in fractures and dislocations of the lumbar spine **(Fig. 7.9)**.

Note: Pelvic and spinal tractions are most often used in treatment of the regional conditions of the neck, spine and lower back. They are discussed in greater details in relevant chapters.

Complications of Fractures

HYPOVOLEMIC SHOCK

Shock due to Hypovolemia

In fractures of major long bones, pelvic fractures, multisystem injuries following road traffic accidents, etc., severe loss of blood may seriously threaten the life of a victim. Delay and apathy is attending a hypovolemic shock could prove fatal.

Source of Hemorrhage

This could be external or internal.

- ❖ **External hemorrhage:** This usually happens in compound fractures, pelvic fractures, etc.
- ❖ **Internal hemorrhage:** It is more often seen is blunt injury of abdomen femur and pelvic fractures, etc. It could be much more in multiple fractures.

Remember

Bloody facts: Do you know a staggering blood loss in fractures:
- Femoral shaft fractures—blood loss could range from 500 to 2,000 mL
- Pelvic fractures—blood loss could range from 1,000 to 2,500 mL

Clinical Features

Look for the classical features of Shock (**Box 8.1**) apart from features of fractures.

Investigations

Laboratory investigations like HB%, blood group, bleeding and clotting time, HIV. HBsAg, etc., are of utmost importance. Plain X-rays of the affected

Box 8.1: Shocking facts—look for the classical features.

- Tongue—pale and dry
- Pale look
- Low BP
- Cold clammy skin
- Cold nose
- Peripheral pulses feeble or absent
- Drowsy or unconscious

limbs and other investigations like MRI, CT scan, etc., are done once the general condition of the patient is stabilized.

Treatment

Speed is the watchword in the treatment of shock and included.
❖ Resuscitation
❖ Immediate fluid replacement by:
  ◆ IV fluids—normal saline, Ringer lactate, etc.
  ◆ Hemaccel
  ◆ Blood—best alternative
❖ Administrations of oxygen
❖ Splinting the fractures
❖ Controlling the bleeding points

ACUTE RESPIRATORY DISTRESS SYNDROME (SYN: FAT EMBOLISM)

Acute respiratory distress syndrome (ARDS) is defined as a post-traumatic distress syndrome occurring within 72 hours of skeletal trauma. It is seen in 10–45% cases of multiple fractures and is an important cause of morbidity and mortality (11%) in multiple fracture and multisystem injuries.

Etiology

Common etiological factor is a long bone fracture in young adults or a pelvic fracture in elderly.

Pathogenesis

Following injury, the bone marrow fats or the platelet agglutination are sucked into the injured vessels and are transported to various sites as emboli giving rise to varied clinical manifestation.

Source of Fat

It could be from two sources:
❖ From bone marrow (accepted).
❖ From plasma by agglutination of chylomicrons which later acts as an embolus (less accepted).

Classification (Sevitt's)

1. **Classical type:** In this variety the onset is less than 24 hours, *tachycardia* is greater than 140/min, *pyrexia* is greater than 40°C, *tachypnea, cyanosis,* changing *cerebral signs* vary from confusion, restlessness and coma. *Petechial rashes* and in *conjunctiva of lower lids, if present is pathognomonic.* In this type, the blood pressure is maintained throughout.
2. **Fulminating type:** Here the sequence of events are very fast and there is no time for the rashes to develop. Patient is comatose within hours and throws repeated seizures. Patient rapidly collapses and death supervenes.
3. **Incomplete type:** The manifestation is between the two types unexplained tachycardia, fever and rash are its features.

Investigations

❖ *X-ray of the chest* may show snowstorm appearance and if seen is pathognomonic **(Fig. 8.1)**
❖ PaO_2 less than 60 mm Hg.

- ❖ Platelet counts less than 1.5 lakhs.
- ❖ ECG shows prominent S-wave.
- ❖ **Gurd test:** Isolation of fat emboli from the blood.
- ❖ There is no pathognomonic laboratory test.

> **Remember**
>
> **The important diagnostic triad in ARDS is represented by the mnemonic TPR**
> - ◀◀ Thrombocytopenia.
> - ◀◀ PaO_2 <60 mm Hg.
> - ◀◀ Rashes.

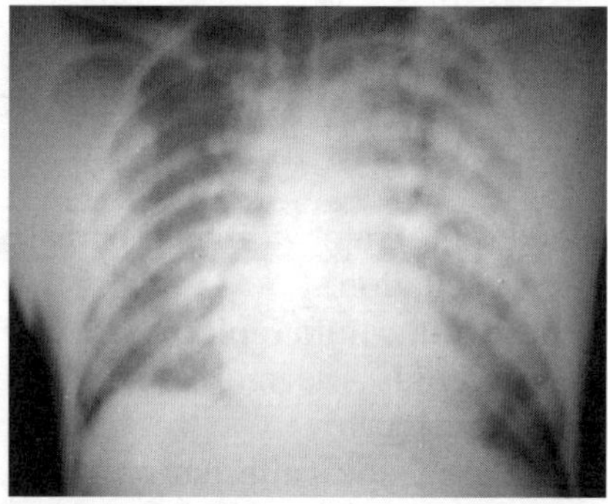

Fig. 8.1: Plain X-ray of the chest showing snowstorm appearance in ARDS.

Management

There are two important steps in the management of ARDS: *Nonspecific* consists of three vital steps:

1. **Keep:** (a) airway patent, and (b) fracture immobilized by POP or external fixators.
2. **Restore:** (a) blood volume, (b) fluid, and (c) electrolyte balance.
3. **Avoid:** (a) careless handling of the injured, (b) unnecessary transportation.

Specific: Again three vital steps are described:

1. **Oxygen administration:** To restore back PaO_2.
2. **Drug therapy:** Steroids are given intravenously. These help gas exchange by decreasing inflammation in the lungs.
   - ◆ *Heparin:* This acts as a lipolytic and antiplatelet agent.
   - ◆ *Low molecular weight dextran:* Acts by increasing plasma volume.
   - ◆ *Intravenous alcohol* is not universally advocated.
   - ◆ *Antibiotics* and other treatment.
3. **Definitive fracture treatment:** Discussed in appropriate sections.

COMPARTMENTAL SYNDROME OF FOREARM

This is one of the most dreaded complications in orthopedics and ranges from mild ischemia to severe gangrene.

Definition

It is an ischemic necrosis of the structures contained within the volar compartment of the forearm.

Incidence and Etiology

It is common in children less than 10 years of age. Supracondylar fracture is the most common cause in children. Crush injuries of the forearm are the most common causes in adults. Occasionally fracture of both bones of forearm may be the cause. More recently intra-arterial injections in drug addicts who lie on their forearm for prolonged periods in narcotized conditions are mooted

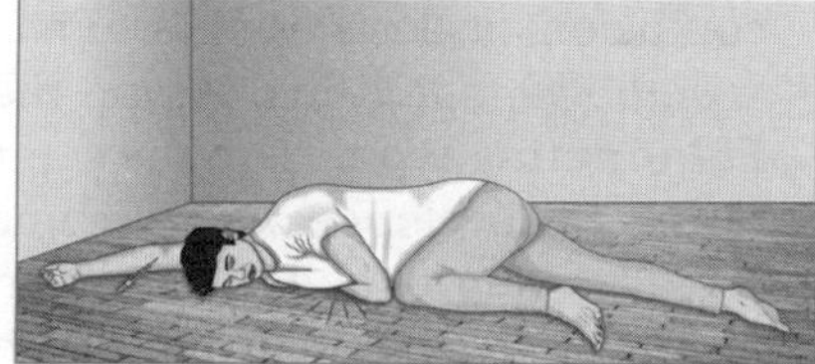

Fig. 8.2: Lying prone on the forearm in an inebriated condition.

to be a cause **(Fig. 8.2)**. Improper application of splints is another important cause.

Usually the flexor muscles of the forearm, especially the flexor digitorum profundus, flexor pollicis longus and rarely flexor digitorum superficialis are involved.

Pathology

It is an inelastic and unyielding deep fascia surrounds the forearm muscles. Rise in the intracompartmental pressure due to any cause is not accommodated and the vessels are compressed resulting in muscle ischemia and consequent fibrosis **(Fig. 8.3)**.

Clinical Features

Impending Volkmann's ischemia: In the acute stages patient gives history of trauma and after an interval of few hours, severe, poorly localized pain develops in the forearm. The volar aspect of the forearm is swollen, red, warm, tender and tense. Fingers are held in flexion and attempt to extend the fingers increase the pain (stretch pain) **(Fig. 8.4)**. Peripheral pulses, which are present initially, disappear later. Median nerve is more commonly affected than the ulnar nerve (See **Box 8.2**).

Note *in compartment syndrome, patient complains of pain out of proportion to the injury.*

Management

Acute Stage

It is a surgical emergency. All encircling tight bandages are removed if present. If there is no improvement, record the pressure within the compartment. If it is more than 30 mm Hg, an emergency surgical decompression is done by fasciotomy **(Figs. 8.5A and B)**. If the pressure is less than 30 mm Hg continuous monitoring is done **(Box 8.2)**.

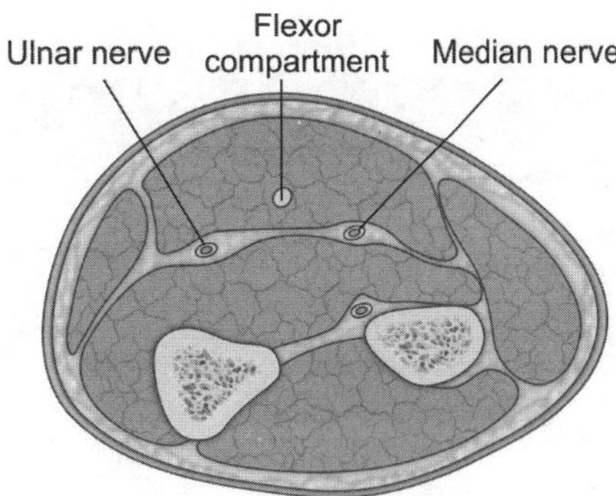

Fig. 8.3: Compartments of the forearm.

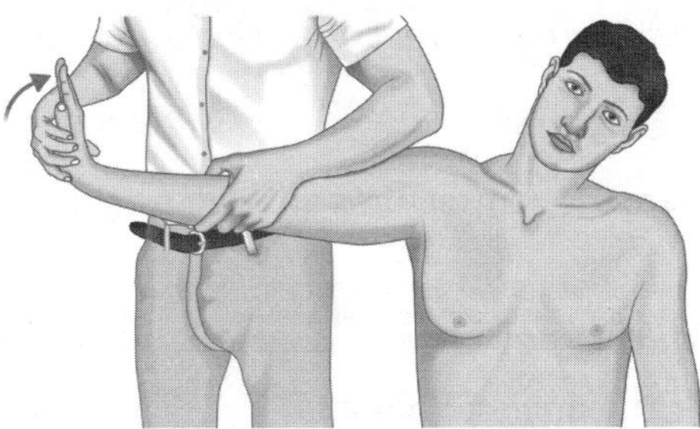

Fig. 8.4: Method of eliciting stretch pain.

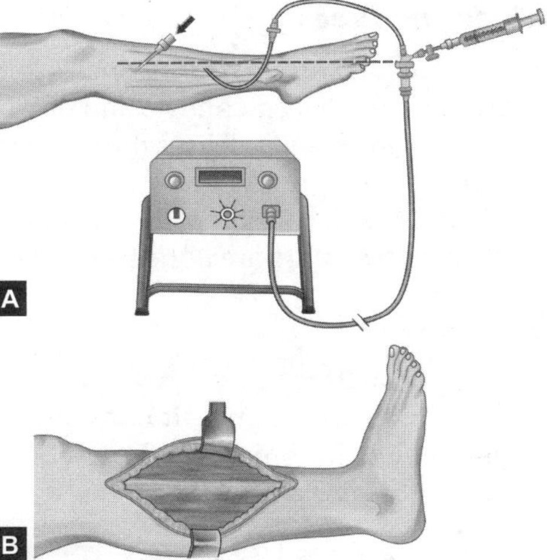

Figs. 8.5A and B: A wide fasciotomy for acute compartmental syndrome.

> **Remember**
>
> **If 5 Ps helps in detection of acute cases, 5 Ps also form clue to the management.**
> - **P**ressure to be relieved either external or internal.
> - **P**ressure to be monitored within the compartment.
> - **P**ulse to be recorded continuously.
> - **P**assive stretch test indicates the severity.
> - **P**utting the fracture back into its position.

Late Cases (Volkman's Ischemic Contracture)

If mild, flexion contractures of flexor digitorum profundus and flexor pollicis longus develops but in severe cases all the finger flexors, thumb and wrist flexors are affected. The forearm is thin and fibrotic. Extensive scar tissue may be present. Peripheral nerves may be affected, amongst them median nerve is the most commonly involved. A *classical claw hand* deformity results. Joint

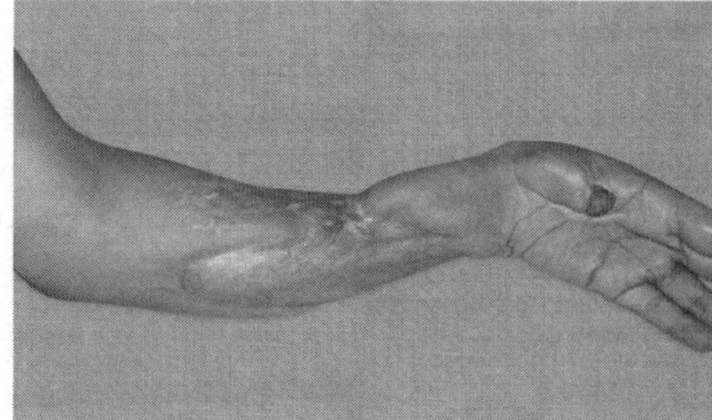

Fig. 8.6: Volkman's ischemic contracture of the forearm.

Box 8.2: Impending Volkmann's ischemia is detected by 6 Ps.

- **P**ain
- **P**allor
- **P**aresthesia
- **P**aralysis
- **P**ulselessness
- **P**ositive passive stretch test

contractures and gangrene may also be seen **(Fig. 8.6)**. Of particular importance is eliciting the *Volkmann's sign* in established VIC. *This test consists of extending the wrist, which exaggerates the deformities, and on flexion, the deformities appear less prominent* **(Fig. 8.7)**.

Treatment

Here the contractures are well established and the treatment plan depends upon the severity of VIC.

Mild Type

- ❖ Dynamic splinting.
- ❖ Physiotherapy.
- ❖ Total excision if single muscle is involved.

Moderate Type

- ❖ ***Max page's muscle sliding operation:*** This consists of releasing the common flexor origin from the medial epicondyle and passively stretching the fingers. This slides the origin of the muscle down and releases the contractures.
- ❖ **Excision of cicatrix.**
- ❖ **Neurolysis:** It consists of freeing the peripheral nerves from the surrounding fibrous tissue.
- ❖ **Tendon transfers** are done if criteria are met.

Severe Type

- ❖ Excision of the scar.
- ❖ Seddon's carpectomy—it consists of excising the proximal row of carpal bones thereby shortening the forearm to overcome the effects of contracted muscles.

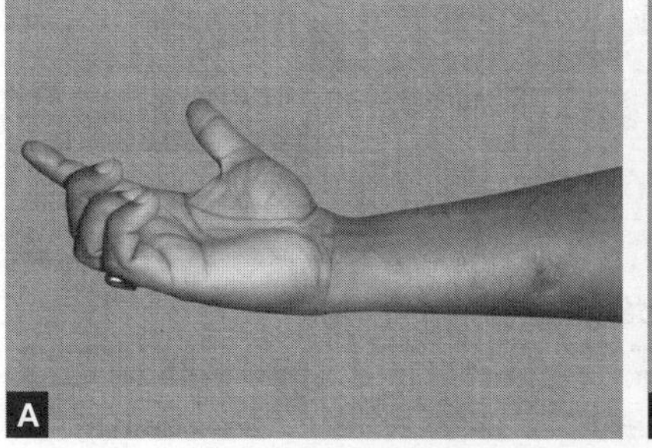

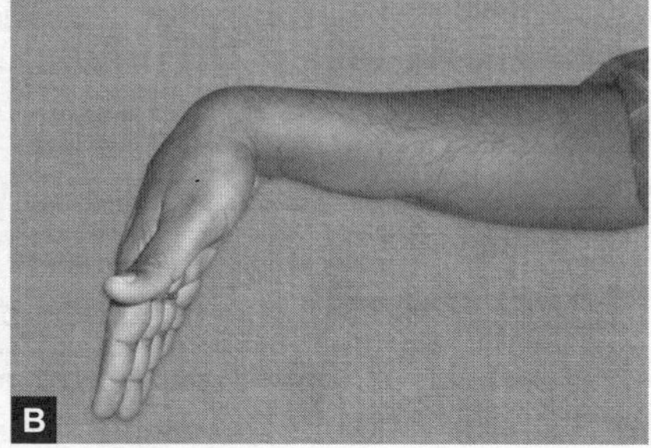

Figs. 8.7A and B: Volkman's sign.

❖ *Arthrodesis* of the wrist in functional position.
❖ *Amputation* for very severe cases of VIC with gangrene.

DELAYED UNION AND NONUNION

The difference between delayed union and nonunion is of degree. In delayed union healing has *not advanced* at the average rate for location and type of fractures but healing can still take place if the limb is immobilized for a longer period. In nonunion there is evidence to show clinically and radiologically that healing has *ceased* and union is improbable and needs surgery. Final status of nonunion is pseudoarthrosis.

Definition (FDA Panel)

Nonunion is said to be established when a *minimum of nine months* has elapsed since the injury and the fracture shows no radiologically visible progressive signs of healing continuously *for 3 months.*

Classification of Nonunion

Muller and Weber depending on the amount of callus adopt two types **(Table 8.1)**.

Table 8.1: Showing types of nonunion.	
Hypervascular nonunion	*Avascular nonunion*
Hypertrophic nonunion (exuberant callus)	Torsion wedge
	Comminuted nonunion
Horse hoof nonunion	Defect nonunion
Oligotrophic nonunion	Atrophic nonunion

Hypervascular Nonunion (Figs. 8.8A to C)

In this, the fracture ends are viable and show biological reaction, hence, stable internal fixation is enough and no bone grafting is required.

Avascular Nonunion (Figs. 8.9A to D)

In avascular nonunion the fracture ends are not viable due to the poor blood supply. No biological reaction is seen, and this needs rigid internal fixation with bone grafting after decortications of nonviable ends.

Causes for Nonunion

Compound fractures, infection, segmental fractures, distraction of fracture fragments, soft tissue interposition.

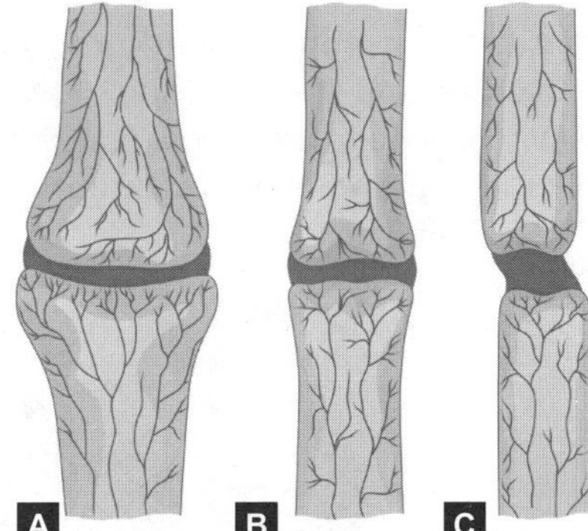

Figs. 8.8A to C: Hypervascular nonunion—elephant foot.

It obstructs the growth of internal callus and thus jeopardizes union. Ill-advised open reduction, insecure and inadequate fixation of fracture.

Apart from these local factors, the general factors, which contribute to poor healing of fractures, are anemia, general debility, cachexia, steroid therapy, osteoporosis, malignancy, etc.

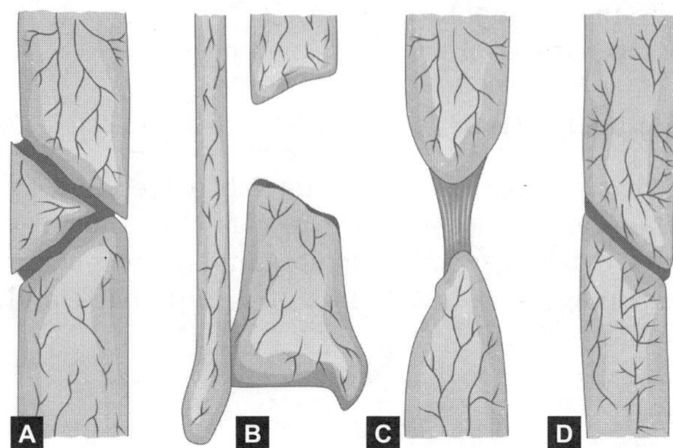

Figs. 8.9A to D: Avascular nonunion.

Clinical Features

Symptoms: The acute symptoms seen in fresh fractures are conspicuously absent in nonunion. There is usually history of no pain or minimal pain. There could be presence of a deformity or loss of function.

Signs: The important clinical signs are painless abnormal mobility, no crepitus, shortening, scars and sinuses, deformity, wasting of limb muscles, etc. **(Fig. 8.10A)**.

Note: In delayed union, patient complains of dull pain at the fracture site and deep palpation clinical tenderness.

Investigations

Radiograph of the part in AP and lateral views **(Fig. 8.10B)**.

Management Principles

* Nonunion is an absolute indication for surgery and it requires open reduction, rigid internal fixation and bone grafting.
* There is no role of conservative treatment.
* Other methods of treatment include electrical stimulation, interlocking nails, Ilizarov, excision, etc.

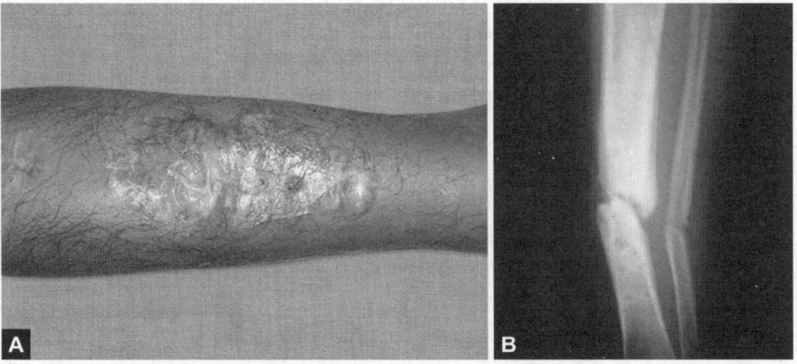

Figs. 8.10A and B: Infected nonunion of tibia.

❖ In delayed union, most of the fractures unite when immobilization is further continued for several weeks. In comprehensive cases, surgery is the treatment of choice.

Other Measures

❖ **Masterly activity:** Do you remember the axiom "leave the sleeping tiger alone"? Well in certain situations nonunion that do not cause significant functional impairments can be left alone (e.g., scaphoid nonunion).
❖ **Resection of the fragments:** Certain non-viable small bone pieces can be safely excised (e.g., distal end of ulna) and in some other situations like nonunion fracture neck femur, the bone is excised and replaced with a prosthesis to make good the loss.

Role of Ilizarov in nonunion: This allows simultaneous correction of all deformities and bone loss. In hypertrophic nonunion gradual compression helps. In avascular nonunion corticotomy, bone transport and compression helps. Ilizarov provides dramatic results but is technically very demanding. It is still the best way to treat cases of infected nonunion.

AVASCULAR NECROSIS (AVN)

Avascular necrosis is a rare but severe complication of certain fractures. It occurs when the blood supply to a segment of bone is affected.

Causes

❖ Extensive stripping of soft tissues, which damage the periosteal blood supply.
❖ In certain bones where the blood supply is unique and unidirectional, e.g., talus, scaphoid, neck of femur **(Figs. 8.11A to C)**.
❖ Other causes like steroid therapy, Caisson's disease, etc., which may cause on embolic block of the blood vessels.

Common sites of AVN are head of femur in fracture neck of femur and dislocations of hip, body of the talus in fracture through the neck of talus, proximal pole of scaphoid in fracture through the waist of the scaphoid.

Problems in avascular necrosis: The loss of blood supply to a major bone segment impairs healing because the avascular segment cannot participate in the reparative process. This defective healing makes the bone weak and susceptible to external forces. This results in collapse of the bone and late osteoarthritic changes.

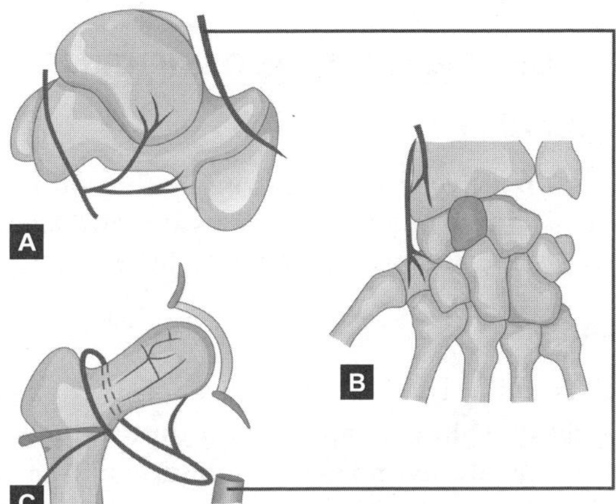

Figs. 8.11A to C: Due to the peculiar blood supply, avascular necrosis is common in the above three bones: (A) Talus; (B) Scaphoid; (C) Head of femur.

Clinical Features

Avascular necrosis of a bone is usually asymptomatic in the early stages. In the later stage patient may complain of pain, limp and slight loss of movements. In very advanced cases patient will show features of osteoarthritis.

Investigations

In the early stages, avascular necrosis can be detected by bone scan, radioisotope study, etc. In the later stages, radiograph shows dense changes in the bone, collapse and osteoarthrotic features **(Fig. 8.12)**.

Treatment

Early stages require no treatment. Protective braces may be given to prevent bone collapse. Surgical decompression has a doubtful role. In the late stages, total hip replacement is advocated for AVN head of the femur. AVN in scaphoid needs open reduction and bone grafting.

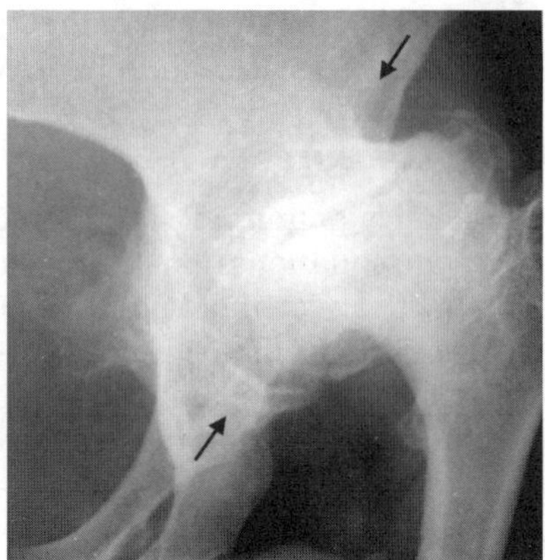

Fig. 8.12: Avascular necrosis of femoral head.

Other Measures

* **Revascularization methods:** Meyer's muscle pedicle graft is a famous example of revascularization procedures for AVN head of femur following fracture of the neck of femur.
* **Resection and replacement (remember R's):** Hemi-replacement arthroplasty with Austin Moore's prosthesis or Thompson's prosthesis is a famous example.
  * Total joint replacement of hip and knee for advanced secondary osteoarthritis following AVN.

TRAUMATIC MYOSITIS OSSIFICANS

Definition

It is a reactive lesion occurring in the soft tissues and at times in the bone periosteum. It is characterized by fibrous, osseous and cartilaginous proliferation of the subperiosteal hematoma. This is later followed by metaplastic changes.

Causes

* **Trauma:** This has a definitive role in the causation of myositis ossificans.
* **Simple blow or repeated minor trauma**
* **Dislocations and avulsion injuries:** Because of the violent stripping of the periosteum and damage to the muscles.
* **Ill-advised massage:** This is by far the most common cause for myositis.

Interesting facts about myositis ossificans
◀◀ It is more common is children due to loose periosteum attachment ◀◀ Patients with head injury, paraplegia are more prone ◀◀ Commonest cause is ill-advised massage.

Pathology: Muscle is commonly involved, but fascia, tendon and periosteum can also be affected. The process is a peculiar alteration within the ground substance of the connective tissue associated with proliferation of undifferentiated connective tissue.

Remember

Myossitis ossificans
Muscles commonly involved are:
- Brachialis anticus.
- Quadratus femoris.
- Adductor muscles of the thigh.

Note: All these muscles take origin from a wide area-suggesting role of periosteum in its genesis.

Clinical Features

In the acute stages, patient may complain of pain, swelling and loss of movements. On examination, there may be tenderness. In the late stages, there is no pain and a bony hard lump may be palpated. This may act as a mechanical block to the movements.

Remember

Areas commonly affected
- Elbow joint common in young athletes.
- Ankle joint—known as footballer's ankle.
- Knee—known as Pellegrini–Stieda disease.
- Shoulder.
- Hip.
- In head injuries it is more common.

Investigations

Radiography has little role in the *acute stages* but in the late stages a bony growth may be evidently seen **(Fig. 8.13)**.

Treatment

Prevention: Remember the famous adage *"prevention is better and than cure".* It suits this conditions completely. Refraining from the ill-advised massage and handling the injured with care prevents this condition from raising its ugly head.

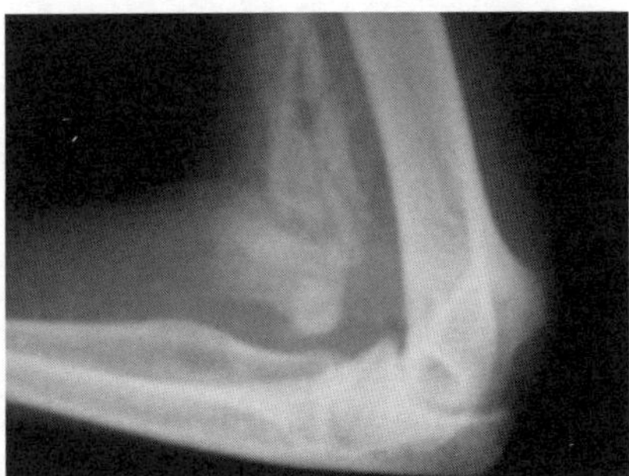

Fig. 8.13: X-ray showing traumatic myositis ossificans.

Curative Measures

- ❖ **Acute stages:** *Conservative* treatment is the method of choice and consists of the following:
  - *Immobilization of the part by splints, etc.*
  - *Drugs*—bisphosphonate therapy, calcitonin and nonsteroidal anti-inflammatory drugs (NSAIDs), it can be recommended.
  - *Physiotherapy:* Active physiotherapy is encouraged and passive stretching is avoided.
  - *Manipulation is done under anesthesia*: It is a double-edged sword and has to be done very carefully. *Adhesions should snap abruptly and should not be broken gradually.*
- ❖ **Chronic stages:** Surgery is the treatment of choice and consists of soft tissue release and excision of bony spur when it is well formed.

Remember

  ◂ The term myositis ossificans is a misnomer because skeletal muscle is often not involved and inflammatory changes are rarely seen.
  ◂ **Myositis ossificans progressiva:** It is a different condition and has nothing to do with the traumatic one. It is a congenital condition affecting all the skeletal muscles.

MALUNION

When fracture fragments heal in an abnormal position, it is called malunion.

Causes

Improper treatment, improper immobilization techniques, treatment by quacks, multiple and multisystem injuries.

Classification

1. **Length malunion:** This commonly results in shortening of the limb and rarely may give rise to lengthening.
2. **Rotatory malunion:** This may cause external or internal rotation deformities.
3. **Angulatory malunion:** This may cause varus or valgus deformities **(Fig. 8.14)**.

Of all the factors mentioned above the one factor, which is not corrected by remodeling, is rotation, while the other three are successfully overcome over the years by remodeling. Hence, all precautions should be taken to correct the rotation element during the initial treatment of fractures.

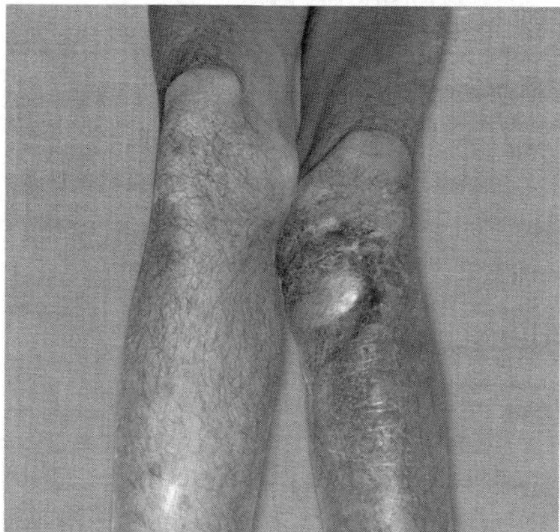

Fig. 8.14: Showing malunion of tibia.

Clinical Features

A patient with malunion of bones may complain of deformity and or loss of function of the affected extremities. There may be shortening and wasting of the involved limbs and restricted movements.

X-rays: Plain X-rays of the affected limb shows the malunion of the bones **(Figs. 8.15A and B)**.

Treatment

Masterly inactivity if patient has no functional problems. Certain malunion is children may be left alone as it is expected to remodel over a period **(Box 8.3)**.

Cosmesis alone does not form a sufficient indication for surgery unless the patient desires

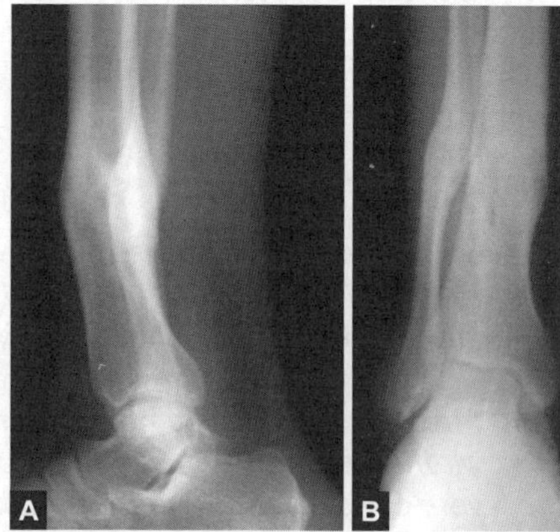

Figs. 8.15A and B: X-ray showing malunion of tibia.

so. Nevertheless, operative treatment is highly justified when malunion affects the function. This can be done by a *corrective osteotomy* at the old fracture site or a *compensatory procedure* may be necessary to restore functions (e.g., Darrach's operation in malunited Colles). Sometimes pain may be the only predominant symptom necessitating *fusion of the joint.*

Box 8.3: Interesting malunion facts (All M's).
◄◄ Malunion is due to:
➢ Mal-reduction
➢ Mal-alignment
➢ Mal-maintenance
◄◄ Made good in children courtesy remodeling
◄◄ Masterly inactivity in most cases
◄◄ Minimal interference if only cosmetic
◄◄ Maximum interference in a functional impairment

OTHER IMPORTANT ACUTE COMPLICATIONS OF FRACTURES

Deep Vein Thrombosis and Pulmonary Embolism

Deep vein thrombosis (DVT) is an important complication seen after fractures of spine, pelvis, femur, tibia, etc. Virchow's triad of venous stasis, vascular damage and hypercoagulability has described the pathogenesis.

Clinical Features

The patient complains of mild to severe calf pain, swelling, difficulty in standing or walking and cramps in the calf muscles or foot. The clinical signs include unilateral leg swelling, increasesd temperature, tenderness, enlarged superficial veins, pitting edema, palpable cord along the involved veins, erythema, etc. **(Fig. 8.16)**.

Homan's sign: When forced ankle dorsiflexion produces calf pain, Homan's sign is said to be positive and is pathognomonic of DVT **(Fig. 8.17)**.

Investigations

Venography helps in definitive diagnosis.

Treatment

Prophylactic methods consist of early ambulation, foot elevation, elastocrepe bandaging, exercises, etc.

Anticoagulant therapy: This consists of aspirin (600–650 mg), heparin (low dose), low molecular weight dextran, low dose warfarin (2.5–16 mg/day daily orally),

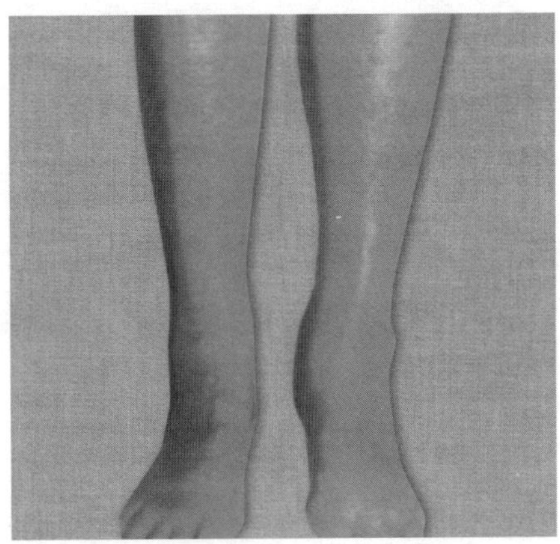

Fig. 8.16: Showing appearance in DVT.

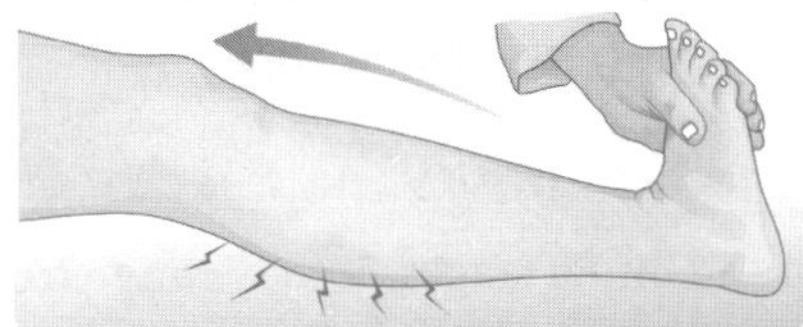

Fig. 8.17: Showing Homan's sign.

etc. Pulmonary thromboembolism is a serious complication of DVT. Patient with pulmonary embolism complains of unexplained dyspnea, pleuritic chest pain, hypoxia, tachypnea, tachycardia, signs of cor pulmonale, etc. Heparin therapy is the treatment of choice. Chronic venous insufficiency is the common long-term complication of DVT.

Disturbing DVT facts

❖ DVT—it can occur as early as 48 hours after injury.
❖ Embolism—it can occur after 4–5 days
❖ Pulmonary embolism-it occur usually after 4–5 days post-accident

INJURY TO BLOOD VESSELS

Blood vessels in close proximity to the bones are injured during fractures and *dislocations* **(Table 8.2)**.

Table 8.2: Involvement of blood vessels in limb injuries.	
Injuries	*Blood vessel involved*
Upper limb trauma	
Fracture clavicle	Subclavian vessels
Proximal humeral fractures	Axillary vessels
Supracondylar fracture of humerus	Brachial vessels
Posterior dislocation of elbow	Brachial vessels
Fracture both bones forearm	Anterior interosseous artery
Lower limb trauma	
Dislocation of hip	Femoral vessels
Fracture femur	Femoral vessels
Supracondylar fracture femur	Popliteal vessels
Dislocation of knee	Popliteal vessels
Proximal tibial fractures	Posterior tibial vessels
Fracture tibia and fibula	Posterior tibial vessels
Ankle injuries	Posterior tibial vessels

Causes of Injury

The blood vessels may be injured in one of the following ways: reflex vasospasm, compression by the fracture fragments or hematoma, incomplete tear, complete tear, partial tear, internal thrombus, tight encircling bandages, etc. **(Fig. 8.18)**.

Effects of Injury

In the initial stages, it may range from mild ischemia to gangrene. In the late stages ischemic contractures may develop.

Clinical Features

Apart from the usual features of fractures, patient may show impending signs of vascular disaster recognized by 5 Ps: **P**ain, **P**ulselessness, **P**aresthesia, **P**allor and **P**aralysis. Cold extremities herald onset of gangrene.

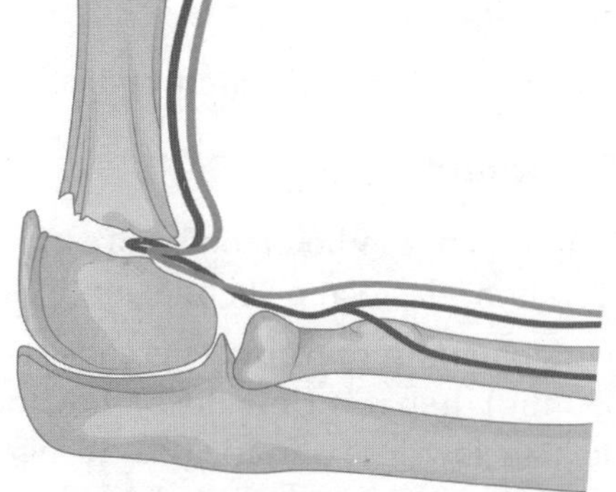

Fig. 8.18: Neurovascular injuries in supracondylar fracture of humerus.

Note: Absence of peripheral pulse is a pointer toward a vascular injury until proved otherwise.

Investigation

It consists of radiograph of the part, Doppler angiogram studies, etc.

Treatment

This consists of prompt reduction of fractures and dislocations and removal of all tight encircling bandages. Thrombectomy, direct end-to-end repair, injection of xylocaine, papaverine, sympathectomy to relieve the vasospasms are some of the commonly recommended methods of treatment. Amputation is considered in irreversible loss of blood supply.

INJURY TO NERVES

About 40% of the bone and joint injuries are associated with peripheral nerve injuries, quite a staggering number **(Fig. 8.19)**.

Types

Two types are described:
- ❖ **Primary:** Here the nerve is injured by the same trauma that resulted in the injury to bone and joint.
- ❖ **Secondary:** This is due to involvement of the nerve in infection, scar, callus, etc.

Incidence

Radial nerve is the most commonly injured peripheral nerve (45%), followed by ulnar nerve (30%), median nerve (15%), peroneal nerve, lumbosacral plexus (3%) and tibial nerve. **Table 8.3** shows the nerve injured in limb trauma.

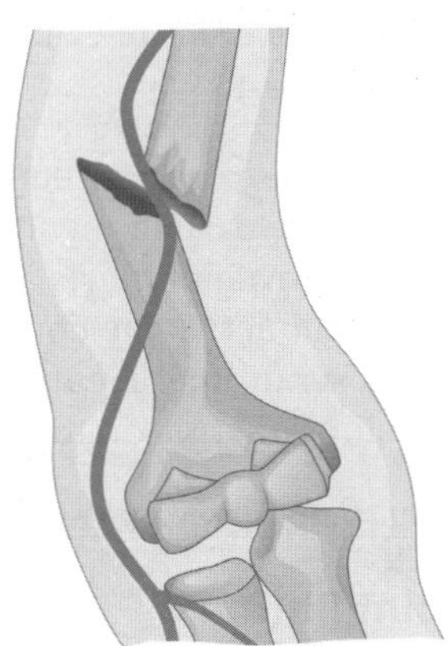

Fig. 8.19: Entrapment of radial nerve in between the fracture fragments of the humerus.

Mechanism of Injury

The nerve may be damaged by the fracture fragments, entrapment between the fragments during fracture reduction, direct injury by the bullets, sharp cutting weapons, etc. In the late stages, the nerve may be trapped in the callus or fibrous tissue.

Types of Nerve Injury

This may be neuropraxia, axonotmesis or neurotemesis depending upon the severity of injury.

Nerve Facts (Table 8.3)

Table 8.3: Nerve facts.	
Trauma	*Nerves injured*
Upper limb	
Fracture clavicle	Brachial plexus
Proximal humeral fracture	Axillary nerve
Fracture humerus	Radial nerve

Contd...

Contd...

Trauma	Nerves injured
Supracondylar fracture humerus	Radial nerve
Posterior dislocation of elbow	Median nerve
Monteggia fracture nerve	Posterior interosseous nerve
Hook of hamate	Deep branch of ulnar nerve
Wrist injury	Median nerve
Lower limb	
Dislocations of hip (posterior)	Sciatic nerve
Anterior dislocation of hip and shaft femur	Femoral nerve
Dislocation of knee	Common peroneal nerve
Proximal tibial fractures and ankle injury	Posterior tibial nerve
Fracture neck fibula	Lateral popliteal nerve

Crush syndrome is seen in severe crush injuries of the limbs and muscles, which results in massive release of myohemoglobin into the circulation, which blocks the renal tubules and leads to myoglobinuria and acute renal tubular necrosis. Prolonged and improper application of tourniquet, acute compartmental syndromes, gas gangrene is some of the other causes of crush syndrome. Treatment is directed towards managing acute renal failure in case patient develops oliguria or anuria.

OTHER IMPORTANT DELAYED COMPLICATIONS

Joint Stiffness

This is due to improper technique of fracture immobilization. This can be troublesome problem. Intra-articular fractures, periarticular adhesions of soft tissues, capsules and muscle contractures are some of the other important causes of joint stiffness. Physiotherapy, exercises, manipulation under anesthesia, surgical excision and lengthening of contractures are some of the important treatment methods.

Reflex Sympathetic Dystrophy

It is an abnormal sympathetic response following fractures. Commonly this is encountered in Colles' fracture.

Osteomyelitis (Fig. 8.20)

It is common in compound fractures (*see the section on osteomyelitis for details*). The other complications peculiar to open fractures are tetanus, gangrene and hypovolemic shock.

Implant Failure

It can occur due to defective manufacturing or biological reactions within the body.

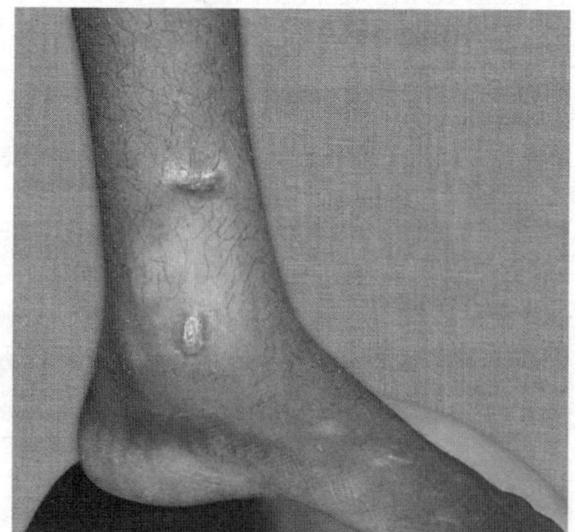

Fig. 8.20: Chronic osteomyelitis.

* **Post-traumatic osteoarthritis** is commonly seen in intra-articular fractures, malunion, etc.
* **Growth alterations** due to epiphyseal injuries in children.

Miscellaneous

The other complications peculiar to open fractures are tetanus, gangrene and hypovolemic shock.

Shortening

After nonunion and malunion, shortening of the long bones is another troublesome complication of fractures. Now the moot point is why do the bones shorten? Well the logical explanations could be one or all the points mentioned below:

In children: It could be due to disturbances in growth following the epiphyseal injuries.

In adults: The causes here are slightly different and it could be due to:
- Loss of small pieces of bone: This can happen in compound, comminuted fractures especially of the tibia.
- Malunion: If there is excess angulation or overlapping during the union, it will translate into shortening.

After Effects of Shortening

- In the upper limbs, it normally goes unnoticed.
- **In the lower limbs:** Here if the shortening is less than 2 cm it goes unnoticed but if it is more than 2 cm, patient has a limb and may develop secondary osteoarthritis of the knee or hip joints over the years due to the altered gait **(Figs. 8.21A and B)**.

Treatment Masterly Inactivity

Shortening of the long bones generally does not require any interference. Even in lower limbs, shortening do not need any treatment. However, interference is required in the following situations: If It is less than 2 cm—shoe raise is given. In addition, if more than 2 cm—limb lengthening procedures usually the Ilizarov's technique is advised.

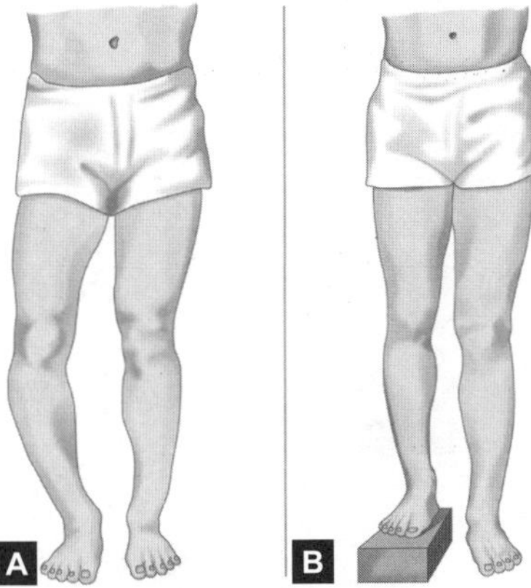

Figs. 8.21A and B: Showing shortening of the leg.

Recap: Complications of Fractures (Table 8.4)

Table 8.4: Complications of fractures.		
Acute	**Chronic**	**Complications peculiar to open fractures**
Shock (hypovolemic or neurogenic)	Delayed union	Infection
	Nonunion	Chronic osteomyelitis
ARDS	Malunion	
Thromboembolism	Shortening	Gas gangrene
Neurovascular injuries	Growth disturbances	Tetanus Hypovolemic shock

Contd...

Contd...

Acute	Chronic	Complications peculiar to open fractures
Radial nerve palsy in fracture shaft humerus	Avascular necrosis	Miscellaneous
	Joint stiffness	Implant failure
Sciatic nerve palsy in post	Post-traumatic arthritis	Reflex sympathetic dystrophy, etc.
Dislocation of hip		
Supracondylar fractures		
Brachial artery injury	VIC	
Acute Volkmann's ischemia	Myositis ossificans	
Crush syndrome		
Deep vein thrombosis		

Injuries to the Joints and Soft Tissues

DISLOCATIONS

Dislocation is defined as a total loss of contact between the two ends of bones **(Figs. 9.1A and B)**. All dislocations are emergencies unlike fractures, for delay in reduction may damage the articular surface, which are deprived of nutrition by the synovial fluid.

Stability of the joint: The stability of a joint comes from the following structures:
1. Shape of the bone ends.
2. **Static stabilizers:** Provided by ligaments.
3. **Dynamic stabilizers:** This is provided by the surrounding muscles.

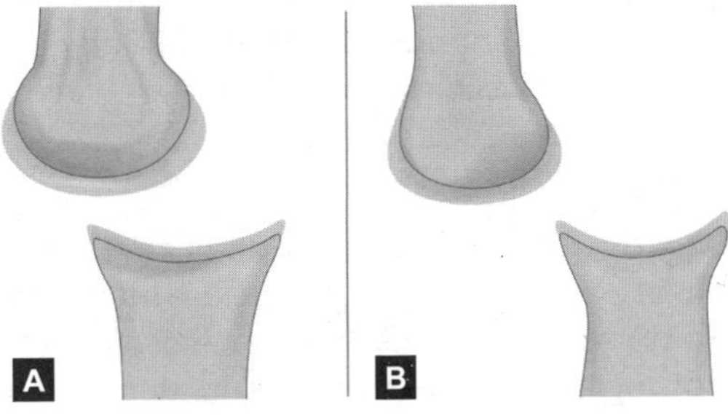

Figs. 9.1A and B: (A) Subluxation; (B) Dislocation.

Pathology

In a dislocation, there could be damage to the capsule, articular cartilage, muscles, and ligaments in varying degrees. There could be osteochondral fractures and avulsion injuries.

Classifications

Types of Dislocation: Congenital or Acquired

Congenital: As in CDH.

Acquired: The following varieties are seen:
- Traumatic—common in young adults due to high-velocity trauma.
- Pathological, e.g., TB hip, septic arthritis, etc.
- Infective, e.g., Tom Smith arthritis in infants.
- Paralytic, e.g., poliomyelitis, cerebral palsy, etc.
- Inflammatory disorders, rheumatoid arthritis, etc.

Traumatic dislocations: This is the most common variety of all dislocations. Considerable force is required to bring the joint out of its position. Capsules are invariably torn and the ligaments are avulsed or torn. There could damage to the articular cartilages, a fragment of which may break and form loose bodies within the joint.

Varieties of Traumatic Dislocations

❖ **Fresh dislocations:** Due to trauma, there could be acute dislocation of a joint. The more common ones are dislocations of the shoulder, patella, and hip, elbow, etc., **(Fig. 9.2).**

❖ **Chronic unreduced dislocation:** In Asian countries, due to poverty, ignorance, illiteracy, apathy fresh dislocations are not promptly reduced and the patient lives with pain and disability. Due to secondary problems like pain, contractures, osteoarthritis, etc., patient may visit a doctor for treatment.

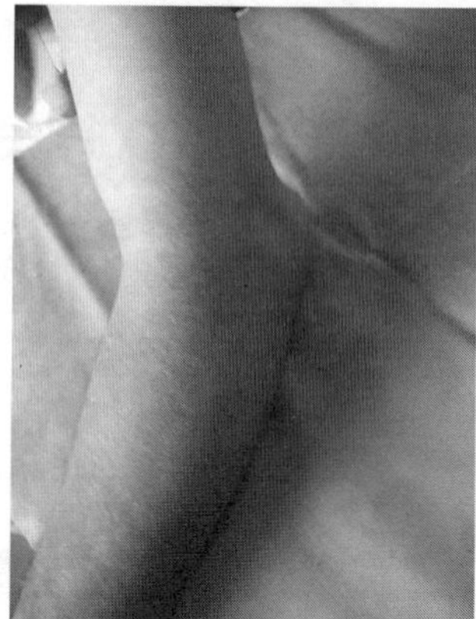

Fig. 9.2: Acquired traumatic dislocation—posterior dislocation of elbow.

❖ **Repeated dislocations:** Due to the inherent instability and other factors, some joints are prone for repeated dislocations. Topping the list in this group is the recurrent dislocations of the shoulder joint and the patella.

❖ **Fracture dislocations:** Here along with the dislocation a piece of the neighboring bone is avulsed from its position or totally broken depending upon the severity of injury, e.g., posterior dislocation of the hip with acetabular fractures.

Dislocation Facts

Why do you think dislocation is an emergency? Reasons: (1) It causes intense pain due to the stretching of the capsules. Unless reduced immediately, pain will not disappear. (2) Nourishment of the articular cartilages is through the synovial fluid, which gets disturbed in a dislocation. If the cartilages are deprived of this nourishment for a longer time, the damages to the cartilages will be permanent resulting in secondary osteoarthritis. Hence prompt reduction is a must.

Clinical Features

Traumatic variety is the most common type of dislocations one encounters in clinical practice. Patient gives history of trauma usually a road traffic accident (RTA) on fall from heights following, which there is pain, swelling deformity and loss of movements. In dislocations of other varieties, clinical symptoms and signs pertaining to that particular disease are seen (e.g., TB).

Typical deformities in dislocations

◄◄ Shoulder—abduction deformity.
◄◄ Elbow—flexion deformity.
◄◄ Hip:
  ➤ Anterior—flexion, abduction and external rotation deformity.
  ➤ Posterior—flexion, abduction and internal rotation deformity.
◄◄ Knee—flexion deformity.
◄◄ Ankle—varus deformity.

Investigations

Radiograph of the affected part should include anteroposterior and lateral views of the joints **(Fig. 9.3)**.

Treatment

Since dislocation is an orthopedic emergency, early closed reduction under general anesthesia is recommended. The part is immobilized for a period of 3–6 weeks to ensure adequate healing.

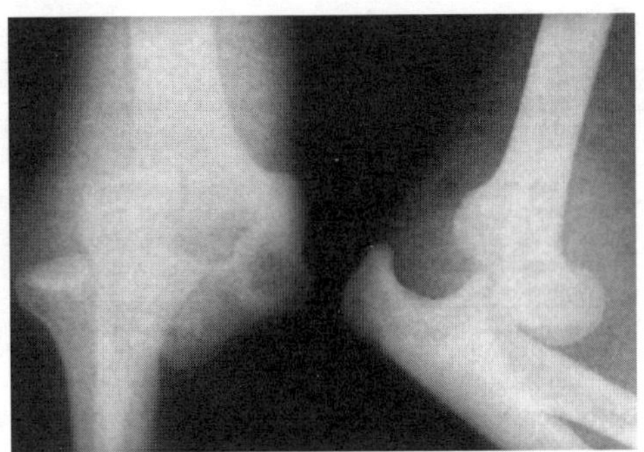

Fig. 9.3: Plain X-ray showing dislocation of the elbow.

Operative reduction is rarely required and is reserved for:

❖ Failure of closed reduction.
❖ Compound dislocations
❖ Irreducible dislocations
❖ Old unreduced dislocations
❖ Recurrent dislocations
❖ Fracture dislocations.

Complications of Dislocations

Acute Injury

Acute Injury to peripheral nerves and vessels can occur, e.g., sciatic nerve palsy in posterior dislocation of hip **(Tables 8.3 and 8.4)**.

Chronic Injury

❖ **Unreduced dislocation,** which is common in Asian countries due to ignorance, delay in seeking treatment, etc.
❖ **Recurrent dislocations**: Due to inadequate and improper healing of soft tissues following initial trauma.
❖ **Traumatic osteoarthritis:** Due to damage to the articular cartilage following impaired nutrition by the synovial fluid.
❖ **Joint stiffness**: Due to capsular and other soft tissue injuries.
❖ **Avascular necrosis**: Due to injury to the vessels.
❖ **Myositis ossificans**: More commonly seen than in fractures due to greater perioseal strip.

SUBLUXATION

Subluxation is defined as partial loss of contact between the two ends of the bones. It poses a problem much less serious than dislocation.

SPRAIN

It is a tear in the ligaments. The severity varies from grade I to grade III **(Figs. 9.4A to C)**. Mild sprains are more common

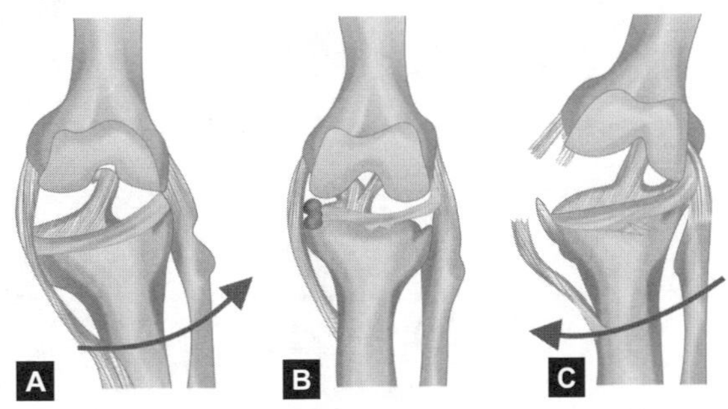

Figs. 9.4A to C: Showing grades of knee medial collateral ligament sprain.

Box 9.1: Price regime.

Treatment: It is essentially conservative and is denoted by the mnemonic
PRICEM:
- P–Pain killers
- R–Rest
- I–Ice compression
- C–Compression
- E–Elevation
- M–Mobilization

and heal by conservative treatment, whereas grade III sprains cause joint instabilities and need to be repaired surgically. Sprains are commonly encountered in knee joints and ankle joints. Mild sprains are treated by the PRICE regime **(Box 9.1)** and immobilization by knee supports **(Fig. 9.5)**.

STRAIN (FIG. 9.6)

It is tearing in the muscles, is more common in young athletes, and usually occurs due to sudden violent contractions. Patient with acute muscular strain complains of organizing from muscle tightness due to spasm and inability to more due to acute pains and spasm **(Fig. 9.7)**.

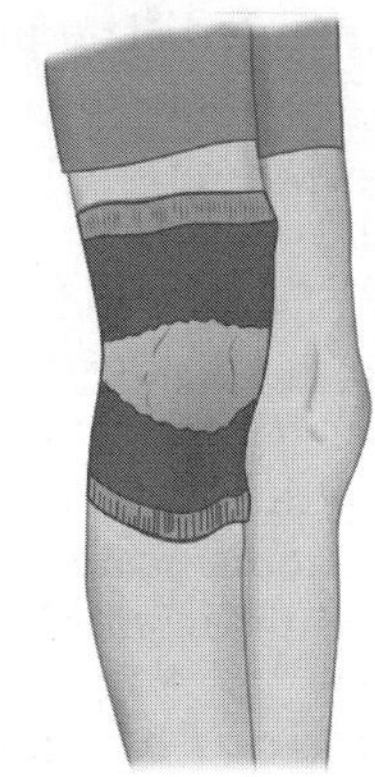

Fig. 9.5: Immobilization of sprained knee by elastic braces.

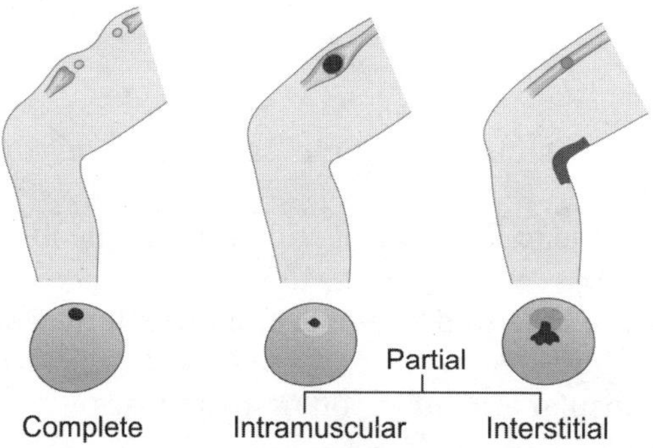

Fig. 9.6: Types of muscles strain.

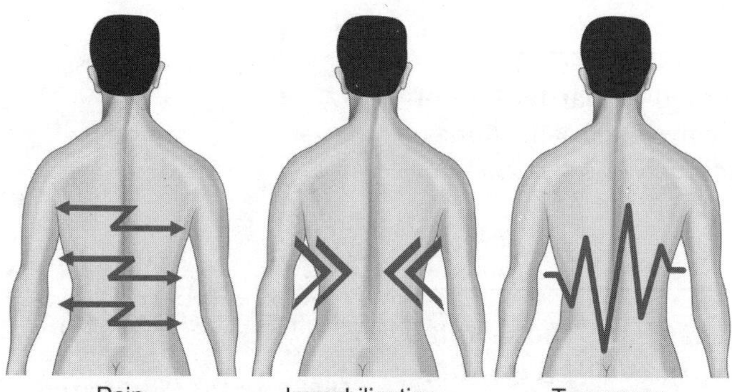

Fig. 9.7: Clinical features of muscle strain.

TENDON INJURIES

Tendon usually does not give way in young unless injured by a sharp cutting object like knife, chopper, etc.

Interesting Facts

- ❖ Common causes of tendon injuries in young adults
  - ◆ Injury by sharp cutting weapons like knife, etc.
  - ◆ Athletic and sports injuries
- ❖ Common causes of tendon injuries in old age
  - ◆ Rheumatoid arthritis
  - ◆ Degenerative changes
  - ◆ SLE
  - ◆ Leprosy
- ❖ Common sites of tendon ruptures
  - ◆ Upper limbs
    - – Supraspinatus tendon
    - – Biceps tendon
    - – Extensor pollicis longus tendon
  - ◆ Lower limbs
    - – Quadriceps tendon
    - – Patella tendon
    - – Achilles tendon

Treatment

In fresh cases, primary repairs or tendon grafting. In old ruptures, if the disability is negligible no treatment is required. In the event of significant disability, tendon transfers may be contemplated.

10
CHAPTER

Fracture of the Clavicle and Scapula

Chapter Outline

- Fracture of the Clavicle
- Fracture of the Scapula

FRACTURE OF THE CLAVICLE

The term clavicle is derived from the Latin root *Clavis* meaning *Key*.

Mechanism of Injury

- **Direct** due to fall on the point of the shoulder. This is the most common mode of injury accounting for 91% of the cases.
- **Direct trauma** over the clavicle due to RTA, etc., accounts for 8% of the cases **(Fig. 10.1)**.
- **Indirect** fall on the outstretched hands accounts for 1% of the cases.

Fig. 10.1: Showing common method of fracture clavicle by direct trauma.

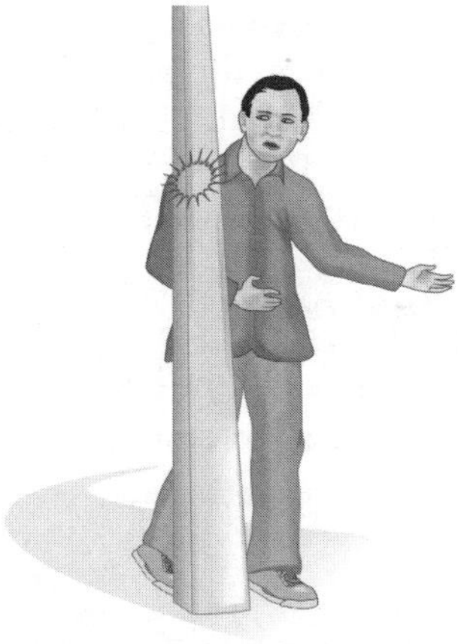

Sites of Fracture

- About 80% of the fracture clavicle occurs at the junction of middle and outer third
- About 1% at medial end of the clavicle
- Lateral end fracture is uncommon.

Clinical Features

Patient presents with pain, swelling, deformity and inability to raise the shoulder on the affected side **(Fig. 10.2)**. Rarely patient may present with pseudo-paralysis of the affected arm.

Radiology

Routine anteroposterior view of the clavicle is sufficient to make a diagnosis most of the times **(Fig. 10.3)**.

Principles of Treatment

Before proceeding to the treatment proper one needs to understand the two distracting forces acting on the fracture fragments in clavicle making the treatment difficult **(Fig. 10.4)**.

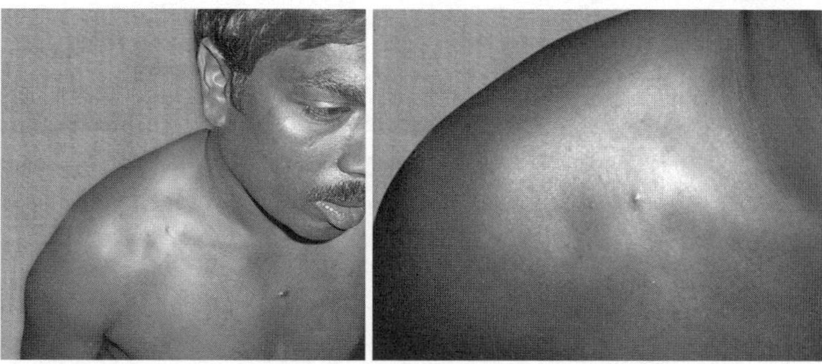

Fig. 10.2: Showing classical deformity in fracture of the clavicle.

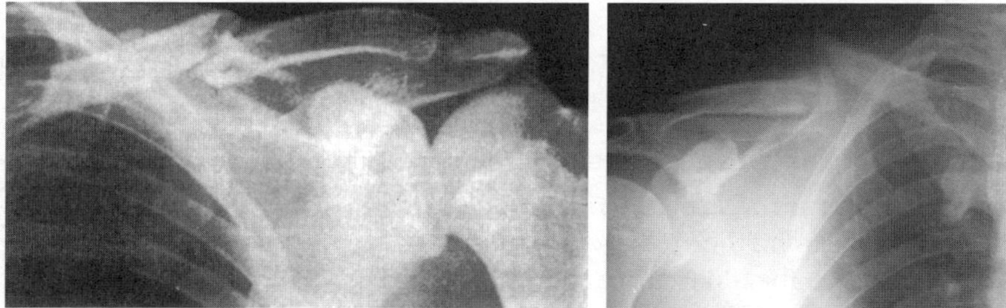

Fig. 10.3: Plain X-ray showing fracture clavicle of middle-third.

Sternocleidomastoid muscle attached at the medial and of the clavicle pulls it up, while the pectoralis major muscles and the gravity pulls the lateral end of the clavicle down. Successful treatment of fracture clavicle depends on how effectively one overcomes these displacing forces. To counter the above two detrimental forces, the shoulder should be elevated and braced back and the arm should be supported while treating fracture clavicle.

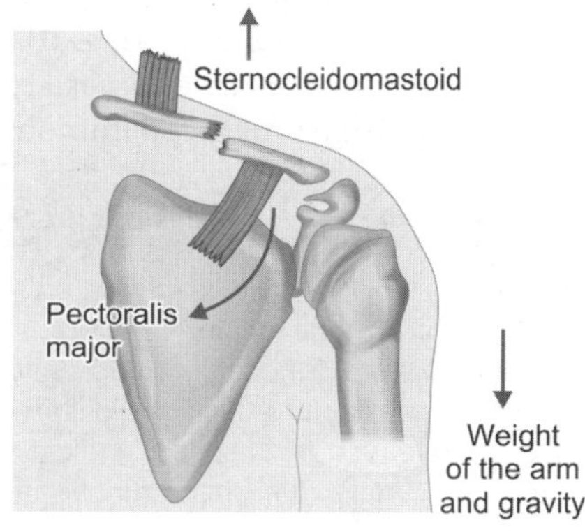

Fig. 10.4: Various displacing forces in fracture clavicle.

Conservative Methods

This is the treatment of choice in fracture clavicle and consists of the following methods:

- ❖ **Cuff and collar sling:** For un-displaced fractures **(Fig. 10.5A)**.
- ❖ **Strapping:** The fracture site using dynaplast gives good results especially in children and young adults **(Fig. 10.5B)**.
- ❖ **Figure of '8' (Fig. 10.5C):** This is popularly used and it acts by retracting the shoulder girdle, minimizes the overlap and allows more anatomical healing.

Surgery is rarely indicated and is considered in the following situations: Open fractures, injury to neurovascular bundle, if the fracture is threatening to penetrate the skin, nonunion, fracture near acromioclavicular joint, and displaced epiphysis in children.

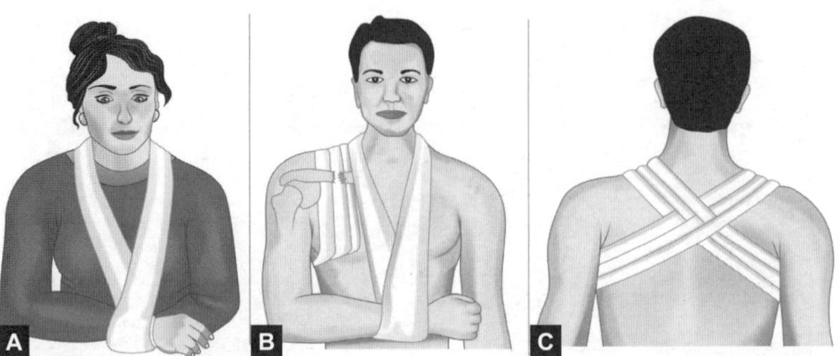

Figs. 10.5A to C: Methods of conservative treatment of fractures clavicle: (A) Strapping and sling suspension; (B) Collar and cuff sling; (C) Figure of 8 bandaging.

Fixations Methods

This could be either by plate and screws **(Figs. 10.6 and 10.7)**, by special intramedullary rods or by K-wire.

Complications of Fracture Clavicle

❖ **Neurovascular injury:** The structures commonly injured are subclavian vessels and the medial cord of the brachial plexus through which the ulnar nerve is derived.
❖ **Malunion** is very common, causes only a cosmetic problem and does not usually impair function. Hence no treatment is required in most situations **(Fig. 10.8A)**.
❖ **Nonunion:** It is rare and requires open reduction, internal fixation and bone grafting **(Fig. 10.8B)**.
❖ **Frozen shoulder:** Due to periarthritis of the shoulder joint following prolonged immobilization.

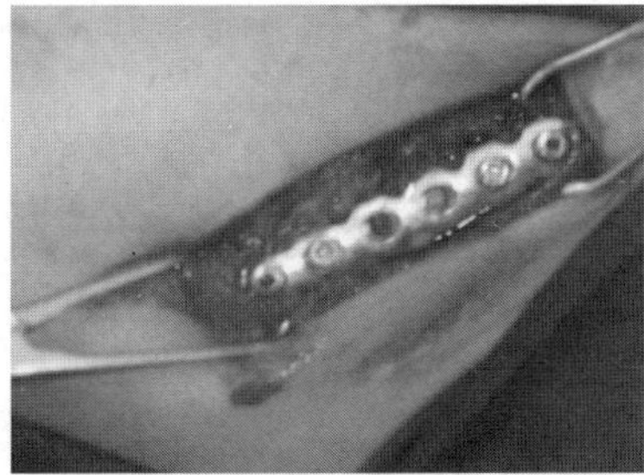

Fig. 10.6: Operative photograph, showing open reduction and internal fixation with plate and screws is rarely indicated in fracture clavicle.

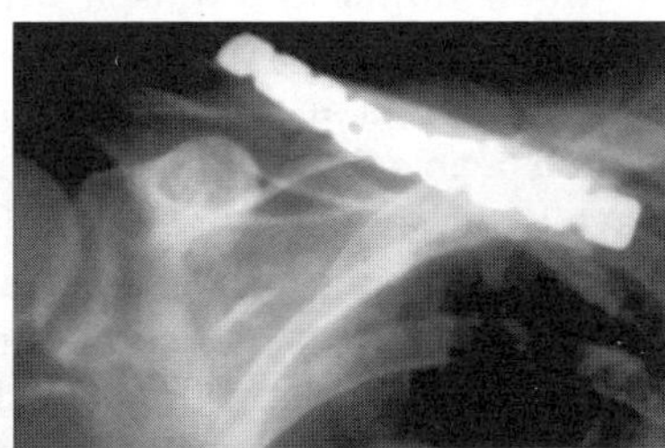

Fig. 10.7: Plain X-ray of the clavicle showing fixation with plate and screws.

Quick facts: Fracture clavicle
◀◀ Most common fracture in children.
◀◀ Common mode of injury is direct.
◀◀ 80% break at junction of middle and distal third.
◀◀ Nearly all fractures are treated closed.
◀◀ Open reduction for specific indications.
◀◀ Malunion is a rule, but no functional disability.

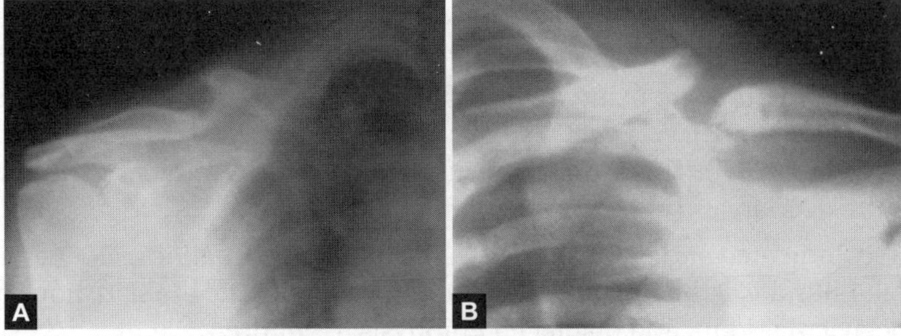

Figs. 10.8A and B: Plain X-ray showing: (A) Malunion of fracture clavicle; (B) Nonunion of fracture clavicle.

FRACTURE OF THE SCAPULA

Scapula is a flat bone thickly covered by muscles. From above downwards, the scapula may be fractured as follows **(Fig. 10.9)**:

- ❖ The coracoid process.
- ❖ The spine of the scapula.
- ❖ The neck.
- ❖ The body.

Mechanism of Injury

The scapula may be fractured due to:
- ❖ Direct injury to the shoulder blade due to fall of heavy objects on the back.
- ❖ Fall on outstretched hands.

Whatever may be the mechanism of injury, scapular fractures are seldom displaced, thanks to the thick muscles surrounding it.

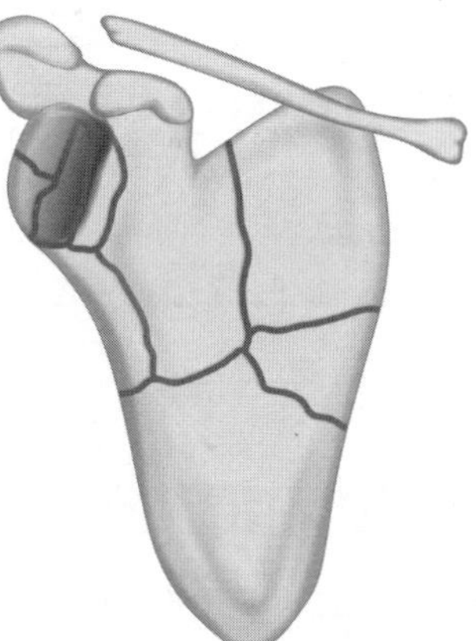

Fig. 10.9: Showing various types of scapular fractures.

11
CHAPTER

Humerus Fractures

FRACTURE SHAFT HUMERUS

Fracture shaft humerus is more common in adults than in children, though it can appear in any age group.

Mechanism of Injury

❖ **Direct force:** As in RTA's, assaults, etc. **(Fig. 11.1)**. This may produce a transverse or comminuted fracture.

❖ **Indirect force:** It is due to fall on an outstretched hand and this will produce an oblique or spiral fracture.

❖ **Birth injuries:** This is the second most common birth fracture after clavicle.

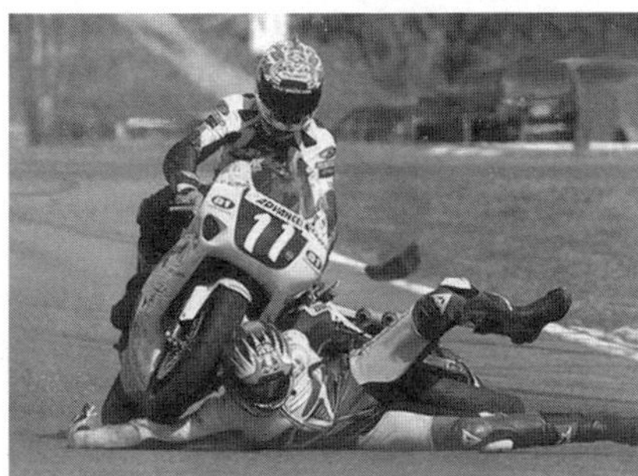

Fig. 11.1: Direct injury in RTA's common cause of humeral shaft fractures.

Anatomic Considerations

The deformity is influenced by the muscles of the upper arm. If the fracture is between pectoralis major and deltoid, the proximal fragment is adducted by pectoralis major, teres minor and latissimus dorsi, while the distal fragment is pulled upwards by the deltoid. If the fracture is below the insertion of deltoid, the proximal fragment is abducted by the deltoid while the coracobrachialis, biceps and triceps **(Figs. 11.2A and B)** pull the distal fragment upward.

Clinical Features

Clinical features show all the signs and symptoms of a fracture **(Fig. 11.3)**. A careful neurological and vascular

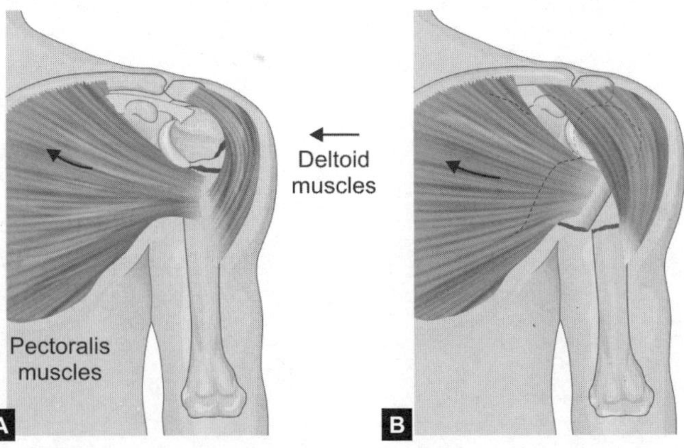

Figs. 11.2A and B: Muscle forces causing deformity in fracture shaft humerus.

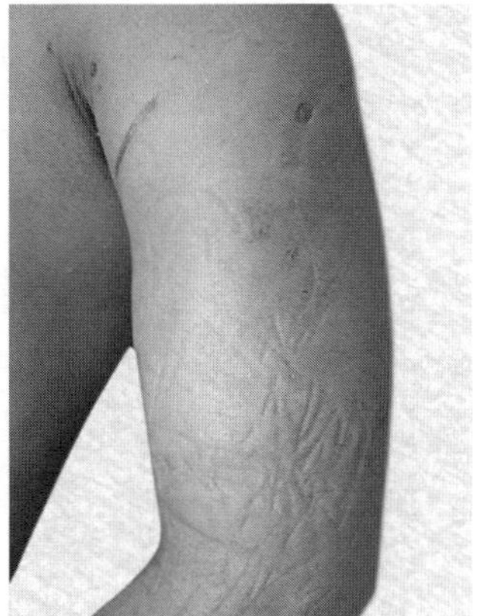

Fig. 11.3: Clinical photograph of fracture shaft of humerus.

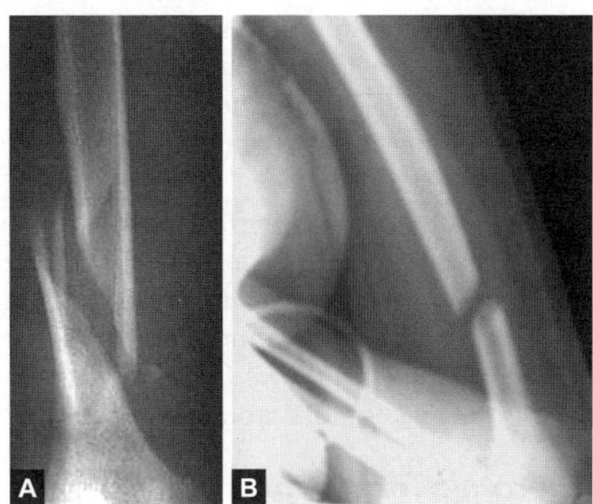

Figs.11.4A and B: Showing spiral fracture and transverse fracture of the humerus.

assessment is important. Injury to radial nerve is common in fractures at the spiral groove or lower one-third of humerus.

Radiology: Radiography of the entire upper arm including both the shoulder joint above and the elbow joint below should be taken. It helps to study the level and pattern of the fracture **(Figs. 11.4A and B).**

Treatment

Conservative Methods (Figs. 11.5A to C)

- ❖ **Undisplaced fractures:**
  - ◆ *Simple U-splint* in birth fractures.
  - ◆ *Simple sling* may be sufficient in young children.
  - ◆ *Chest arm bandage:* Here the arm is strapped to the side of the chest with bandages. It can be considered in children less than 5 years of age.
- ❖ **Displaced fractures:**
  - ◆ *Hanging cast:* This is useful in older children and adolescents. Here gravity aids in reduction of the fracture. They are not suitable if the level of fracture corresponds to the upper limit of the cast, because of the deforming effect of the proximal end of the cast. It is indicated in comminuted fractures of the distal third. If the cast is too heavy it may cause distraction and consequent delayed or nonunion.

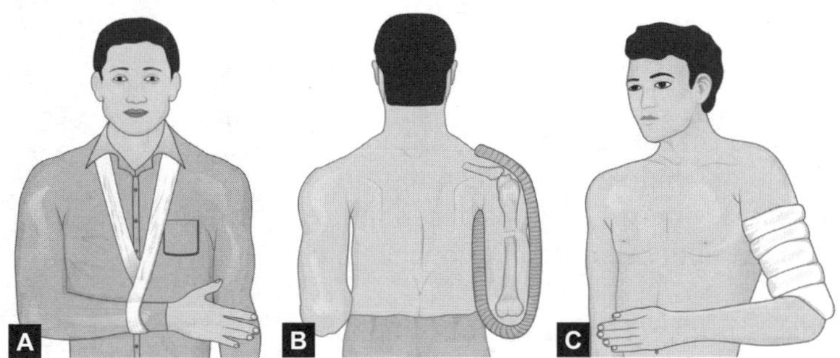

Figs. 11.5A to C: Showing different conservative treatment methods in fracture shaft of humerus:
(A) Hanging cast; (B) U-slab; (C) Caste brace.

- *A plaster U-splint* is sufficient in most of the situations of fractures of the proximal and middle third portions of the humerus. The method of application of a U-slab is shown in **Figure 11.6**. U-slab covers the following areas of the upper arm:
  - *Inner arm of the U:* Supports the inner side of the arm just beneath the axilla.
  - *U-turn:* Supports the medial epicondyle, olecranon tip and the lateral epicondyles.
  - *Outer arm of the U:* Supports the outer aspect of the arm, shoulder, and extends up to the base of the neck.

Operative Treatment

Fortunately, the incidence of surgical treatment in humerus fracture is reduced to a miniscule few cases with the following specific indications:

- Failed conservative treatment.
- Multiple fractures and unstable fractures.
- Multi-system injuries.
- Radial nerve palsy after closed reduction.

Methods

- DCP plating for fractures at all levels **(Figs. 11.7 and 11.8)**.
- Intramedullary fixation at middle third fractures.
- Recently interlocking nailing is also being tried with varied success **(Figs. 11.9A to C)**.

Complications

- **Radial nerve injury:** This is common in lower one-third fractures and is usually of a high variety. It may also be damaged in the spiral groove. Closed fractures need observation, splinting of wrist and fingers. If a radial nerve deficit occurs after closed manipulations, immediate exploration is necessary.
- **Vascular injury:** Injury to the brachial vessels is unusual. It requires repeated assessment and prompt treatment.
- **Malunion:** In humeral fractures, angular deformity of 20° is acceptable in the middle and distal one-third; while in the proximal one-third, 30° is acceptable. Thick muscles in the upper arm usually conceal the mal-union.
- **Nonunion:** This is not very common but may be seen due to overweight hanging cast. This requires open reduction, rigid plating and bone grafting.

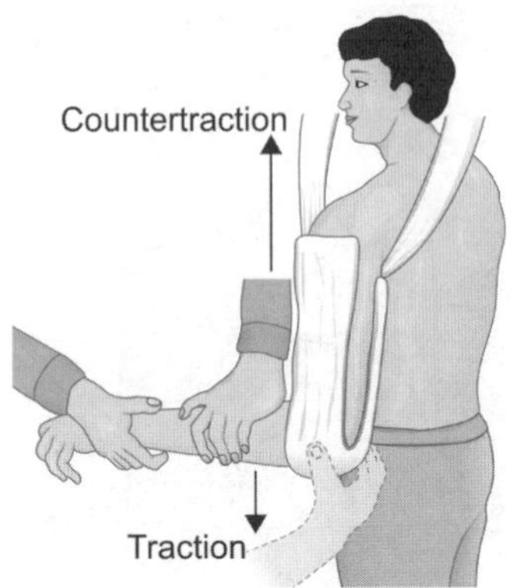

Fig. 11.6: Method of closed reduction and application of a U-cast.

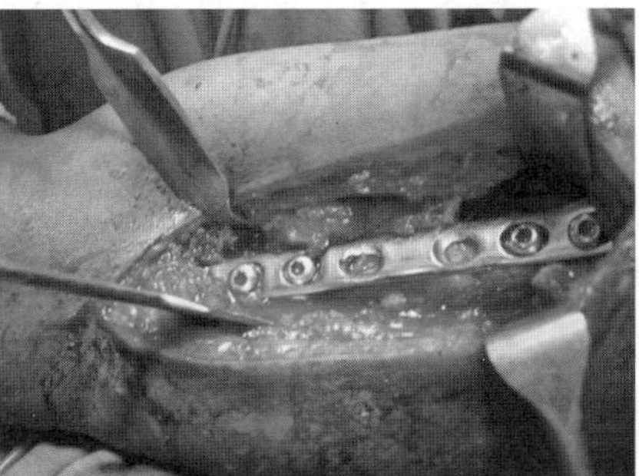

Fig. 11.7: Operative picture of the surgical fixation of fracture shaft humerus with DCP plate and screws.

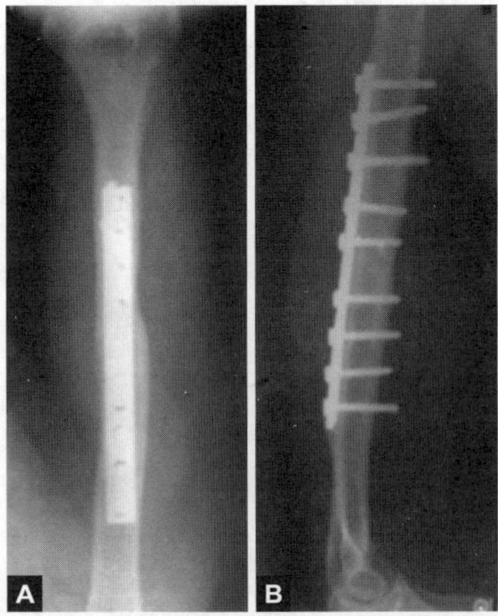

Figs. 11.8A and B: Plain X-ray showing surgical fixation of fracture shaft humerus with DCP plate and screws.

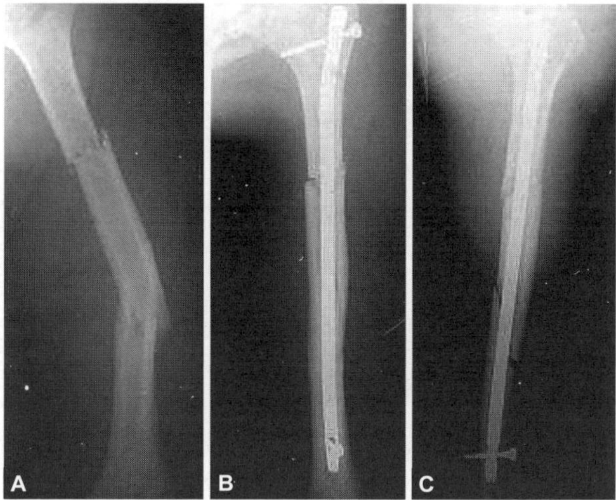

Figs. 11.9A to C: Surgical fixation of segmental fracture humerus with interlocking nails.

HUMERAL FRACTURES OF SPECIAL INTEREST

❖ **Greater tuberosity fracture of the humerus:** This fracture is more commonly seen in adults and is due to the fall on the joint of the shoulder. Rarely could it be due to avulsion of the supraspinatus muscle **(Fig. 11.10)**. Patient complains of pain, swelling and inability or difficulty to abduct the shoulder. Plain X-rays help to study the displacement and angulation of the tuberosity **(Fig. 11.11)**. Conservative treatment is by cuff and collar, sling, etc., suffices for un-displaced or minimally displaced fractures. Abduction splints or ORIF is reserved for displaced fractures. Frozen shoulder could be a trouble some late compliances.

❖ **Surgical neck fractures:** These are commonly seen is frail elderly women and is due to trivial fall on the point of the shoulder. However, unlike fracture neck of femur, this fracture is frequently impacted and generally heals well by simple conservative methods take sling. Displaced fractures **(Fig. 11.12)** required closed reduction and percutaneous K-wire fixation or rarely open reduction and rigid internal fixations. Axillary nerve injury may occur and is identified by the loss of sensation in the regiment bandage area. Frozen shoulder is another important complication.

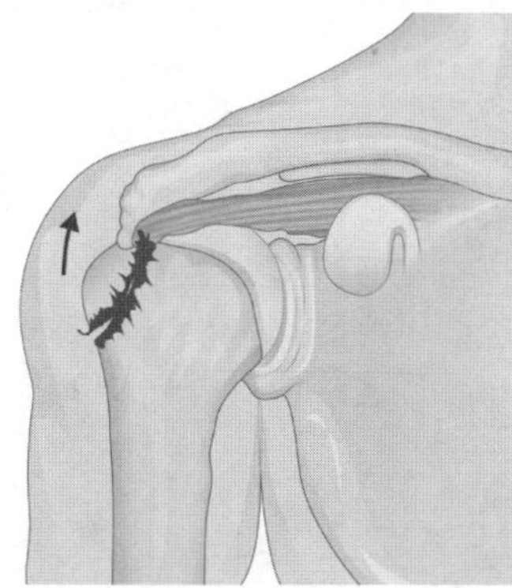

Fig. 11.10: Showing avulsion fracture of greater tuberosity of humerus.

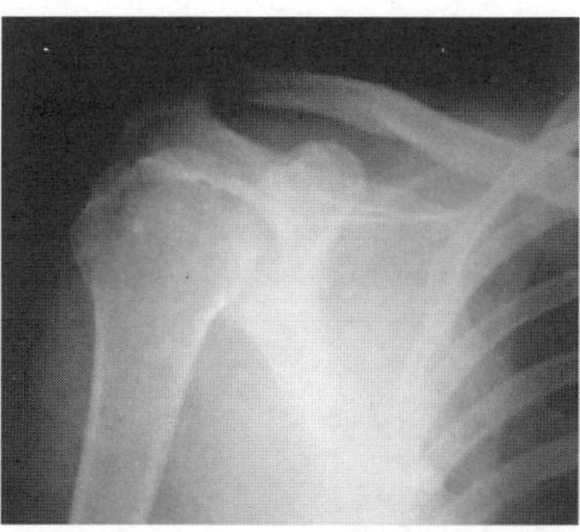

Fig. 11.11: Plain X-ray showing avulsion fracture of greater tuberosity of humerus.

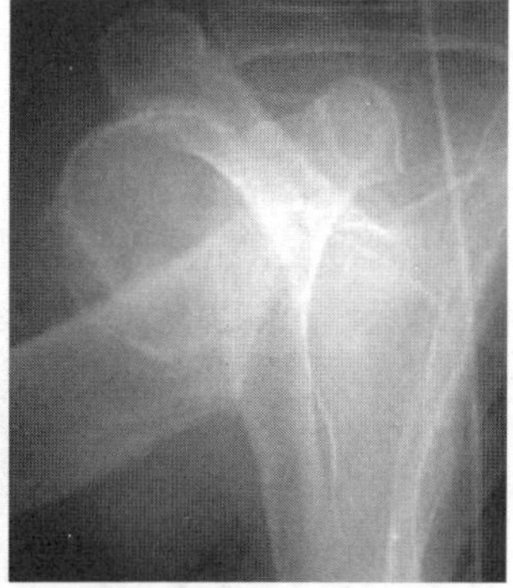

Fig. 11.12: Showing displaced surgical neck fracture of humerus.

Fractures of Both Bones of Forearm

Injuries of the forearm present an interesting combination of injuries like fracture bones forearm, Monteggia fractures, Galeazzi fractures, Essex-Lopresti fracture, etc.

FRACTURE BOTH BONES OF FOREARM

This is a difficult problem especially in adults. The complex muscle arrangements already described makes retention of the fracture fragments very difficult. The fracture could be due to either direct or indirect trauma.

Clinical Features

Patient presents with pain, swelling, deformity and other features of fractures. Tenderness can be elicited and the functions of the forearm, elbow and wrist are usually affected (**Fig. 12.1**).

Radiology (Figs. 12.2A to C)

It plays an important role in the diagnosis of this fracture and a routine AP and lateral views including both elbow and wrist joints helps.

Treatment

Conservative treatment consists of closed reduction by traction and countertraction methods under general

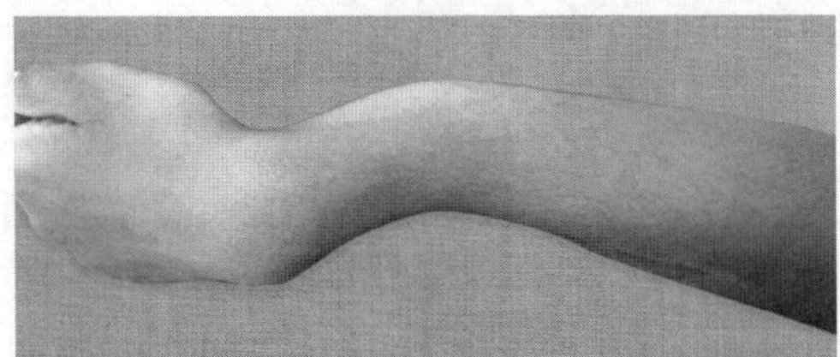

Fig. 12.1: Showing deformity due to fracture both bones of the forearm.

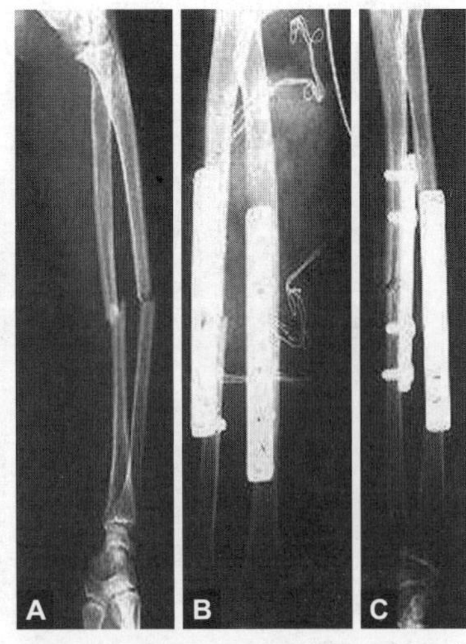

Figs. 12.2A to C: Fracture both bones of forearm fixed rigidly with DCP plates and screws.

anesthesia followed by an above elbow plaster cast immobilization and is usually successful in children.

Surgery: In adults open reduction and internal fixation is often indicated because it is difficult to regain length, apposition, axial and normal rotational alignment in adults by closed reductions. Open reduction is by two approaches, one for the radius and the other for the ulna. The choice of implants for ulna is either a medullary nail or plate and screws but for fracture radius, rigid compression plating is usually desired. Cancellous bone grafting is done if the comminution is more than one-third of the circumference of the bone **(Figs. 12.2A to C)**.

Complications of Fracture Both Bones of Forearm

- ❖ **Volkmann's ischemia:** Because of the tight fascial compartment, a patient with fracture both bones forearm is more prone to develop acute compartmental syndrome.
- ❖ **Delayed union and nonunion:** This can be encountered due to soft tissue interposition, inadequate immobilization, etc. It has to be treated by open reduction, rigid internal fixation and cancellous bone grafting.
- ❖ **Malunion:** Due to the complex muscular forces it is difficult to retain the position of both bones in perfect alignment after closed reduction. It is in this situation that malunion commonly results. It is treated by corrective osteotomy, plating and bone grafting.
- ❖ **Cross union:** This is due to malunion of a radial fracture in a medially deviated position, which occupies the interosseous space and blocks pronation and supination. If the cross union takes place in the middle third of the forearm, it can be left alone as the forearm is held in midpronation with less functional damage. Elsewhere it needs corrective osteotomy and rigid internal fixation.

MONTEGGIA FRACTURE

It is fracture upper third of ulna with dislocation head of the radius. *This is usually called a* **"treacherous lesion"** *because the dislocation is often missed.* Monteggia first described it in 1881.

Mechanism of Injury

Monteggia fractures are caused by fall on the outstretched hands with hyperpronation (common) or hyperextension **(Fig. 12.3)**. A direct blow over the forearm can also result in such an injury.

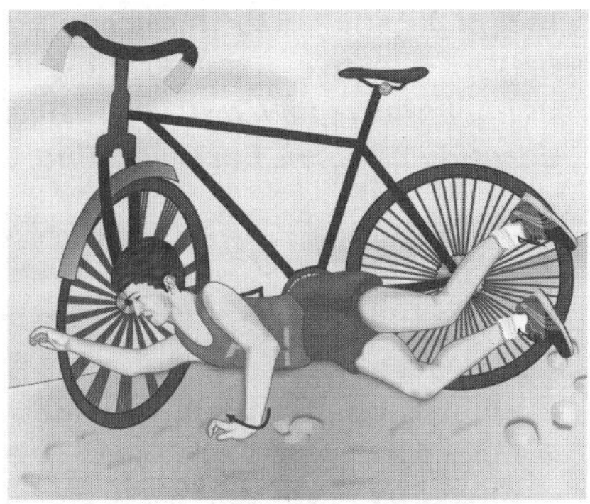

Fig. 12.3: Showing mechanism of injury in Monteggia fractures.

Clinical Features

All varieties of Monteggia fractures may show marked pain and swelling over the forearm and the elbow **(Fig. 12.4)**. There may be severe loss of forearm function. Depending upon the type of Monteggia fractures, the head of the radius and the fracture angulations of the ulna may be felt anteriorly, either posteriorly or laterally. Features suggestive of injury to the posterior interosseous nerves may also be present.

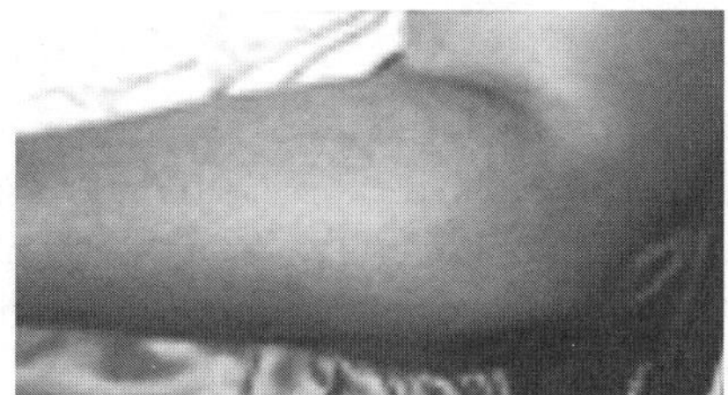

Fig. 12.4: Clinical photograph showing Monteggia fractures.

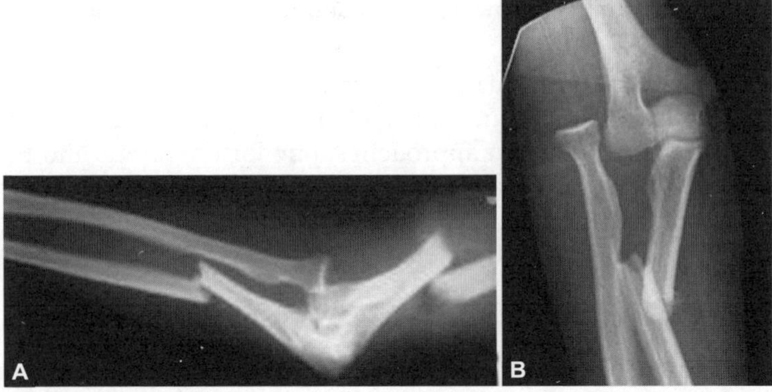

Figs. 12.5A and B: Radiograph showing monteggia fracture: (A) Anterior; (B) Lateral.

Radiology (Figs. 12.5A and B)

This plays a very important role in the diagnosis of these fractures. A routine anteroposterior and lateral views of the forearm including the elbow joint above are the recommended views. These views help to study the fracture angulations and the direction of the dislocation of the head of the radius.

In order to avoid missing the diagnosis of dislocation of the head of radius, in a few doubtful cases, McLaughlin's line is employed as described below **(Fig. 12.6)**. A straight line drawn along the center of the shaft of the radius cuts the capitula in the center irrespective of the position of the elbow. *If this does not happen, then a strong suspicion of the missing dislocation has to be borne in mind.*

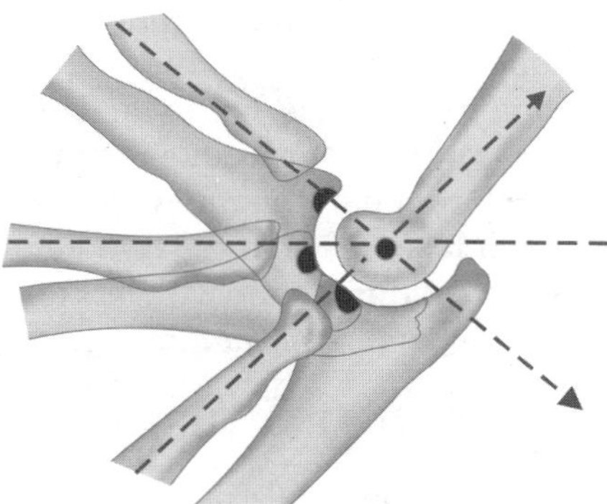

Fig. 12.6: Showing McLaughlin's line.

Monteggia fractures, why called as treacherous

◄◄ Because dislocation of the head of the radius is often missed.

Reasons
- ◄◄ **Missed by patient:** As he reflexly pulls the elbow after fall and reduces the dislocation unknowingly.
- ◄◄ **Missed by quack:** Due to ignorance
- ◄◄ **Missed by physician:** Fails to order to include the elbow in radiographs of forearm bone fractures
- ◄◄ **Missed by radiologist:** If he/she fails to utilize the McLaughlin's line

Treatment

In children, closed reduction under general anesthesia is tried first. If successful, the forearm is immobilized in an above elbow plaster cast or slab for a period of 4–6 weeks. If closed reduction fails, then open reduction of the head of the radius and repair of the annular ligament is carried out. In adults, open reduction and rigid internal fixation for ulnar fracture with plate and screws is the treatment method of choice.

Complications of Monteggia Fractures

- ❖ Unreduced dislocation head of the radius.
- ❖ Posterior interosseous nerve palsy.
- ❖ Malunion of fracture ulna.
- ❖ Nonunion of fracture ulna.
- ❖ Myositis ossificans.
- ❖ Synostosis between radial head and proximal ulna.
- ❖ Tardy posterior interosseous nerve palsy.
- ❖ Proximal migration of radius.
- ❖ Dislocation of inferior radioulnar joint.
- ❖ Cubitus valgus deformity.

GALEAZZI FRACTURE

(Also called "Piedmont fracture" after Piedmont Orthopedic Society).

This is a fracture of radius at the junction of middle and distal third with associated subluxation or dislocation of the distal radioulnar joint. Subluxation of this joint may be present initially or occur during treatment. *French people* call this fracture **reverse Monteggia**. Campbell called it as *fracture of necessity* since it always requires open reduction and internal fixation (ORIF).

Incidence: This is three times as common as Monteggia fracture.

Mechanism of Injury

- ❖ Fall on an outstretched hand with marked pronation of the forearm.
- ❖ Direct blow on the dorsolateral side of the forearm.

Clinical Features

There will be history of pain, swelling, deformity and other features of a fracture. Tenderness can be elicited and the functions the wrist are usually not affected **(Fig. 12.7)**.

Radiology

It plays an important role in the diagnosis of this fracture and a routine AP and lateral views including distal radius ulnar joints helps **(Fig. 12.8A)**.

Treatment (Galeazzi Fracture)

Closed reduction is usually not successful due to the deforming forces of the muscles. Hence, ORIF is the preferred method of treatment **(Figs. 12.8B and C)**. Intramedullary nails and small plates do not provide adequate fixation, long plate and screws are thus used and the dislocated distal radioulnar joint may be fixed with K-wire.

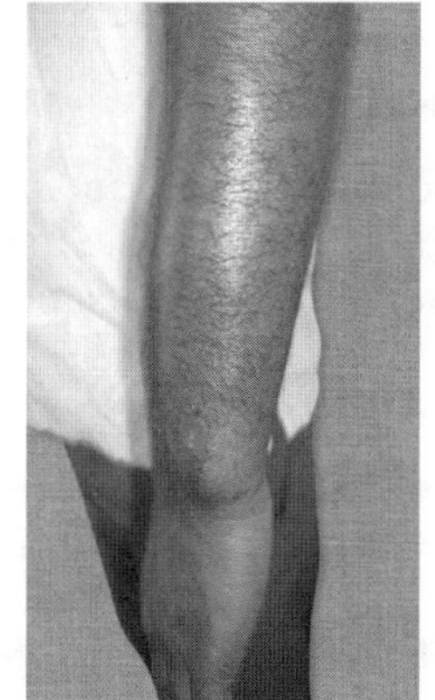

Fig. 12.7: Clinical photograph showing Galeazzi's fracture.

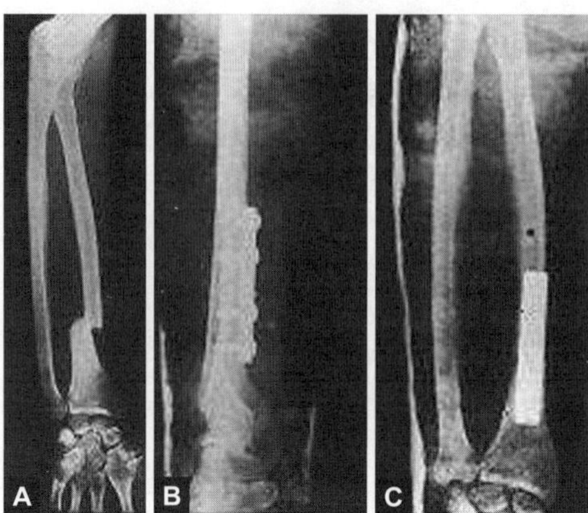

Figs. 12.8A to C: (A) Galeazzi fracture; (B and C) ORIF with DCP plate and screws (preferred method).

ISOLATED FRACTURE OF ULNA

In a remarkable show of unity, the twin bones of the forearm. Radius and ulna stay together and usually break together. Nevertheless, in some strange instances the shaft of the ulna may break singly due to a direct blow and is infamously called **"night stick fracture"**.

Interesting Fact

Mystery behind night stick fracture: A burglars night out may end up in a nightmare if he is caught with the booty by a patrolling police officer. When he tries to ward off the raining blows from the cops lathi, a direct blow over the medial border of the forearm could result in this fracture. Hence the name **(Fig. 12.9)**.

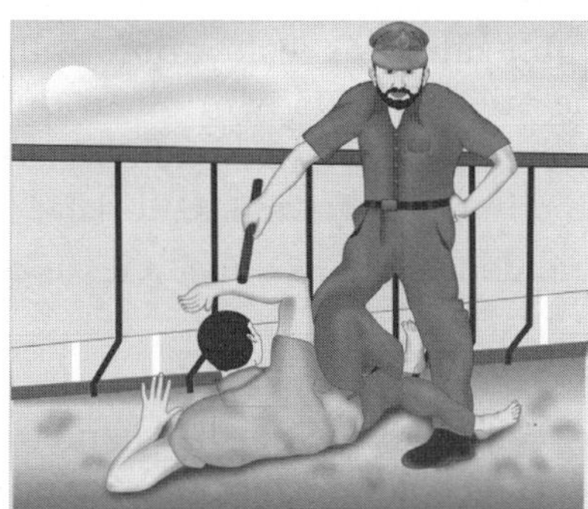

Fig. 12.9: Showing the common mechanism of night stick fracture.

Radiograph

Radiograph of the forearm helps is the diagnosis **(Fig. 12.10)** and the management is by open reduction and rigid internal fixation with plate and screws.

Complications

❖ Nonunion and malunion are notorious complications.
❖ Angulations of the fracture and subluxation of the distal radioulnar joint can also occur.
❖ Rarely entrapment of extensor carpi ulnaris tendon in distal radioulnar joint is encountered.

Essex-Lopresti Fracture

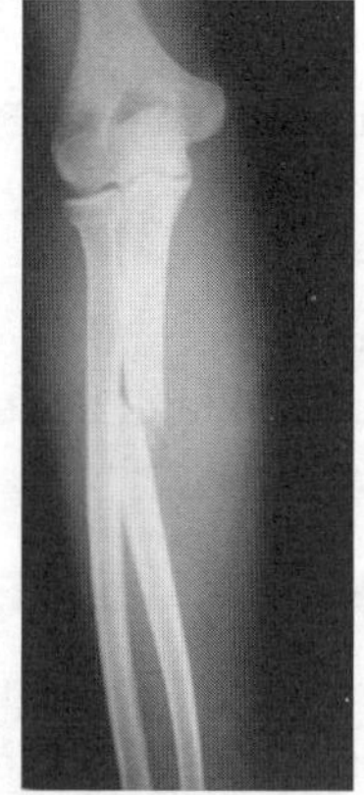

Fig. 12.10: Showing isolated fracture ulna.

This is a fracture of the radial head with injury to the distal radioulnar joint. It is a relatively rare fracture and in order to avoid missing it, radiograph of the wrist joint should be taken in all cases of fracture of the head of the radius. If there is, disruption of distal radioulnar joint, excision head of the radius is likely to aggravate the proximal migration of the radius. Hence, if fracture radial head needs excision, it has to be replaced by silastic prosthesis **(Fig. 12.11)**.

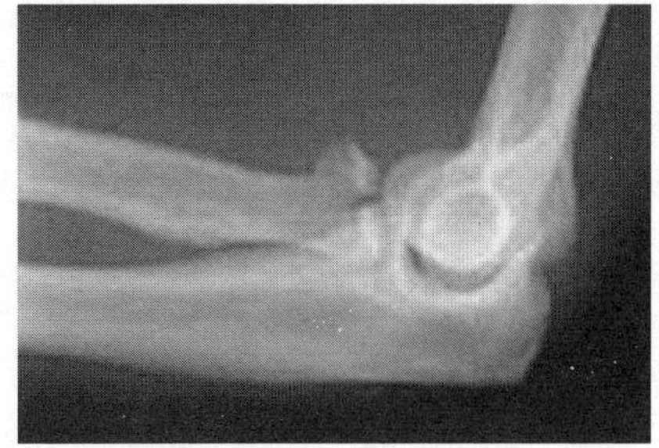

Fig. 12.11: Showing Essex-Lopresti fracture.

Wrist Fractures

COLLES' FRACTURE

This is also called as **"POUTTEAU'S"** fracture in many parts of the world. It was first described by Abraham Colles in the year 1814. It is not just fracture lower end of radius but a fracture dislocation of the inferior radioulnar joint. The fracture occurs about 1" (about 2.5 cm) above the carpal extremity of the radius. Following this fracture, some deformity will remain throughout the life but pain decreases and movements increase gradually.

Mechanism of Injury

The common mode of injury is fall on outstretched hands with dorsiflexion ranging from 40 to 90° (average 60°). The force required to cause this fracture is 192 kg in women and 282 kg in men.

Clinical features

Usually the patient is an elderly female in her 60s and the history given is a trivial fall on an outstretched hand **(Fig. 13.1)**. The patient complains of pain, swelling, deformity and other usual features of fracture at the lower end of radius. Though **_dinner fork_** deformity is a classical deformity in a Colles' fracture, however, it is not found in all cases but seen only if there is a dorsal tilt or rotation of the distal fragment. However, the styloid process test is more reliable. There are six classical displacements in a Colles' fracture; however, the most common is the **dorsal displacement (Fig. 13.2)**.

Styloid process test (Fig. 13.3A): Normally the radial styloid process is lower by 1.3 cm when compared to the ulnar styloid process. In Colles' both radial and

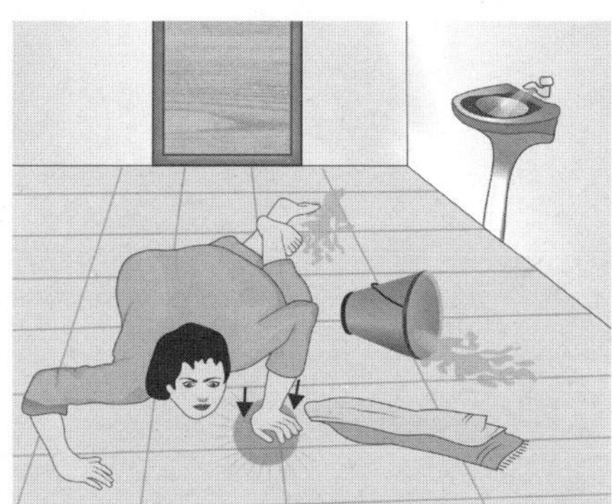

Fig. 13.1: Showing the common mechanism of Colles' fracture is old women.

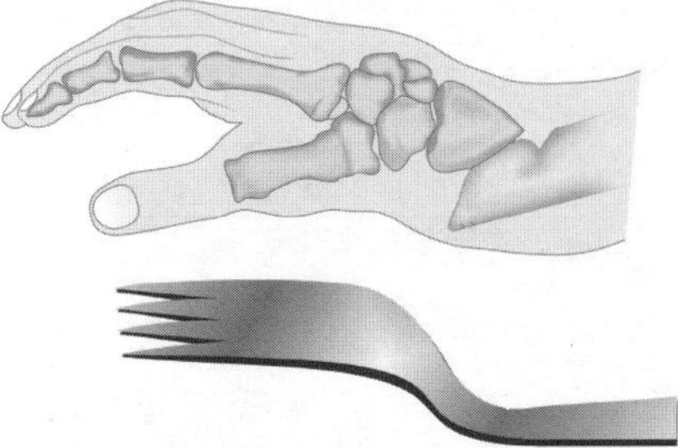

Fig. 13.2: Colles' fracture (a dinner fork deformity).

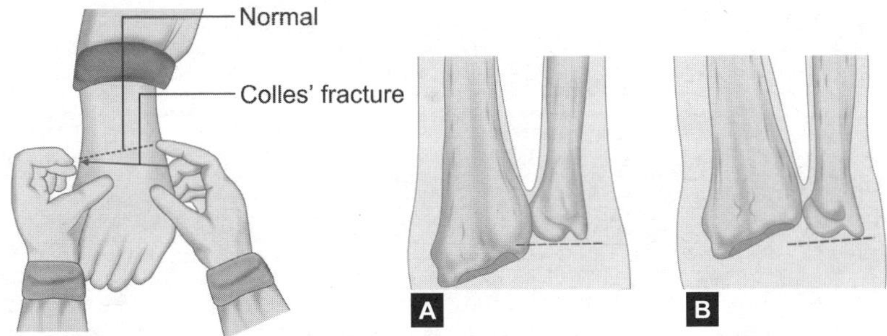

Figs. 13.3A and B: Styloid process test: (A) Normal; (B) In Colles' fracture. It also suggests positive (A) and negative (B) ulnar variance.

ulnar styloid processes are at the same level and are found in all displacements of Colles' fracture **(Fig. 13.3B)**. *Hence, this is a more reliable sign than the dinner fork deformity.*

Note: *D*inner fork deformity **(Fig. 13.2)** is seen only in *d*orsal displacement and *d*orsal tilt in a Colles' fracture (note the *d's*).

Radiology

Radiograph of the wrist both AP and lateral views of the affected wrist and lower end of the radius help in evaluating the fracture reasonably accurately **(Figs. 13.4A and B)**.

Treatment Methods

Aim: The aim of treatment is to restore fully functional hand with no residual deformity. The treatment methods include conservative methods, operative methods and external fixators.

Conservative methods: Here fracture reduction is carried out by closed methods under general anesthesia (GA) or local anesthesia (LA) and a

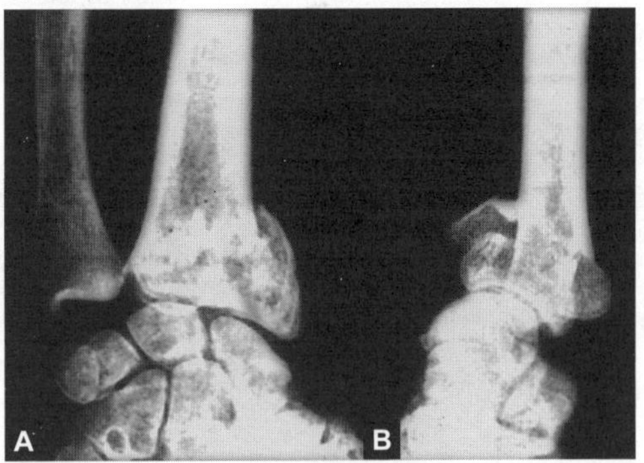

Figs. 13.4A and B: Colles' fracture: (A) AP view; (B) Lateral view.

plaster cast is applied **(Fig. 13.5)**. The plaster cast is removed after 6–8 weeks and physiotherapy is begun. However, the common method of immobilization is the **"Colles cast"** (a below elbow plaster cast) **(Figs. 13.6A and B)**.

The common causes for failure of reduction are incomplete reduction of the palmar fracture line and dorsal comminution of the lower end of radius.

Closed Reduction and Percutaneous Fixation

However, more recently, for comminuted Colles' fracture, closed reduction and percutaneous K-wire fixation under C-arm or X-ray control is being increasingly used as the treatment method of choice. The technique is simple and the results seem to be good **(Figs. 13.7A and B)**.

Operative methods: This consists of ORIF with plate and screws **(Fig. 13.8)**. However, operative treatment is rarely required for Colles' fracture except in a few special situations.

Indications: Operative treatment may be required in the following situations: extensive comminution, impaction, median nerve entrapment and associated injuries in adults.

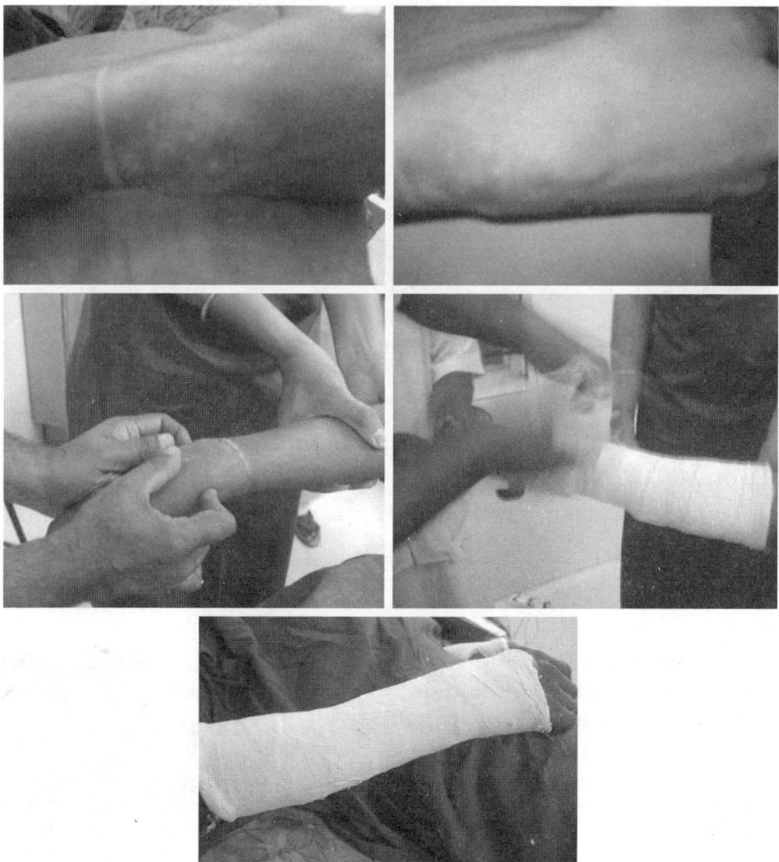

Fig. 13.5: Showing the steps of closed reduction and application of a below elbow cast in displaced Colles' fracture.

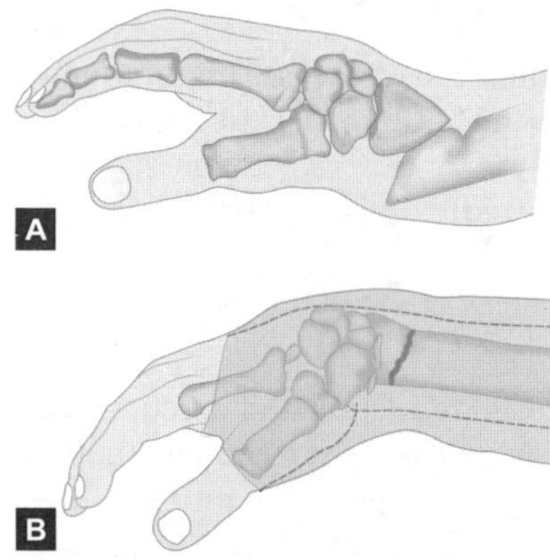

Figs. 13.6A and B: Showing retention of a Colles' fracture by a Colles' cast (a below elbow cast).

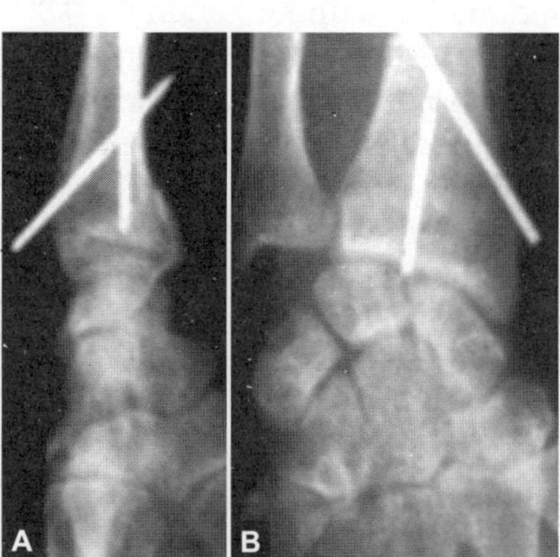

Figs. 13.7A and B: Showing percutaneous fixation of a Colles' fracture.

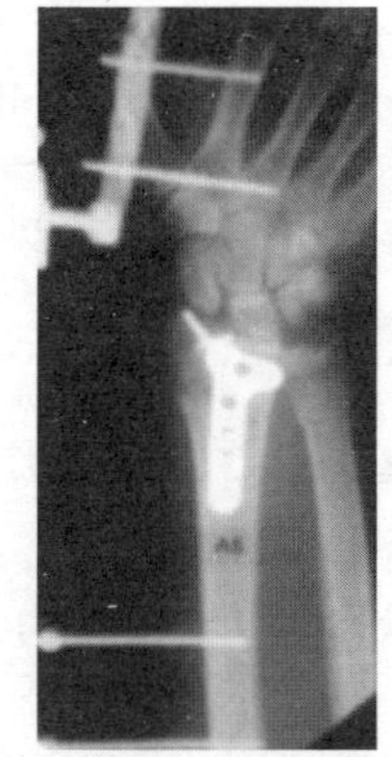

Fig. 13.8: Showing plate fixation of a Colles' fracture.

External fixators: These are found to be extremely useful in highly comminuted fractures, unstable fractures, compound fractures and bilateral Colles' fracture **(Fig. 13.9)**.

Complications: Colles' fractures may be associated with many complications. However, a few significant ones are discussed here.

Malunion

This is the most common complication of Colles' fracture. It may be due to improper reduction, inadequate immobilization or recurrence due to comminution, etc. **(Fig. 13.10)**. No treatment may be required if there is no functional impairment.

Rupture of Extensor Pollicis Tendon

This occurs due to the attrition of the tendon as it glides over the sharp fracture surfaces. This usually occurs after 4–6 weeks and may be repaired or left alone with no residual disability.

Sudeck's Osteodystrophy

This is due to abnormal sympathetic response which causes vasodilatation and osteoporosis at the fracture site **(Fig. 13.11)**. The patient complains of pain, swelling, painful wrist movements and red stretched shiny skin. Treatment consists of immobilization of the affected part with plaster splints, injection of local anesthetics near the sympathetic ganglion in the axilla or cervical sympathectomy in extreme cases.

Frozen Hand Shoulder Syndrome

This is a troublesome complication, which develops due to unnecessary voluntary shoulder immobilization by the patient on the affected side for fear of fracture displacements. It is said that the patient has performed a *mental amputation* and kept the limb still.

Carpal Tunnel Syndrome

Malunion of Colles' fracture crowds the carpal tunnel and compresses the median nerve.

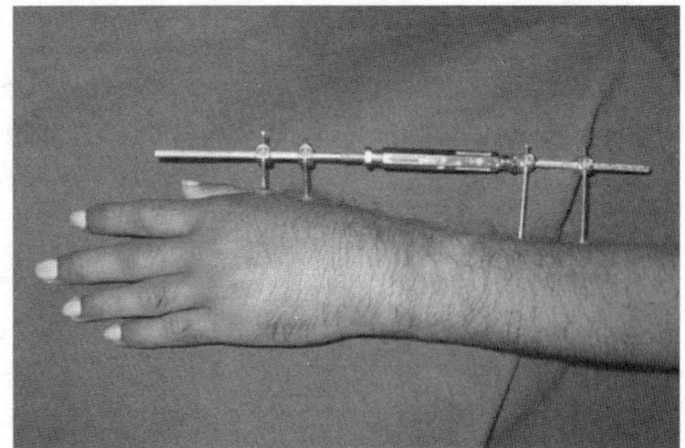

Fig. 13.9: Showing external fixation of a Colles' fracture.

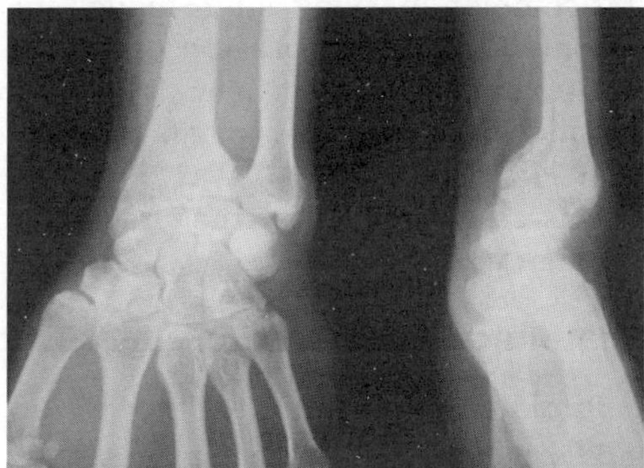

Fig. 13.10: X-rays showing malunion of Colles' fracture.

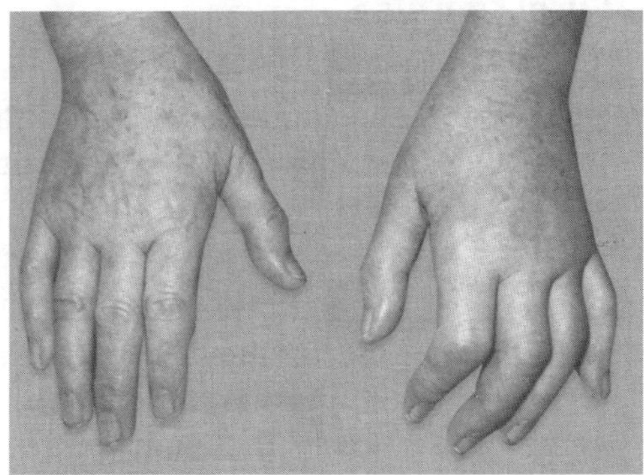

Fig. 13.11: Sudeck's dystrophy.

Nonunion

This is extremely rare in Colles' fracture because of the cancellous nature of the bone which enables the fracture to unite well. However, soft tissue interposition may cause this problem. The treatment consists of open reduction, rigid internal fixation and bone grafting.

SCAPHOID FRACTURE

Scaphoid fractures usually result from fall on outstretched hands. Frequently misdiagnosed, it is known for complications like early avascular necrosis, late carpal instability and arthritis. Hence, prompt and correct treatment is mandatory. Lack of callus in fractures in this region makes judgment about the progress of union difficult.

Etiology and Mechanism of Injury

It is common in young adults though it can be seen in patients of 10–70 years of age.

❖ The common mode of injury is fall on an outstretched hand with hyperextension and slight radial deviation at the wrist.
❖ It is associated with other fracture of carpus and forearm bones in about 17%.

Anatomical Classification (Fig. 13.12)

❖ Proximal pole fracture (20%).
❖ Waist fracture (70%).
❖ Distal body fracture (10%).
❖ Tuberosity fracture

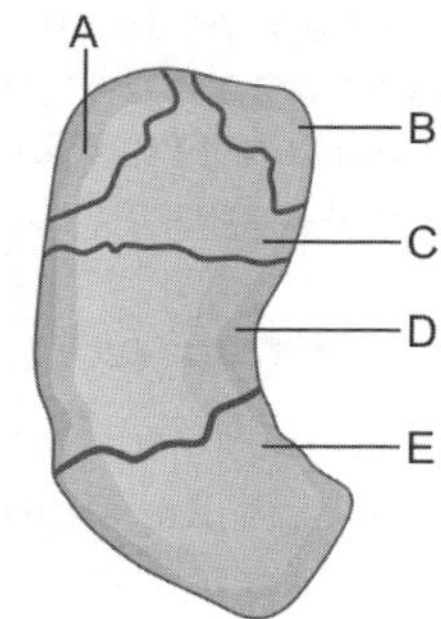

Fig. 13.12: Showing different levels of scaphoid fracture: (A) Fractures of the tuberosity; (B) Distal articular fracture; (C) Distal one-third fractures; (D) Waist fractures; (E) Fractures of the proximal pole.

Clinical Features

Patient complains of pain and swelling of the wrist. Tenderness in the anatomical snuffbox is a characteristic finding. The movements of the wrist may be painful.

Radiology

Routine radiograph of the wrist with the AP and lateral views. AP views in the radial and ulnar deviated positions helps to identity this fracture **(Fig. 13.13)**.

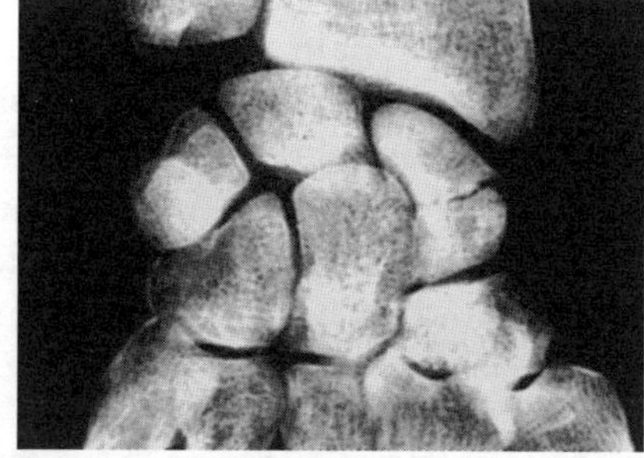

Fig. 13.13: Radiograph showing fracture scaphoid.

However, few cases the X-rays may not show a fracture in the initial stages. Hence repeat X-ray should be done after 2–3 weeks.

Treatment Methods

❖ **Undisplaced fracture:** The treatment for this fracture is essentially conservative. It consists of a below elbow cast applied up to the level of the metacarpal heads of the index, middle, ring and little fingers. In the thumb, it extends up to the level of the PIP joints. The wrist is held in sight dorsiflexion and radial deviation. The whole position assumes a **"glass-holding"**. Position and is popularly called the **"scaphoid cast"** (Fig. 13.14).

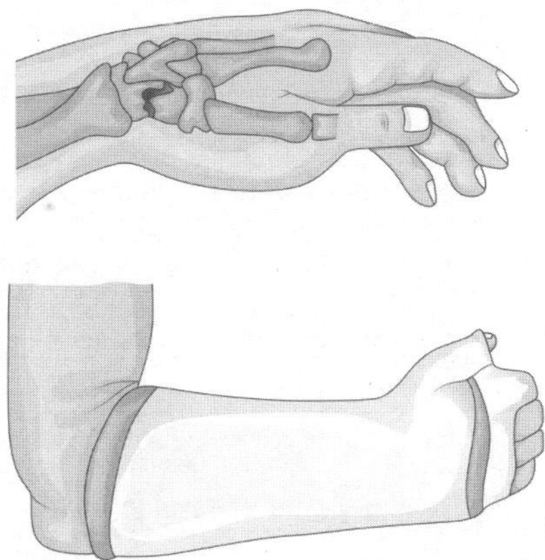

Fig. 13.14: Showing scaphoid fracture which commonly occurs at the wrist being treated by a "scaphoid cast".

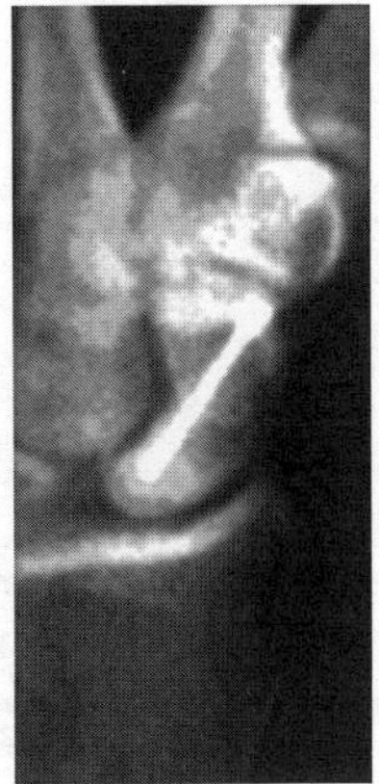

Fig. 13.15: Radiograph showing Herbert screw fixation for fracture scaphoid.

❖ **Displaced fractures:** Initially closed reduction under general anesthesia or regional anesthesia and immobilization with scaphoid cast is tried. If it fails, open reduction and internal fixation with Herbert screws is indicated **(Fig. 13.15)**.

Note: Union rate in:

❖ Undisplaced fracture: It is 95% at 10 weeks time.
❖ Displaced fracture: It is 54%.

Complications

❖ Nonunion due to delayed diagnosis, displacement and associated carpal injuries.
❖ About 40% cases are undiagnosed in the initial stages of fracture.
❖ Incidence of avascular necrosis is as high as 40%.

14
CHAPTER

Injuries of the Hand

Hand is the most dexterous part of the human body. Anatomically though made up of small bones functionally performs a wide array of unbelievable functions. Few important injuries of the hand are discussed here.

BENNETT'S FRACTURE

Bennett's fracture is a fracture dislocation of the base of the first metacarpal bone of the thumb with either subluxation or dislocation of the first carpometacarpal joint. It was described by Edward Bennett in 1882. It is an **intra-articular** fracture.

Mechanism of Injury

The common mechanism of injury is an axial blow directed against the partially flexed metacarpal, in most cases during **"fist fights"**.

Clinical Features

Patient complains of pain and swelling at the base of the thumb. Tenderness could be elicited. Movements of the thumb are painful and restricted.

Plain X-ray of the wrist helps to make an accurate diagnosis **(Fig. 14.1)**.

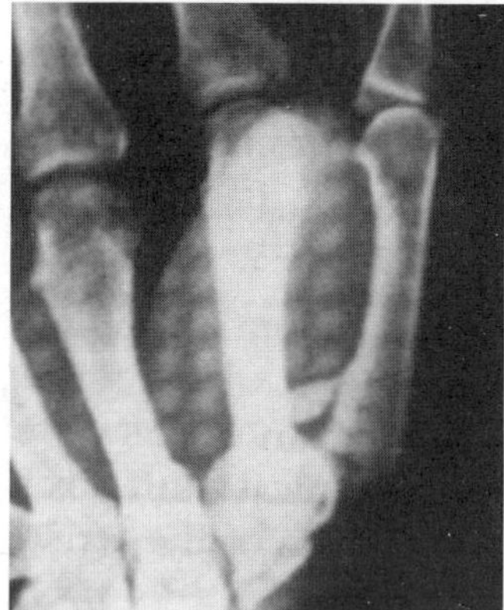

Fig. 14.1: Radiograph showing Bennett's fracture.

Treatment

Like all other intra-articular fractures, it needs accurate reduction and retention to prevent future post-traumatic osteoarthritis. A single attempt at closed reduction is tried first and a percutaneous fixation under C-arm or X-ray control with K-wire is usually performed.If it fails, ORIF with K-wire or a small screw is carried out.

Complications

Patient may complain of inability to make a firm grip. This could be possibly due to post-traumatic osteoarthritis.

ROLANDO FRACTURE

This was first described by Rolando in the year 1910. Though this is also a fracture of the base of the first metacarpal, but unlike Bennett's fracture, it is **extra-articular** in nature. Absence of the notorious distracting muscle forces as in Bennett has, makes this fracture simpler to treat. Closed reduction and retention with a thumb spica for 2–3 weeks is the recommended method of treatment.

Quick facts: Rolando fracture in comparison with the Bennett's fracture

- ❮❮ Extra-articular
- ❮❮ No displacing muscle forces
- ❮❮ Since extra-articular perfect reduction is not a must.
- ❮❮ Conservative treatment suffices.

DORSAL METACARPOPHALANGEAL JOINT DISLOCATION (KAPLAN LESION)

Kaplan described a hyperextension injury due to buttonholing of the metacarpal head through the volar capsule into the palm. Here there is an interposition of volar plate between the base of the proximal phalanx and the head of the metacarpal.

Incidence

This is commonly seen in the index finger, thumb and little finger in that order of frequency. It is rarely seen in the middle and ring fingers.

Clinical Features

Pain, swelling deformity, puckered palmar skin (characteristic) loss of the movements of the affected finger. etc., are some of the important clinical features **(Figs. 14.2A and B)**.

Plain X-ray

Presence of sesamoid bone within the MCP joint is pathognomonic of this condition **(Fig. 14.3)**.

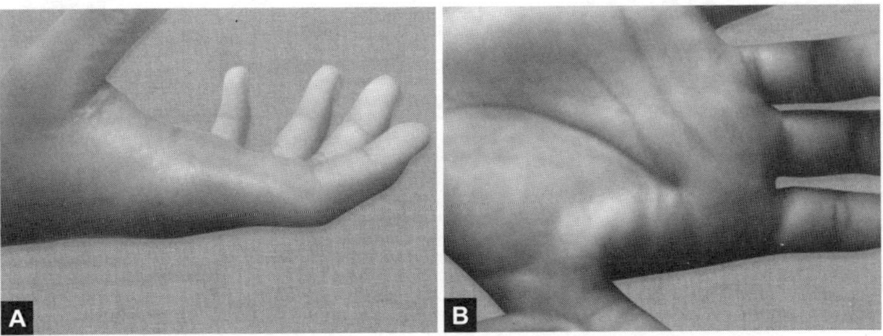

Figs. 14.2A and B: Dislocation of II MP point (Kaplan's lesion).

Treatment

A single attempt at closed reduction is made and if this fails surgical reduction either by the volar (Kaplan's operation) approach or by dorsal approach is done.

MALLET FINGER

(Syn: Baseball finger, Drop finger)

Mallet finger is a common finger injury and is due to **avulsion** or avulsion fracture of the extensor tendon from its insertion at the base of the distal phalanx.

Mechanism

This injury occurs when the finger is forcibly flexed, while the extensor tendon is taut, e.g., while tucking the bed, catching a ball, striking an object with extended finger, etc. **(Figs. 14.4A and B)**.

Clinical Features

Pain, swelling, tenderness, flexion deformity of the tip of the finger and inability of the patient to actively extend the finger at the distal PIP joint **(Fig. 14.5)**.

Plain X-ray

Plain X-ray of the affected finger in the lateral view may show an avulsion fracture **(Fig. 14.6)**.

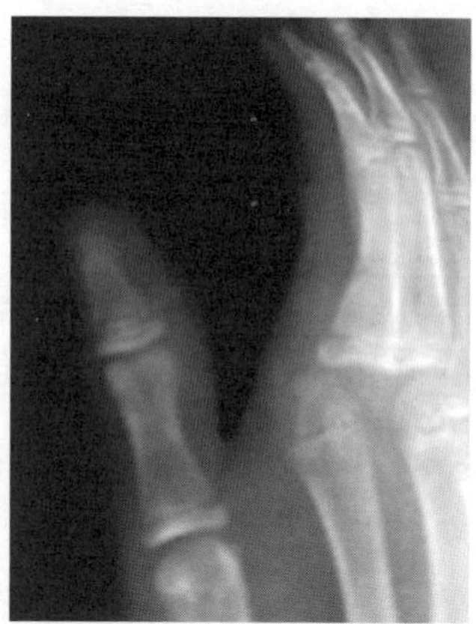

Fig. 14.3: Plain X-ray showing Kaplan's lesion.

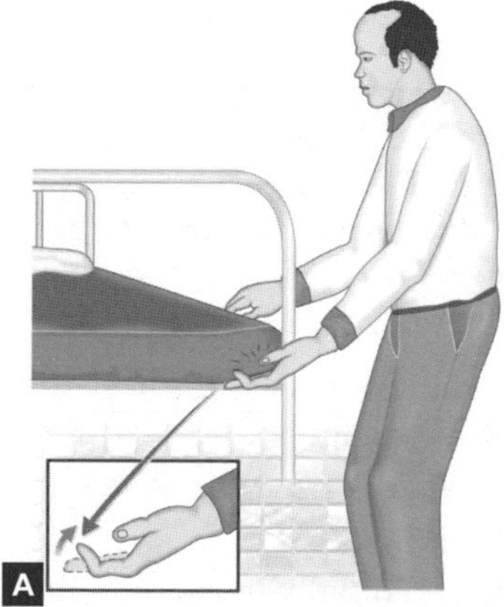
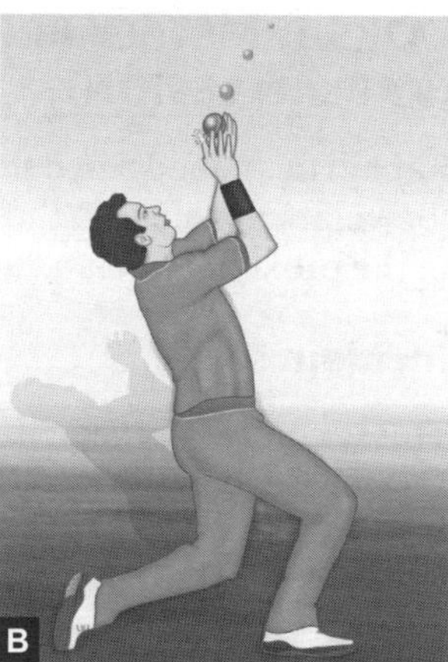

Figs. 14.4A and B: Showing common mechanism of mallet injury.

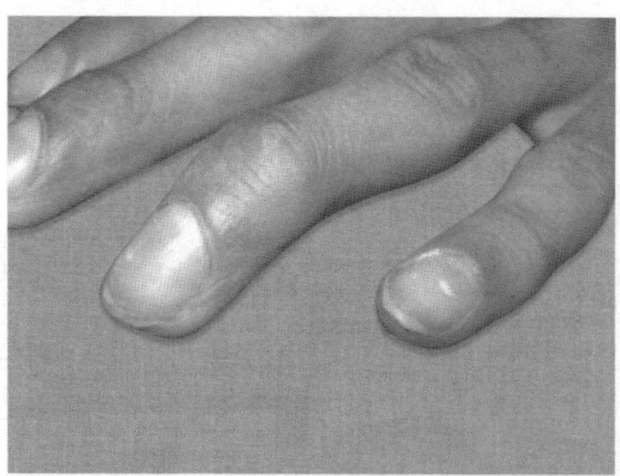

Fig. 14.5: Clinical photograph showing mallet finger.

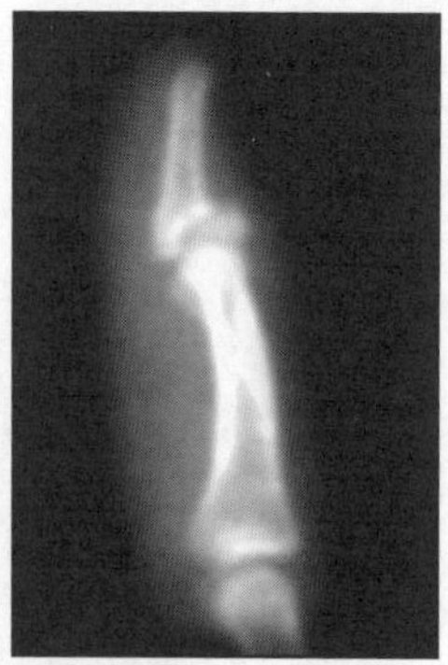

Fig. 14.6: Plain X-ray showing avulsion fracture in mallet fracture.

Treatment

Distal interphalangeal joint is immobilized in hyperextension by using:

- Simple volar unpadded aluminum splint, which provides three-point pressure.
- Dorsal padded aluminum splint.
- A stack plastic mallet finger splint **(Figs. 14.7A and B)**.

Jersey finger: It is due to avulsion of flexor digitorum profundus from its insertion on distal phalanx. This is the opposite of **'mallet finger'** and the patient is unable to flex the distal interphalangeal joint. It is seen in football and rugby players **(Fig. 14.8)**.

Metacarpal Bone Fractures

- **Metacarpal shaft fracture:** The common causes for these injuries are direct hit on the dorsum of the hand as in assault, boxing, fall, road traffic accident (RTA), etc. They are easily diagnosed by plain X-ray of the hand **(Fig. 14.9)**. These fractures should be accurately reduced with no rotational malalignment and immobilized with either plaster (common) or percutaneous **(Fig. 14.9)** or open K-wire fixation (less common).
- **Metacarpal neck fracture** of the fifth metacarpal neck is known as **boxer's fracture**. It occurs when a closed fist hits against a hard object, in this case, the jaw of the opponent! **(Figs. 14.10A to C)**.
- **Metacarpal head fractures:** These are also known as *'fight bite'* fractures as they occur when the patient strikes an opponent's teeth in a fist fight. They are frequently intra-articular and need open reduction and internal fixation with K-wire **(Figs. 14.11A to C)**.

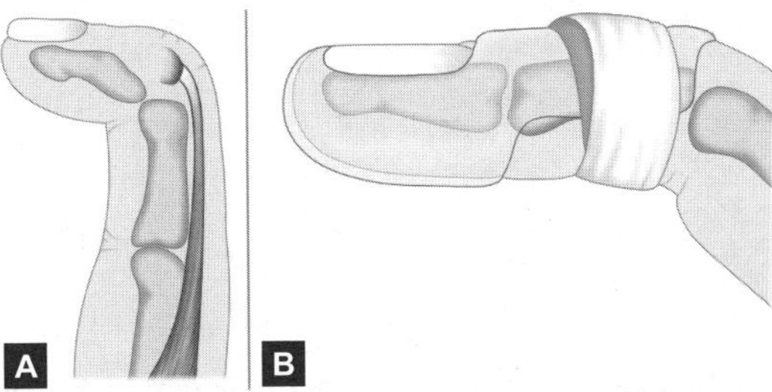

Figs. 14.7A and B: Showing: (A) Mallet finger; (B) Treatment by a dorsal splint.

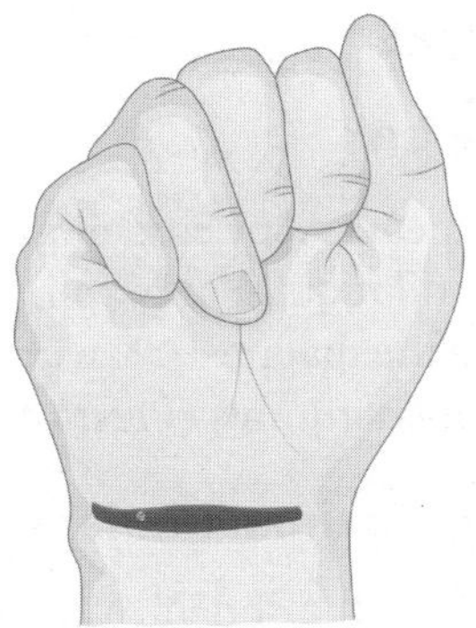
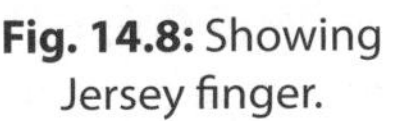

Fig. 14.8: Showing Jersey finger.

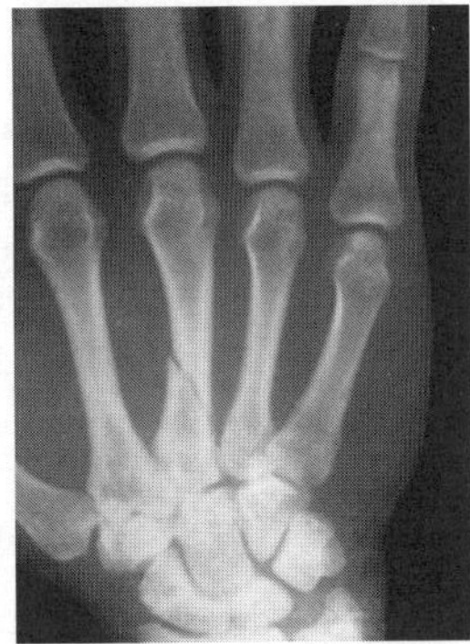

Fig. 14.9: Plain X-ray showing metacarpal fracture.

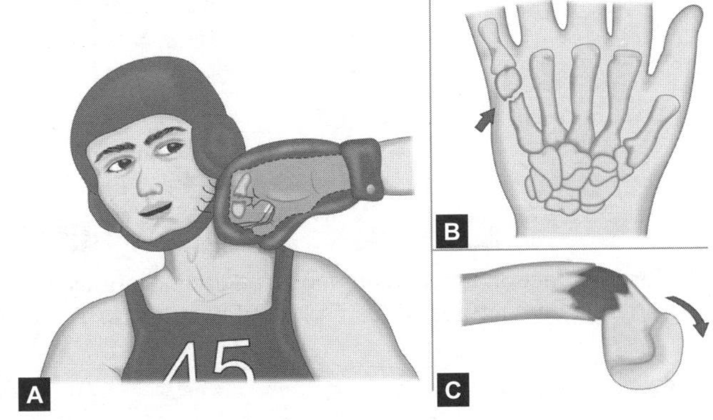

Figs. 14.10A to C: Showing common mechanism of fracture neck of 5th metacarpal bone (Boxer's fracture).

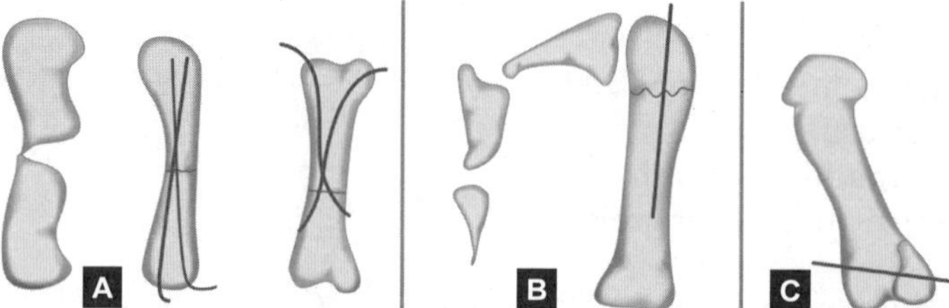

Figs. 14.11A to C: Metacarpal fractures treated by closed reduction and percutaneous pinning: (A) Unstable fracture fixed with criss-cross K-wires; (B) Neck fracture fixed by intramedullary fixation; (C) Bennett's fracture fixed with K-wire.

PHALANGES FRACTURE

Fracture of Distal Phalanx

These fractures are usually caused by crushing injuries; they are frequently comminuted and require only splinting. Plain X-ray of the hand helps to make the diagnosis. K-wire fixation may be required for unstable or open injuries **(Figs. 14.13A to C)**.

Fracture of Middle or Proximal Phalanx (Fig. 14.12)

These are due to direct blow on the dorsum of fingers. The fracture is angulated towards the palm. Rotational malalignment should be strictly avoided. Undisplaced fractures are best managed by conservative methods by buddy taping (here, the unaffected finger is used as the supporting external splint) **(Fig. 14.10)**, while highly unstable oblique fracture require open reduction and K-wire fixation **(Figs. 14.13A to C)**. Severely comminuted fractures are aligned best by external fixators.

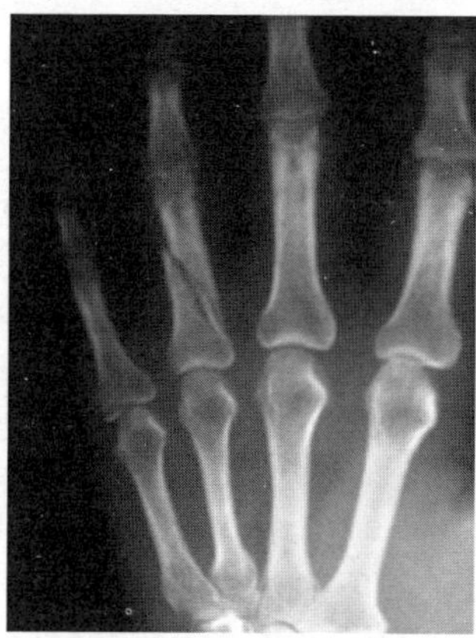

Fig. 14.12: Plain X-ray showing oblique phalangeal fracture.

Complications

The important complications of finger bone fractures are nonunion, malunion, tendon adhesions, joint stiffness, infection, etc.

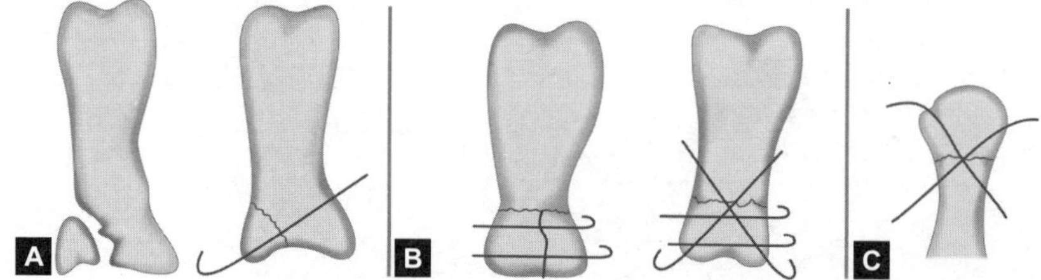

Figs. 14.13A to C: Closed reduction and percutaneous fixation of various phalanges fractures: (A) Unstable short oblique fractures; (B) Comminuted fracture; (C) Condylar fracture.

Fracture Pelvis and Trunk

FRACTURE OF PELVIS

Stability of the Pelvis

It depends on both bony and ligamentous structures. Anterior portion of the pelvic ring neither participates in normal weight-bearing nor is it essential for maintenance of pelvic stability. The posterior arch is formed by the sacrum, SI joints and iliac bone and is the weight-bearing portion of the pelvis. The posterosuperior SI ligaments provide most of the ligamentous stability of the SI joints **(Fig. 15.1)**.

Stable Pelvic Fracture

These fractures do not involve the pelvic ring and they are minimally displaced.

Unstable Pelvic Fracture

They involve the pelvic ring and are widely displaced. Pelvic fractures pose a problem different from others. Here the emphasis is on recognition of potential complications associated with these fractures, the notable ones being injuries to the major vessels and nerves of the pelvis and major viscera like intestines, bladder and the urethra, severe intrapelvic hemorrhage from fracture of pelvic ring. Mortality from pelvic fracture varies from 10 to 50%. Proper fracture management decreases the blood loss and controls the hemorrhage. A to F management as proposed by Mac Murthy in multiple trauma patients is important in management of the pelvic fractures.

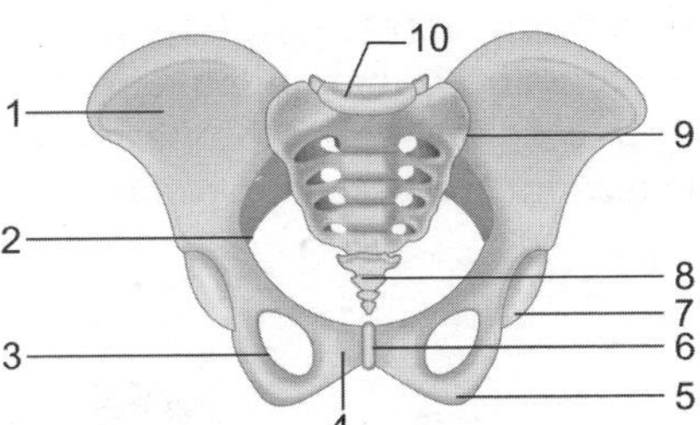

(1: Iliac bone; 2: pelvic ring; 3: Obturator fossa; 4: Rami; 5: Ischial tuberosity; 6: Pubic symphysis; 7: Acetabulum; 8: Coccyx; 9: Sacroiliac joint; 10: sacrum)

Fig. 15.1: Showing anatomy of pelvis.

Vital practice points

A to F management of Mac Murthy:
A. Airway management
B. Blood and fluid replacement
C. Central nervous system management
D. Digestive system management
E. Excretory system management
F. Fracture management

History

Pelvic fractures usually occur due to high-velocity trauma following a road traffic accident (RTA) or due to fall from a height. The relative incidences are as follows:

- RTA—80.7%.
- Fall—16.1%.
- Compression fracture—rest.

Mechanism of Injury

There are four mechanisms by which pelvic ring fractures are produced:

- Anteroposterior compression **(Fig. 15.2B)**.
- Lateral compression **(Fig. 15.2A)**.
- Vertical shears forces.
- Inferior forces (e.g., fall on buttocks) **(Fig. 15.11)**.

The first two mechanisms are common in RTA and may cause stable or unstable fractures. Vertical shear forces are due to fall from a height and will cause grossly unstable fractures. Fortunately, most pelvic fractures are stable and respond to non-operative treatment. Unstable fractures need manipulative reduction and stabilization by external fixators and sometimes by internal fixation. A proper evaluation of the fracture by radiograph and CT scan helps to determine the best course of management.

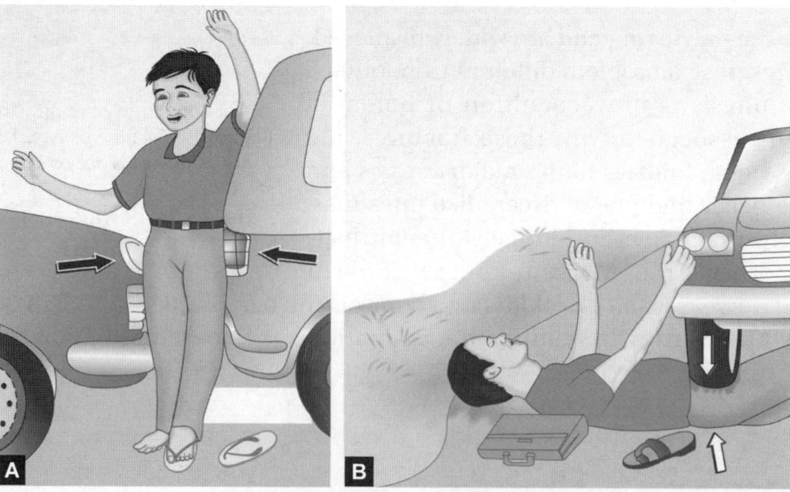

Figs. 15.2A and B: Common mechanism of pelvic fractures is RTA: (A) Lateral compression injury; (B) Anteroposterior compression injury.

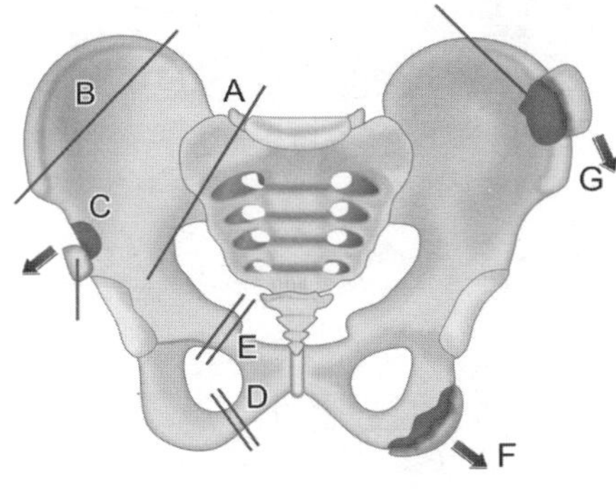

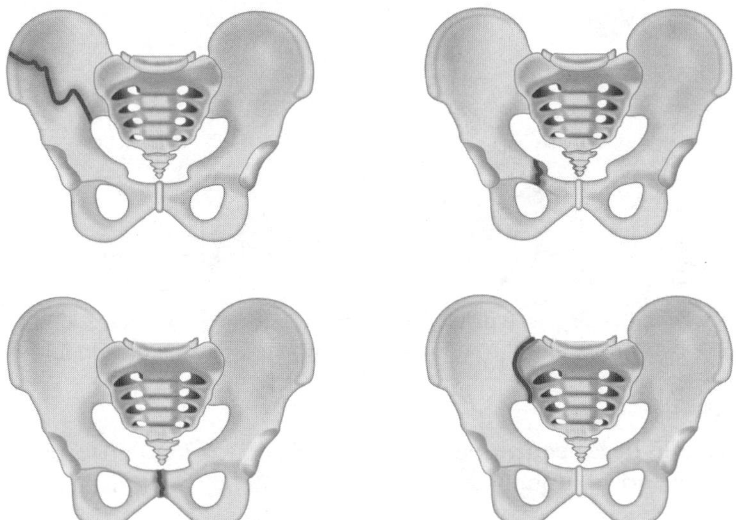

Fig. 15.3: Showing avulsion fractures and fractures of individual bones not affecting the pelvic ring: (A) fracture of the sacrum, (B) fracture of the iliac wing, (C) avulsion fracture of anteroinferior iliac spine, (D) inferior rami fracture, (E) superior ramus fracture, (F) avulsion fracture of ischial tuberosity, and (G) avulsion fracture of anterosuperior iliac spine.

Fig. 15.4: Showing stable pelvic fractures.

Classification

Broadly speaking the pelvic fractures can be placed under two categories.

Fractures not Affecting the Integrity of the Pelvic Ring

Direct blow fractures, which are commonly seen in iliac bone and avulsion fractures frequently encountered in the young, come under this group. Avulsion fractures are commonly seen in anterosuperior and inferior iliac spines and ischial tuberosity **(Fig. 15.3)**. Ring and single break fractures in the pelvic ring. These fractures are stable **(Fig. 15.4)**.

Fractures Affecting the Integrity of the Pelvic Ring

These are single or double break fractures in the pelvic ring and could be stable or unstable. A stable fracture is one, which resists displacing forces. Obviously, fractures, which cannot resist usual forces, are called unstable fractures and these pose a major therapeutic challenge **(Figs. 15.5A to C)**.

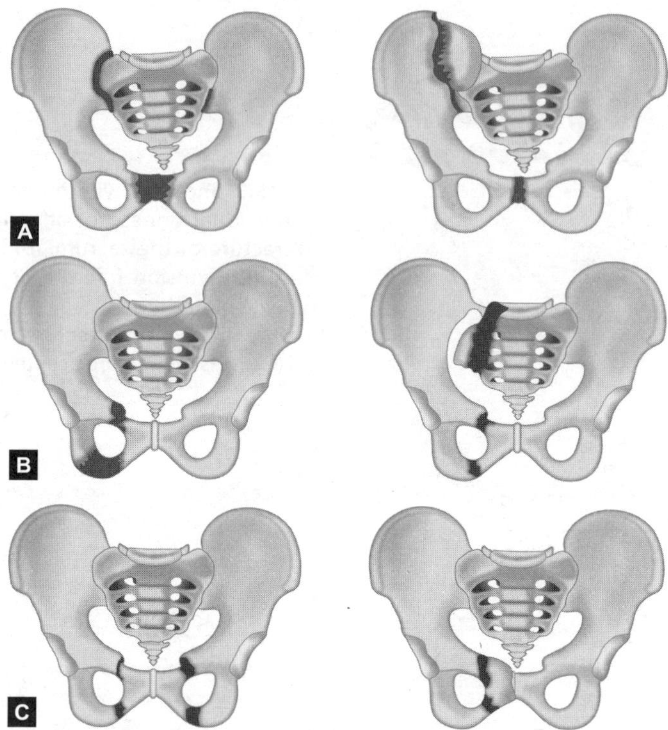

Figs. 15.5A to C: Showing the displaced pelvic fractures: (A) Dislocation of pubic symphysis and SI joint; (B) Fracture ipsilateral pubic rami with subluxation of SI joint; (C) Straddle fracture (double vertical fracture).

Many classifications have been proposed for pelvic fractures. Key and Conwell's classification is by far the simplest and commonly used classification. It has prognostic importance too.

Relative incidence
◄◄ Fracture pubic bones are the most common >69%. Single ramus more common than multiple rami fracture.
◄◄ Malgaigne—11.8% fracture.
◄◄ Multiple crush injuries—10.8% fracture.
◄◄ Wing of ilium—5.4% fracture.

Clinical Features

Symptoms: Patient most often gives a history of high-velocity trauma and usually presents in a state of hypovolemic shock. Features of intra-abdominal injuries and genitourinary injuries are frequently present.

Signs: The patient may present with all signs of shock, tenderness over the fracture site and perineal injuries.

Clinical Tests

❖ Compression test: When a compressive force is applied through the two iliac bones patient complains of pain in pelvic fracture **(Fig. 15.6)**.

❖ Distraction test: When distraction force is applied to the two iliac bones at the anterosuperior iliac spine, patient complains of pain **(Fig. 15.7B)**.

❖ Direct pressure test: Direct pressure over the symphysis pubis elicits pain **(Fig. 15.7A)**.

Following this, an examination for abdomen and pelvis injuries is carried out and next urethral catheterization or urethrogram is done.

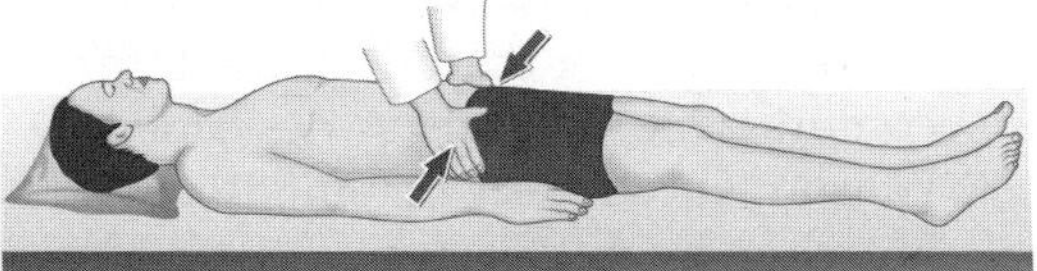

Fig. 15.6: Showing compression test in pelvic fractures.

Radiography: Different radiographic views are recommended to study the fracture configuration, displacements, etc., in pelvic fractures:

❖ Plain AP view.

❖ Oblique view—45° oblique projections.

❖ Internal and external rotation view.

❖ Inlet view—40° caudad view.

❖ Outlet view—40° cephalad view.

Further radiographic studies include CT scans and 3-dimensional imaging.

Management

General principles: One should remember that pelvic fractures are usually due to high-velocity trauma and is associated with multiple fractures and multiple system injuries. Resuscitation and correction of hypovolemic shock takes precedence over the management of fracture per se. Nevertheless, once the general condition is stabilized attention should be given to treat the fracture, which will prevent further blood loss and damage to visceral organs.

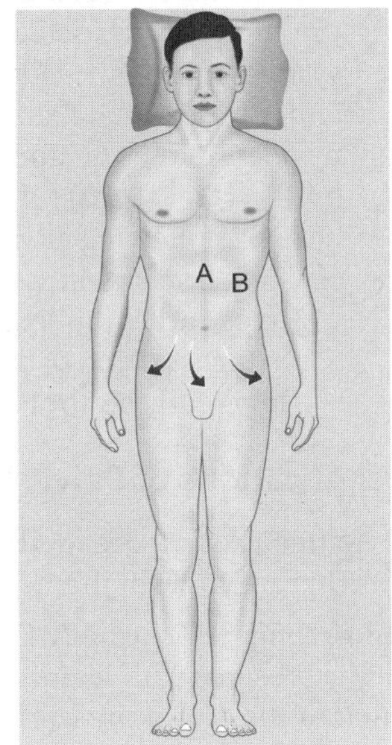

Fig. 15.7: Showing: (A) Direct pressure test; (B) Distraction test.

Treatment points
Three main pitfalls in the treatment of pelvic fracture:
1. Treating only fracture overlooking visceral injuries.
2. Over treating a stable fracture.
3. Treating an unstable fracture.

Treatment Methods

❖ **If the patient is in shock:** Resuscitation and other general measures, to improve the general condition of the patient. Blood transfusion and other medical and surgical emergency measures are carried out.

❖ **Management of pelvic fractures:**

  ◆ *Avulsion fractures:* Conservative treatments like bed rest, traction; physiotherapy, etc., give good result. They rarely need surgery.

  ◆ *Undisplaced fractures:* Respond to bed rest, traction, pelvic slings **(Fig. 15.8),** nonsteroidal anti-inflammatory drugs (NSAIDs), etc.

  ◆ *Displaced fractures: If* the displacement is <2.5 cm conservative treatment like the ones mentioned above usually suffices. Nevertheless, if the displacement is >2.5 cm reduction and later retention of the displacement is necessary. Reduction by lateral compression methods as described by Watson Jones is very helpful. Retention is either by spica cast, canvas sling **(Fig 15.8)** or external fixators.

* *Role of external and internal fixators:* The above methods usually suffice but the fractures associated with multiple system injuries need to be stabilized either by external fixators **(Fig. 15.9)** or by open reduction and internal fixation (ORIF) **(Fig. 15.10)**. These two methods have the following advantages:
  - Gives firm stability.
  - Helps early mobilization.
  - Reduces period of bed rest.
  - Helps early control of osseous bleeding.

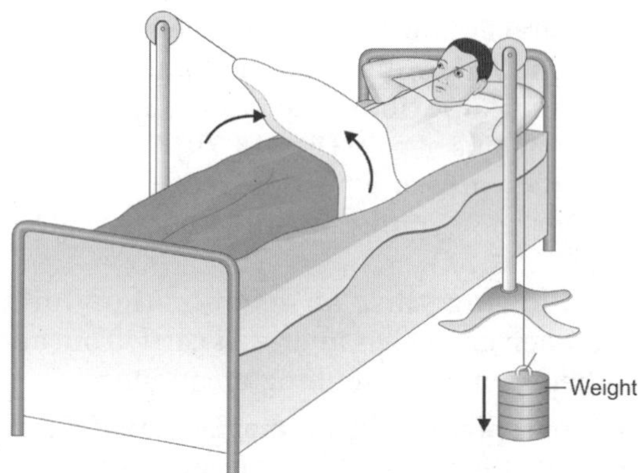

Fig. 15.8: Pelvic sling as a mainstay of conservative treatment in fracture pelvis.

Complications of Pelvic Fracture

Pelvic fracture is a dreaded injury as it is associated with a plethora of complications. The following are some of them:

Hemorrhage: It is usually intra-abdominal and the incidence is around 20 per cent. Patient usually presents with features of shock. If the pulse is >100/min it suggests 20% blood volume deficit, if the blood pressure is <100 mm systolic it suggests 30% volume deficit. Diagnostic peritoneal lavage and open paracentesis has an accuracy rate of 98% in intra-abdominal injuries. CT scan is also sensitive and specific. Treatment is by laparotomy and is indicated if there is continuing blood loss, visceral perforation, expanding palpable suprapubic hematoma.

Injuries of lower urinary tract: Rupture of urethra and rupture of urinary bladder are the common lower urinary tract injuries frequently seen in separation of pubic symphysis and fracture pubic rami. It has an average incidence of 13%. The dictum is *"All pelvic fractures must be assumed to have urinary tract injuries until proved otherwise."*

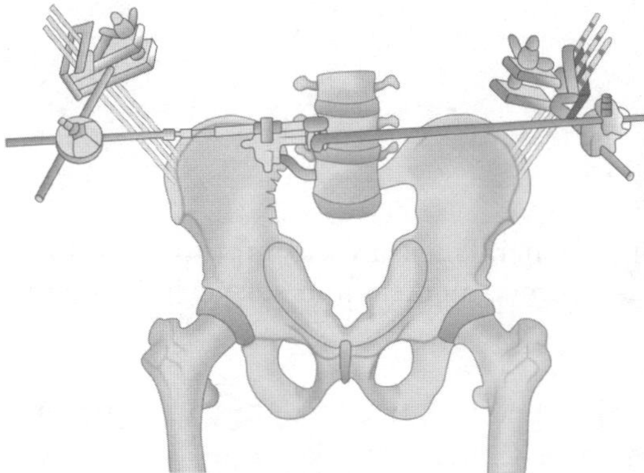

Fig. 15.9: Showing treatment by external fixation methods in pelvic fractures.

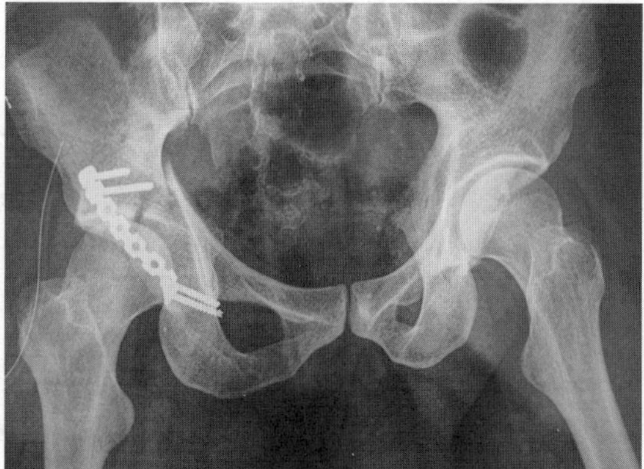

Fig. 15.10: ORIF of displaced pelvic fractures.

Presence of hematuria is not pathognomonic but its presence calls for three radiographic studies like retrograde urethrogram, cystogram and IVP. Rupture of anterior urethra is seen in straddle fractures and is not very common. Rupture of posterior urethra is relatively more common and is limited to male. Suprapubic cystostomy, direct repair, rail road repair, urethroplasties are some of the treatment methods.

Bladder injuries are seen in 4% of the cases and are associated with symphysis pubis injuries and rami fracture. 80% injuries are extraperitoneal and calls for direct surgical intervention as quickly as possible.

Other injuries: Testicular injuries and vaginal lacerations, bowel, rectal and urethral injuries are all common and require immediate surgical intervention.

Other Complications

Loss of reduction, sepsis, thrombophlebitis, delayed union, nonunion, post-traumatic arthritis, fat embolism, major arterial injuries, abdominal wall injury, neurological injuries usually L5, S1 roots due to sacral fracture are the other common complications.

Recap

Pelvic fractures:
- A fracture feared for its complications.
- RTA accounts for 80% of cases.
- Fracture broadly classified into not affecting and affecting integrity of the pelvic ring.
- Fracture pubic rami, usually single, is the most common pelvic fracture (69%).
- Usual presentation is hypovolemic shock.
- Correction of hypovolemia and other general measures takes precedence over fracture management.
- Conservative treatment usually gives good results.
- External and internal fixation is done for specific indications.
- Intra-abdominal and genitourinary injuries are common possibilities and need early recognition and prompt treatment.
- Mortality is 20%.

Note: Mortality in closed pelvic fractures is 10–30% and open fractures are 40–50%.

COCCYX FRACTURES

Coccyx in human beings in present the extinct that. It is formed by the fusion of five vertebral bones injury to the coccyx is relatively the common.

Mechanism

It is commonly due to direct fall on the buttocks **(Fig. 15.11)**. Patient usually complains of chronic pain in between the buttocks. The treatment is essentially conservative in nature with periods of bed-rest and symptomatic treatment for pain and inflammation.

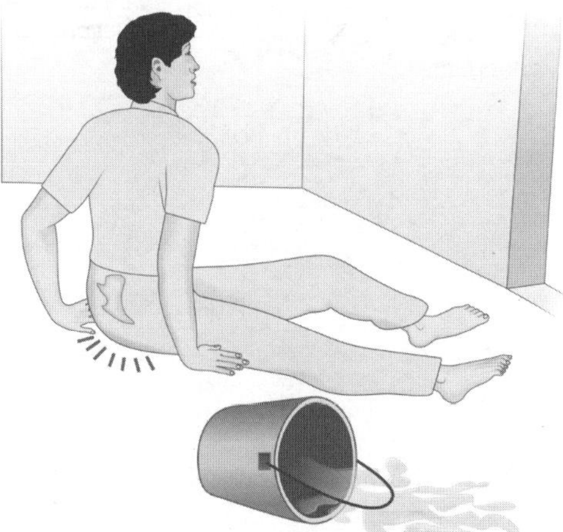

Fig. 15.11: Showing mechanism of injury in coccyx fractures.

Radiology

X-ray of the pelvis helps in the diagnosis.

Conservative Management

- To relieve pain, thermotherapy likes ultrasound and TENS.
- To relieve prolonged pressure on the buttocks, sitting on a ring cushion and sitting on alternate buttocks is advised.
- Isometric exercises to the glutei maximus muscle in sitting, lying and prone positions are advisable.
- *Seitz bath helps to relieve pain.

Note: These injuries are difficult to tackle.

Reasons:
1. Due to the position of coccyx which is deep and covered by thick muscles on either side.
2. Due to the pressure from sitting. Hence long sitting posture needs to be controlled.

RIB FRACTURES

These are relatively rare injuries and are usually due to direct trauma. The rib usually breaks at the angle which is a point of maximum convexity **(Fig. 15.12)**.

Intercostals muscles provide natural immobilization to the fractured ribs and hence no aggressive management is required. Strapping **(Fig. 15.13)**, ultrasound or TENS, etc., are effective in reducing the pain. Occasionally a local infiltration of hydrocortisone helps.

Very rarely the fracture fragments may pierce the pleura causing pneumothorax, hemothorax, etc. These are dangerous injuries and needs to be managed aggressively.

Rehabilitation

This essentially consists of deep breathing exercises, which are progressively made more vigorous to improve the mobility of the thorax.

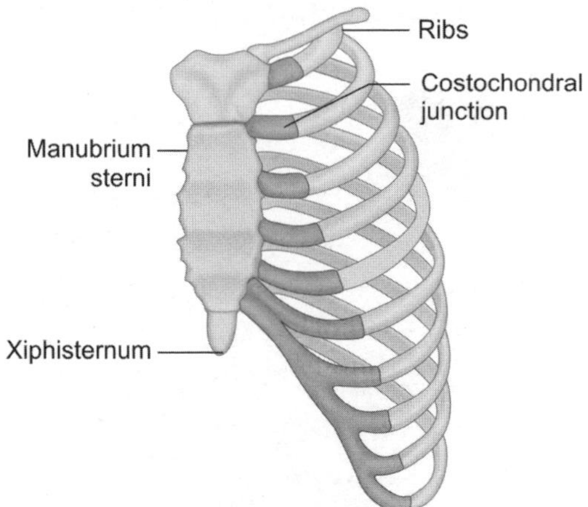

Fig. 15.12: Showing anatomical features of ribs.

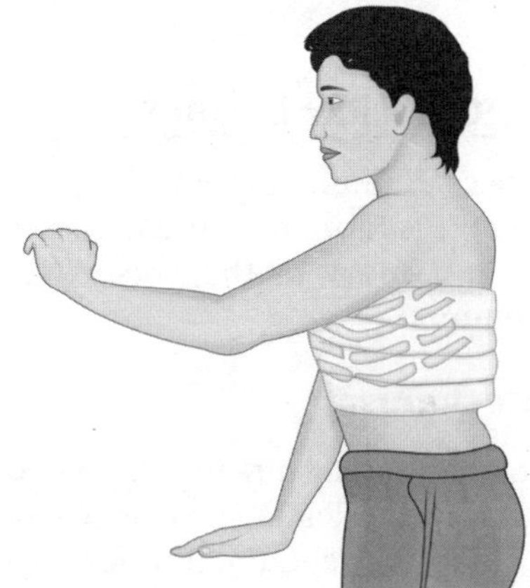

Fig. 15.13: Showing strapping method for treatment of fracture ribs.

---

*Seitz bath—this consists of sitting in a shallow tub of warm water. Commonly advocated in piles patients after surgery.

16
CHAPTER

Injuries of the Spine

CERVICAL SPINE INJURIES

Injuries of the cervical spine are dangerous and if associated with neurological damage the results can be devastating. Though diagnostic and treatment methods have vastly improved over years, still injuries of the cervical spine pose the greatest challenge to the skill and acumen of orthopedic and neurosurgeons. Jefferson pointed two areas commonly involved in cervical spine injuries, C_1-C_2 and C_5-C_7. According to Meyer C_2 and C_5 are commonly involved. Neurological damage is seen in 40% of cases. In 10% of cases, radiographs are normal.

Causes

❖ Fall from height—it is the most common cause in developing countries.
❖ Diving injuries—diving into water with insufficient depth or in an inebriated condition.
❖ Road traffic accidents (RTAs)—common cause in developed countries, e.g., whiplash injury **(Fig. 16.1)**.
❖ Gunshot injuries, etc. These injure the cervical spine and the cord directly.

Mechanism of Injury (Figs. 16.1 and 16.2)

❖ **Pure flexion force**—compression fracture of vertebral body from C_5-C_7, e.g., fall from height.
❖ **Flexion rotation force**—fall on one side of shoulder or head, disruption of facet joint and capsule is seen in C_5-C_7.
❖ **Axial compression**—fall of an object on the head results in load compression, e.g., explosive comminuted fracture of C_5 body (burst fracture, i.e., from C_5-C_6).
❖ **Extension force**—avulsion fracture of superior margin of vertebral body, e.g., whiplash injury.

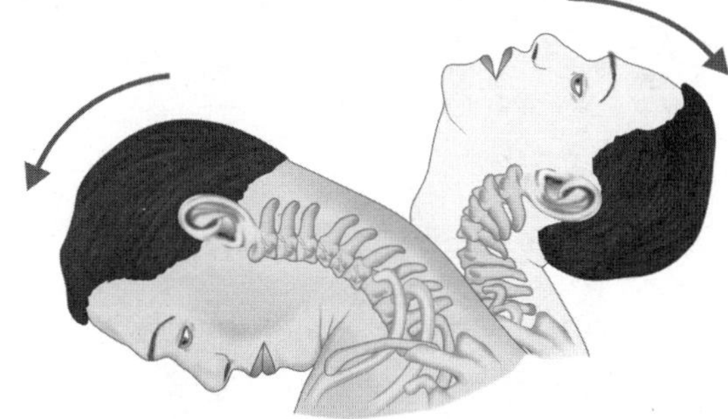

Fig. 16.1: Whiplash injury: Due to sudden deceleration, forceful hyperextension is followed by flexion of the neck.

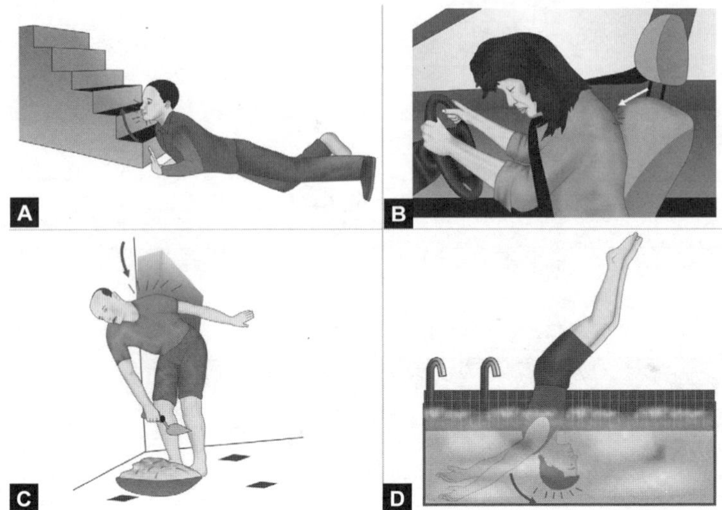

Figs. 16.2A to D: Showing common mechanism of spine injuries: (A) Hyperextension injury; (B) Flexion extension injury; (C) Flexion rotation injury; (D) Flexion injury.

- ❖ **Lateral flexion**—fracture pedicle, fracture transverse process and facet joints, etc.
- ❖ **Direct injuries**—fracture spinous process and body due to assault, gunshot injury, etc.

Clinical Features

Patient usually gives history of trauma following which there will be pain, swelling and inability to move the neck. There will be tenderness over the involved spinous process and there could be a palpable gap. There may be signs of neurological involvement and is examined the following way as shown in **Figures 16.3 to 16.10**. After examining the sensory system, the lowermost functioning muscle is documented and a functional level is established. Next, the sacrally innervated skin is

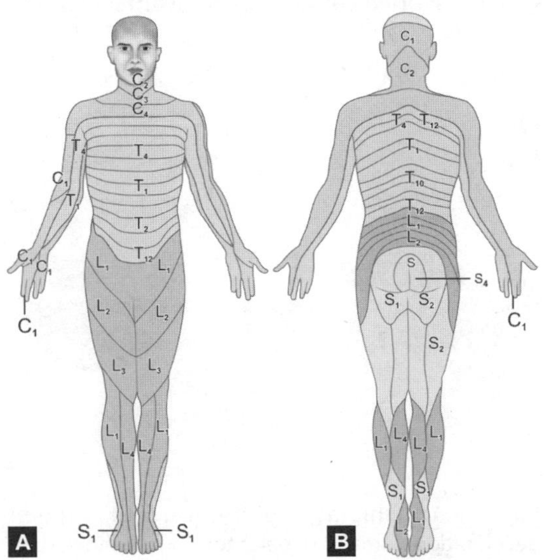

Figs. 16.3A and B: Dermatomal levels: (A) Anterior; (B) Posterior (Look for loss of sensations).

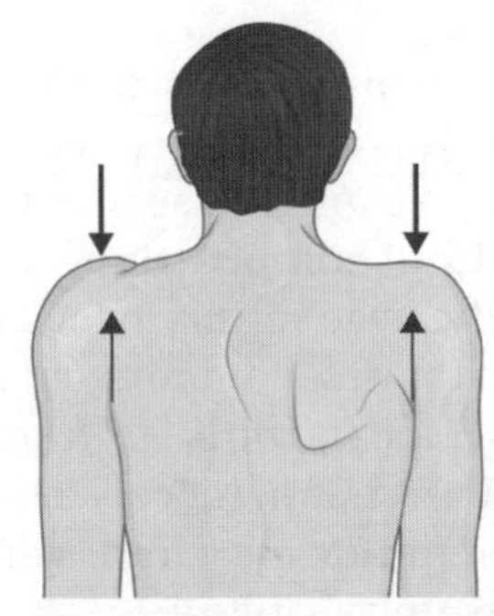

Fig. 16.4: Examination of C_3-C_4 (trapezius muscle).

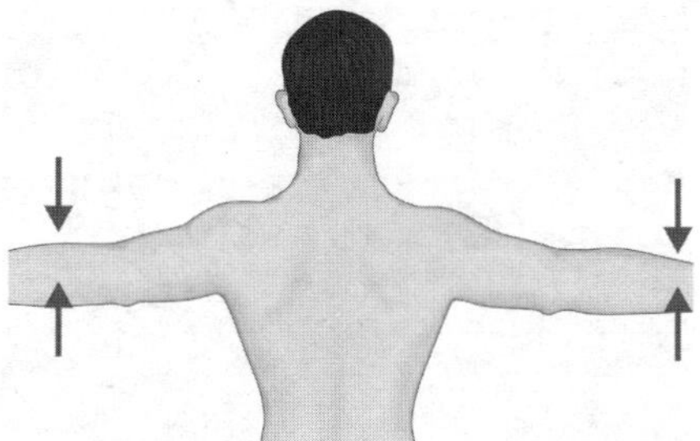

Fig. 16.5: Examination of C$_5$-C$_6$ roots (deltoid muscle).

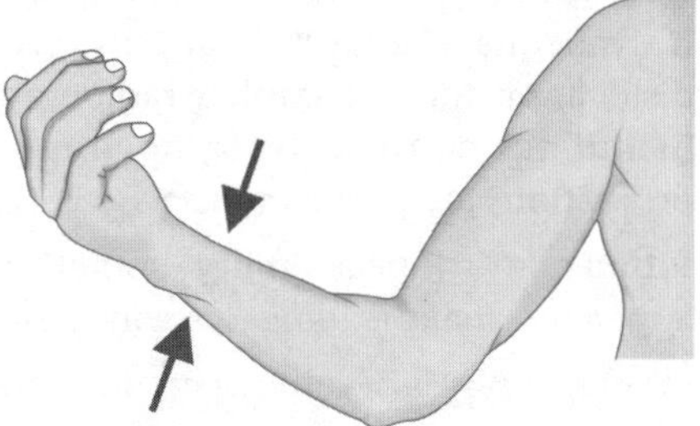

Fig. 16.6: Examination of C$_5$-C$_6$ roots (biceps muscle).

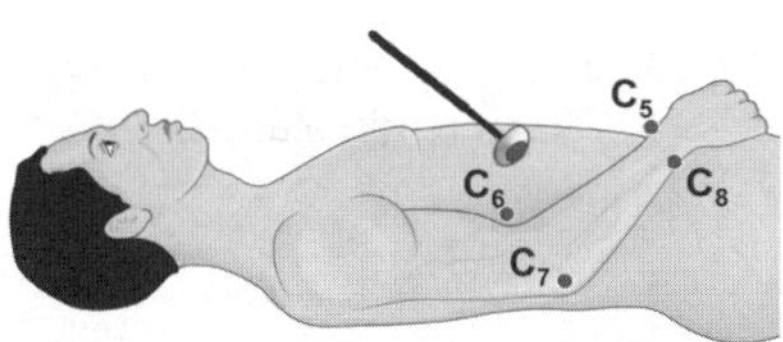

Fig. 16.7: Examination of upper limb reflexes.

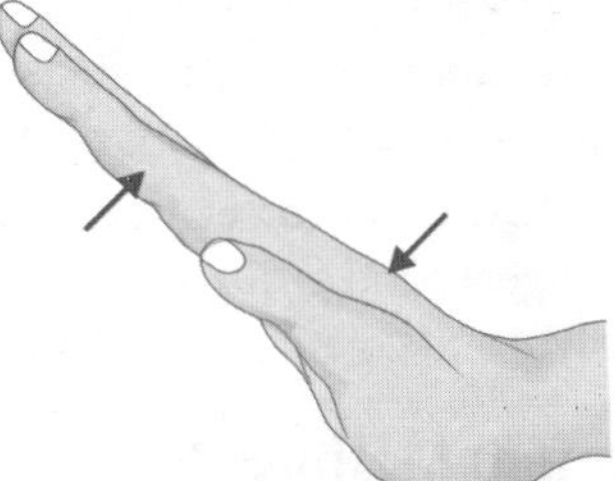

Fig. 16.8: Examination of C$_7$-C$_8$ (wrist extensors).

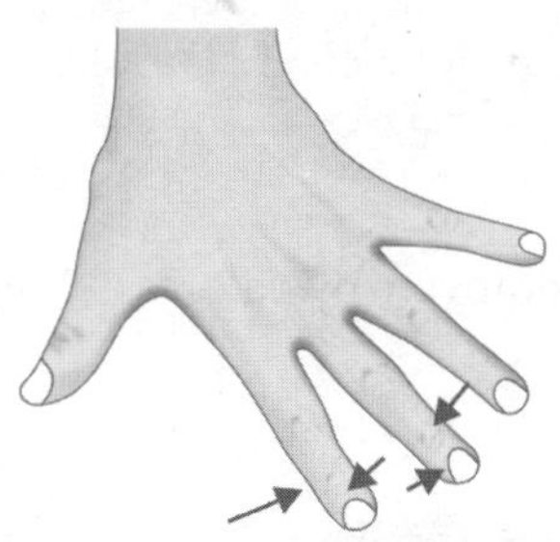

Fig. 16.9: Examination of C$_8$-T$_1$ (dorsal interosseous muscle).

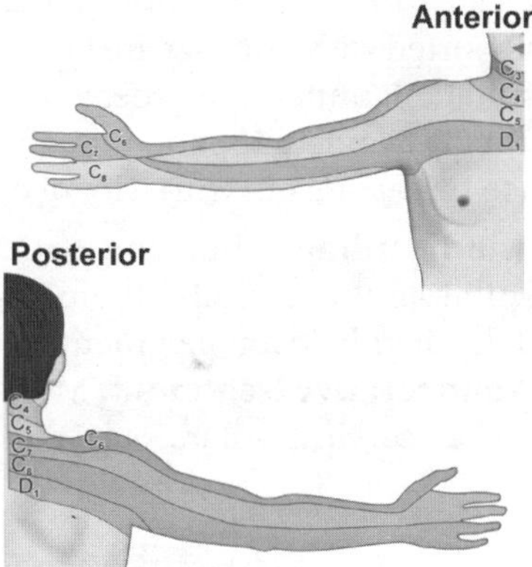

Fig. 16.10: Showing dermatomal pattern of cervical nerve roots.

examined. Perianal, anal, scrotal, labia and plantar surface of the toes are examined. *Perianal sensation may be the only sign to indicate an incomplete lesion.*

Other Examinations

Rectal sensation—loss of sensation around the anus *rectal motor*—sphincter contracts, over the gloved finger. *Bulbocavernosus reflex* involves S1, S2 and S3 nerve roots. Squeeze the glans penis, anal sphincter contracts around the gloved finger.

Radiography: Lateral view is important **(Fig. 16.11)**. If an adequate lateral radiography reveals no fracture or dislocation, then a complete radiographic examination including anteroposterior, open mouth and oblique projections are performed.

Pitfalls: In "whiplash injury", sometimes the X-ray may appear normally leading to errors in diagnosis.

Myelography is of value in incomplete lesion who fails to show progressive improvement.

CT scan makes an accurate diagnosis of hidden fracture. It is not helpful in assessing the soft tissue injury.

MRI evaluates cord injuries better. MRI is found to be very reliable and helpful in assessing the bony, soft tissue damages and injury to the cord very accurately.

General laboratory investigations—like Hb percentage, blood group, bleeding time, clotting time, electrolyte states, etc., are done.

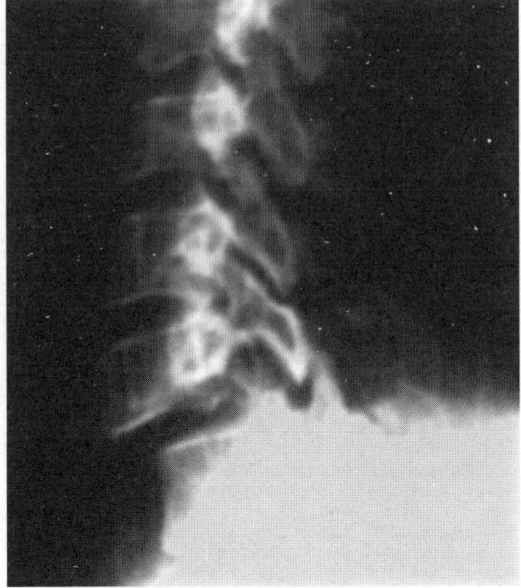

Fig. 16.11: Radiograph showing cervical fracture dislocation.

Treatment Methods

At the accident site: Resuscitation and transport is important. *In a person lying still without using his neck after an RTA, a cervical spine injury is always suspected until proved otherwise.* The patient is transported with utmost care over a stretcher to the hospital. All unnecessary neck movements should be totally avoided. If patient needs resuscitation it has to be carried out with a lot of care.

At the hospital: When the patient reaches the hospital, in the causality the patient is stabilized and the definitive management is done as follows:

❖ **Nonoperative treatment:** Most cases can be treated nonoperatively by halo vest, Minerva jacket, cervical collars, etc. **(Figs. 16.12A to C)**.

Treatment facts
Goals of treatment of cervical spine injury: ◂ Realign the spine. ◂ Prevent further neurological damage. ◂ Aid neurological recovery. ◂ Obtain and maintain spinal stability. ◂ Aim at early functional recovery.

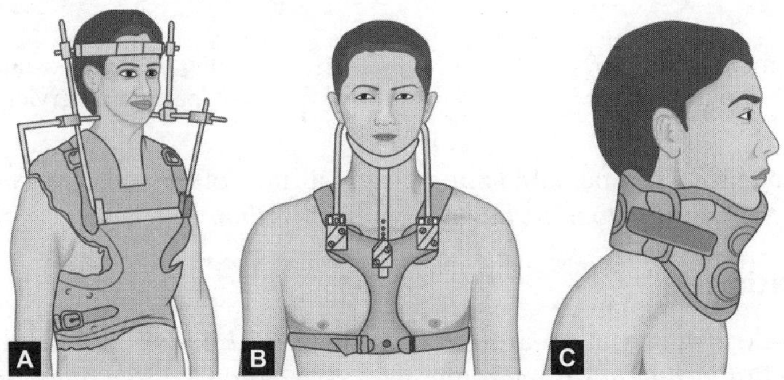

Figs. 16.12A to C: Methods of cervical immobilization: (A) Halo-vest traction; (B) Four post-cervical collar; (C) Cervical collar.

❖ **Indications:** Stable cervical spine fractures with no neurological injury. A rigid cervical brace or halo for 8–12 weeks is usually sufficient.
❖ **Skeletal traction:** Reduction with traction is done for unstable fracture. *Urgency of reduction is based on neurological loss* **(Fig. 16.13)**.

Traction is given for 3–6 weeks and once satisfactory reduction is achieved, patient is mobilized with a collar, corset or jacket **(Fig. 16.14)**.

Surgical Treatment

Indications: Unstable injury with or without neurologic damage require surgery.

Methods: In most patients early open reduction and internal fixation (ORIF) is indicated to obtain stability. Cervical spine is stabilized through an anterior or posterior approach. Usually a posterior approach is used with triple wire stabilization and fusion with iliac bone grafting. This allows rapid mobilization of patient in a cervical orthosis.

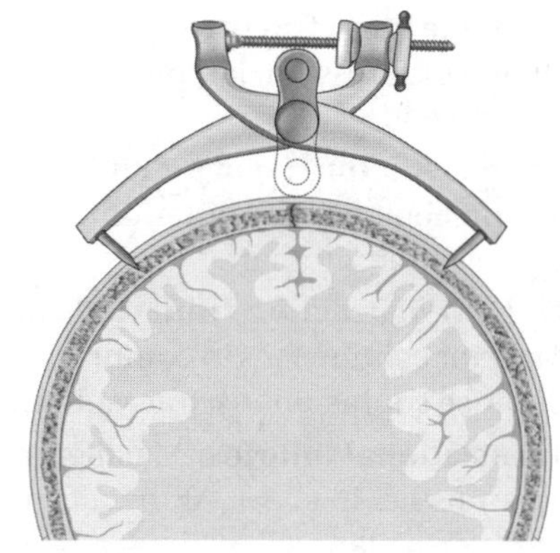

Fig. 16.13: Crutchfield tongs.

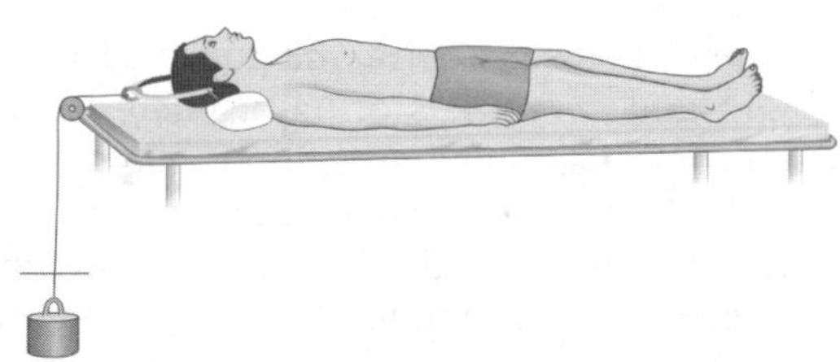

Fig. 16.14: Showing skeletal traction applied through Crutchfield tongs.

THORACIC AND LUMBOSACRAL SPINE INJURIES

Thoracolumbar spine is generally regarded as extending from 10th thoracic vertebrae to second lumbar vertebrae and is the transitional area between the kyphotic upper thoracic spines to the lordotic lumbar spine. The general anatomy of the vertebral column is more or less the same as in other areas of spine. The three-column concept has already been described. Anterior column is the load bearing structure and the posterior column functions as motion limiters as well as load-bearing structures. Mercifully, the thoracolumbar injuries spare the upper limbs and vital functions. Though a lesser challenge than cervical injury nevertheless it poses problems, no less risky than the former.

Mechanism of Injury

❖ Fall from a height.
❖ RTAs: Seat belt injury (chance fracture).
❖ Other causes like gunshot injuries, assault, etc.

Types of Lumbar Fractures (Figs. 16.15A to D)

Wedge compression: Isolated failure of anterior column due to forward flexion. No neurological deficit.

Stable burst fractures: Anterior and middle columns fail. No loss of integrity of posterior elements.

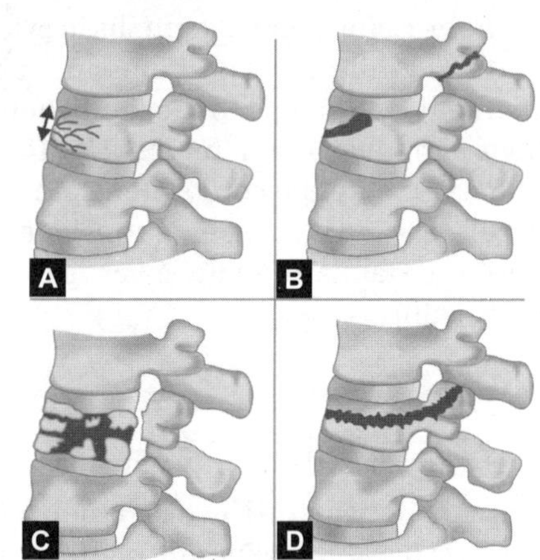

Figs. 16.15A to D: Thoracolumbar fractures (A) Flexion compression fracture; (B) Burst fracture; (C) Flexion distraction fractures (seat belt fractures); (D) Lateral compression fractures.

Unstable burst fractures: Anterior and middle column fail in compression. Posterior column fail in compression, lateral flexion or rotation. Post-traumatic kyphosis and neural symptoms are present.

Chance fracture (seat belt injury): Horizontal avulsion fracture of vertebral bodies caused by flexion about an axis anterior to the anterior longitudinal ligament. A strong tensile force pulls entire vertebrae apart.

Flexion distraction injury: Flexion axis is posterior to the anterior longitudinal ligament. Anterior column fails in compression. Middle and posterior column fail in tension. It is unstable because supraspinous, interspinous and ligamentum flavum fail.

Translational injuries: Malalignment of neural canal, which has been much disrupted. All 3 columns fail in shear. At the affected level, one part of sacral canal has been displaced in the transverse plane.

Clinical Features

Patient gives history of trauma due to RTA or fall from height and complains of pain; posterior swelling, tenderness, palpable interspinous gap or a step may be felt. Neurological involvement may vary from paraplegia to individual nerve root involvement. Spinal shock is present for 24 hours during which all the reflexes are lost. Cauda equina paralysis is present if the lesion is below L1.

Investigations

Radiography of the affected spine (Figs. 16.16): This is the preliminary investigation and all three views (AP, lateral and oblique) are taken.

CT scan and MRI: Both CT scan and MRI have found to be more useful than radiographs in evaluation of spinal trauma. While CT scan helps in studying the bony elements, MRI helps in the study of both bone and soft tissue elements **(Fig. 16.17)**. The damage to the cord is detected fairly accurately and is now being considered as the "gold standard" in the investigation of spine injury.

MANAGEMENT

This is discussed under two heads.

Management at the site of accident: This consists of careful handling of the patient suspected to have spine injury. Consider all patients with spine injury to have neurological damage and shift them to the hospital with utmost care and caution avoiding all unnecessary movements.

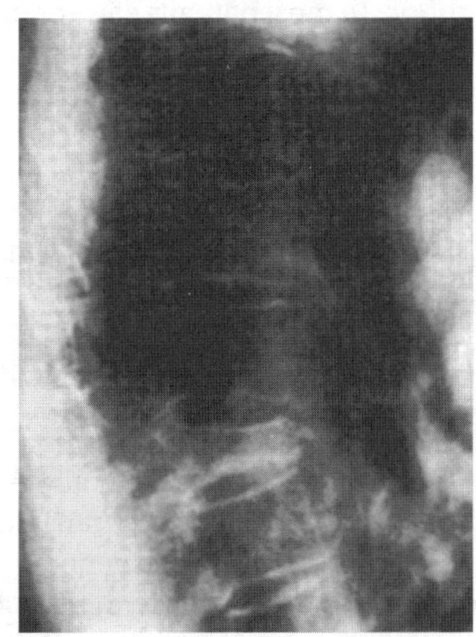

Fig. 16.16: Radiograph showing flexion compression fracture of T_{12} vertebra.

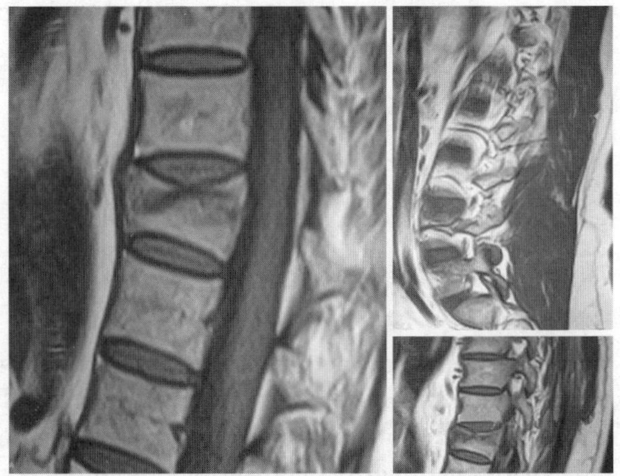

Fig. 16.17: CT scan showing fracture to T_6 vertebra.

Definitive treatment at the hospital: This varies depending upon the nature of injury and the presence or absence of neurological damage.

- ❖ **"Practice":** Caution in handling the neck.
- ❖ **"Examination":** The general condition and other systems like CNS/CVS/RS/PA/GI tract, etc. Also, examine from head to toe, the presence of other fractures, head, chest injuries, blunt injury abdomen and pelvic fractures.
- ❖ **"Evaluate"** the spine injury by gentle careful clinical examination. This has to be supplemented by proper investigations like X-ray, CT-scan, MRI, etc.
- ❖ **"Assess":** Carefully assess the level and extent of neurological damage by examining the dermatome, myotome and reflexes.
- ❖ **"Plan":** After evaluating and assessing the damage, plan the line of treatment. The treatment options include nonoperative, traction and operative methods. Now let us carefully took into various treatment modalities:

Treatment Methods

- ❖ **For stable fracture without neurological deficit:** Less than 30% anterior wedge, lateral, central compression fracture of the vertebral body is considered as stable fracture. In these injuries there is no fracture of the posterior cortex of the vertebral body, and there is no disruption of the neural arch.

  Treatment: This is essentially conservative and consists of bed rest, NSAIDs and external spine supports like brace, corsets, etc. If the vertebral body compression is less than 30%, only corset is used and if the compression is more than 30% but less than 50% a plaster jacket along with a corset is preferred **(Figs. 16.18A to D)**.
- ❖ **For stable fracture with neural deficit:** It has to be first determined whether the neurological deficit is complete (loss of motor power, sensory loss and absent reflexes) or incomplete (only cord or only spinal nerve roots).

  If neurological damage is incomplete, IV steroids are given for 4 days later anterior decompression and anterior interbody fusion in the first stage is done. Posterior segmental spinal stabilization by pedicle screws, Hartshill rectangle frame, Luque instrumentation, etc., can be done one week later. Laminectomy has fewer roles as it makes the spine less stable.

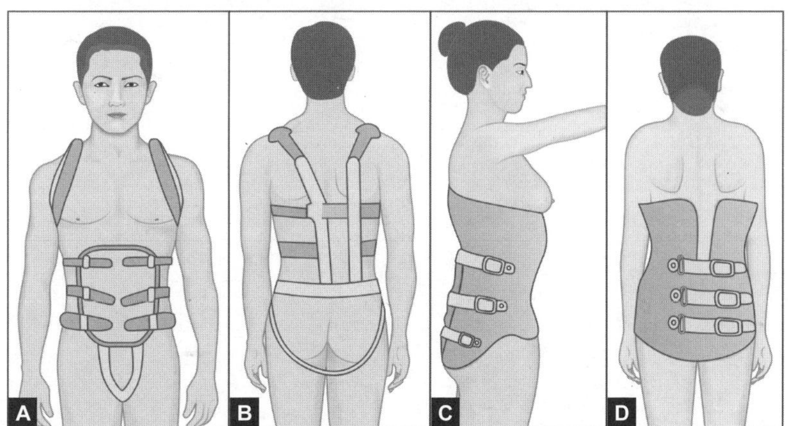

Figs. 16.18A to D: Showing treatment of stable thoracolumbar fractures with brace.

- ❖ **Unstable fracture without neurological deficit:** This is best treated by early open reduction, internal fixation, fusion and is done preferably within 12–24 hours. It is done with spinal cord monitoring. Internal fixation is either by VSP plates, Hart shill frame, Harrington instrumentation, etc.
- ❖ **Unstable fracture with neurological deficit:** Systemic Decadron 4–6 mg/every 6 hours IV for 3 days is given. Early open reduction and internal fixation and fusion are done in incomplete neurological deficit cases **(Figs. 16.19A and B)**. This is also desirable in complete neurological deficit to permit early-uninhibited rehabilitation. Segmental spinal stabilization with Luque or Hart shill frame is recommended.

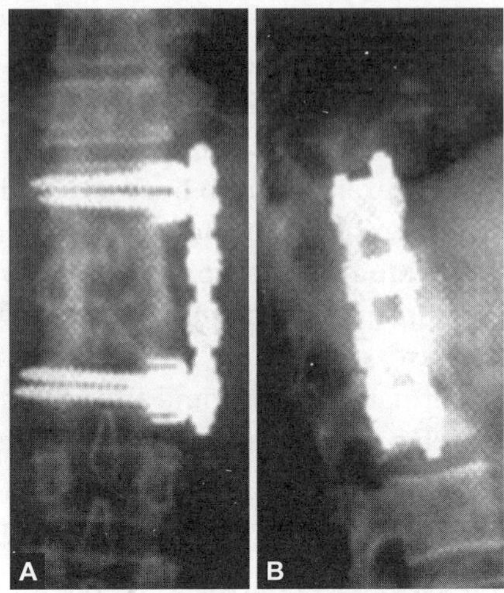

Figs. 16.19A and B: Radiograph showing posterior spinal stabilization.

17
CHAPTER

Hip Trauma

Injuries to the hip are one of the most catastrophic events for both the patient and the treating orthopedic surgeons. Being the biggest weight-bearing joint in the body, it is prone to lots of complications. It needs a great clinical acumen to put the house in order as far as hip joint is concerned.

FRACTURE NECK FEMUR

Etiology

- It is common in older patients with osteoporosis or osteomalacia (12%) and in them usually it is fracture through a pathological bone.
- It is common in elderly women secondary to senile osteoporosis. It also causes marked comminution of the posterior cortex and thus decreases the quality of reduction.

Mechanism of Injury

Majority are due to trivial fall **(Fig. 17.1)**, because of direct blow over the greater trochanter. Major trauma in young adults like road traffic accident (RTA) fall, etc.

Classification

Many classifications are proposed for fracture neck femur. It is broadly divided into intracapsular or extracapsular fractures **(Figs. 17.2A and B)**.

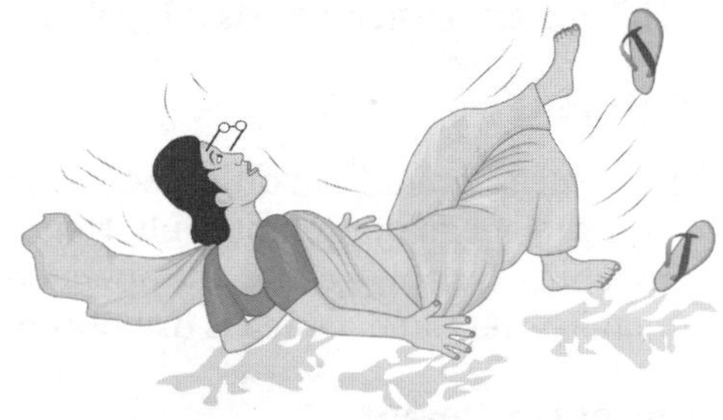

Fig. 17.1: Fracture neck femur is common in elderly females due to trivial fall like a slip in the bathroom.

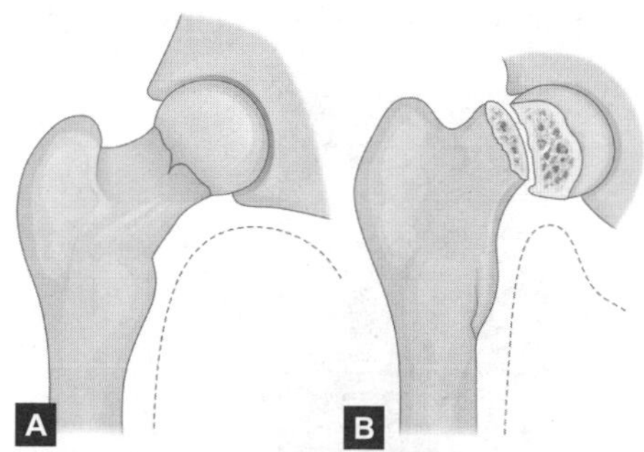

Figs. 17.2A and B: Showing intracapsular fracture of neck femur: (A) Undisplaced; (B) Displaced broken Shenton's line.

Broad Classification

* Intracapsular—from subcapital area to the middle of the neck **(Figs. 17.3A)**.
* Extracapsular—from base of the neck to the pertrochanteric region **(Figs. 17.3B)**.

Clinical Features

Usually, patient is an elderly female and gives history of trivial trauma, such as slip and fall in a bathroom **(Fig. 17.1)**. Patient complains of pain and restriction of movements of the affected hip. On examination, there is tenderness over the anterior hip joint line. There is minimal shortening and external rotational deformity of the affected limb due to the fracture being intracapsular. The capsule prevents the muscular forces from displacing the fracture fragments grossly. Active straight leg rising is difficult. In impacted fracture neck of femur, patient complains of groin pain, antalgic gait and restriction of hip movements.

Investigations

Radiography consists of routine AP and lateral views of the hip joint. The following points are noted.
* The extent of fracture line whether complete or incomplete.
* The fracture angle.
* Break in the Shenton's line.
* Posterior wall comminution of the neck is best seen in the lateral view.
* Prominent lesser trochanter.
* The degree of osteoporosis (Singh's index).

Treatment

Fracture neck femur is an orthopedic emergency, which needs to be reduced and fixed within 24 hours to get an optimum result. Hence, *speed is the watchword* in managing fracture neck femur and invariably needs to be operated because of the small proximal fragment an accurate reduction is required, which is usually not possible by conservative methods.

Aims of Treatment

* Early anatomical reduction, which helps, prevents further vascular damage.
* Impaction of the fracture fragments.
* **Rigid internal fixation:** Enables revascularization from the surrounding soft tissues and uninjured bones, which helps in early callus formation.

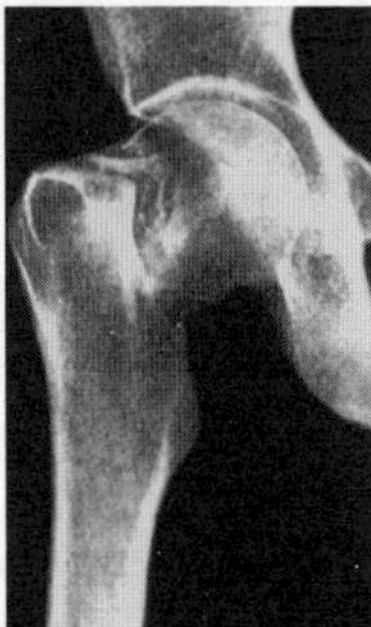

Fig. 17.3A: Radiograph showing intracapsular fracture neck femur.

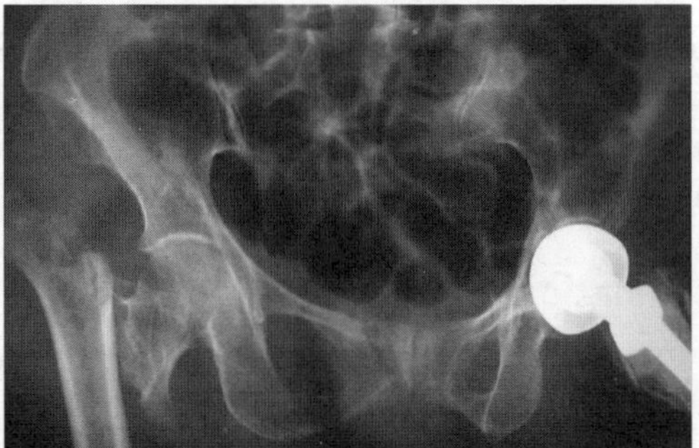

Fig. 17.3B: Extracapsular trochanteric fracture.

Treatment Plans

Aim of surgery

Goal of surgery is anatomical reduction, impaction and stable internal fixation.

Multiple pins (Knowles, Moore) for impacted fracture, percutaneously for medically unfit persons **(Fig. 17.4A)**, and for fractures in children **(Fig. 17.4B)**.

ASNIS: This is a system of cannulated screws that provide improved pullout and bending and torque strengths as compared to Knowles pins. These are the commonly preferred screws for the intracapsular variety **(Fig. 17.5A)**.

Fixed angle nail: It has fallen into disrepute because the nail is rigid and may penetrate the joint **(Fig. 17.5B)**.

Sliding or telescoping nails (dynamic hip screws): It has replaced the fixed angle nail. The nail offers collapsibility which ensures continuous impaction at the fracture site and which lessens the chance of nail penetration through the femoral head. *This is the most commonly employed fixation method for fracture neck femur* especially the extracapsular variety **(Fig. 17.5C)**.

Meyer's muscle pedicle graft: A mention has to be made about the posterior muscle pedicle grafting technique. Muscle pedicle graft from the gluteus maximus or quadratus femoris (Meyer's technique), is particularly useful in posterior wall comminution. Dr Bakshi of Kolkata has popularized this technique.

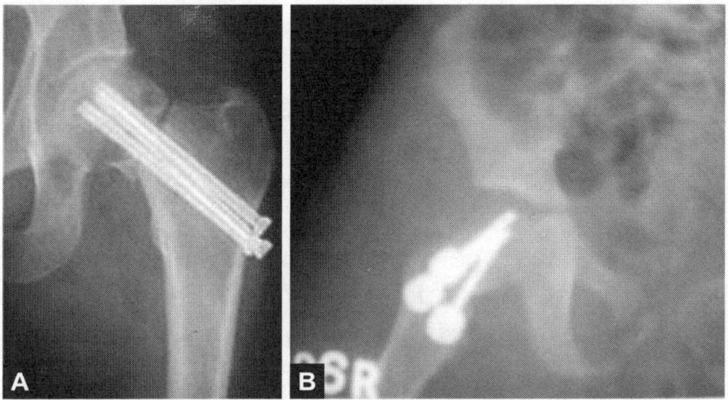

Figs. 17.4A and B: Radiograph showing intracapsular fracture neck femur fixed with (A) Multiple cannulated screws; (B) Moore's pins in children.

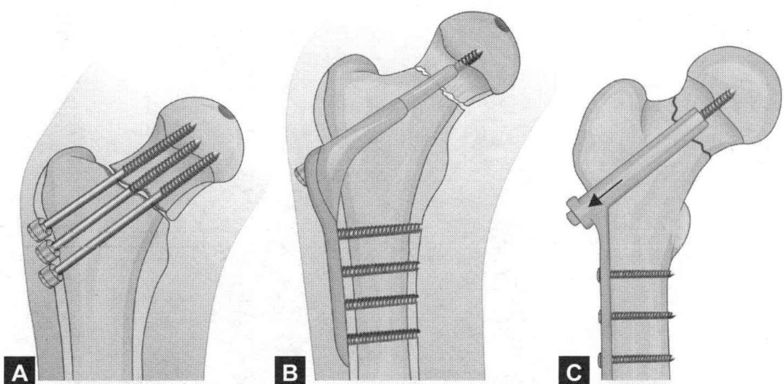

Figs. 17.5A to C: Showing methods of internal fixation of intracapsular fracture neck of femur: (A) Multiple pins; (B) Blade plate fixation; (C) Dynamic hip screw.

Other treatment options: These include hemi replacement arthroplasty, osteotomy and very rarely THR. However, they are not recommended as the primary modality of treatment in fresh fracture neck of femur . They are also indicated in special situations, such as nonunion, AVN, etc., and are discussed below.

SUBTROCHANTERIC FRACTURE

Subtrochanteric region is defined as an area between the lesser trochanter and a point 5 cm distal to it. Subtrochanteric fracture is a difficult fracture due to problems, such as malunion, delayed union, nonunion, shortening, angular deformity, rotational malalignment, etc. **(Fig. 17.6)**.

Mechanism of Injury

It is usually due to direct trauma due to RTA or fall and is common in young individuals.

Clinical Features

The patient presents with pain, swelling, shortening, complete external rotation deformity and other usual features of fractures.

Radiology (Fig. 17.7)

Radiograph helps to study the level and pattern of fracture and thereby helps plan the treatment.

Treatment

Conservative Methods

There are advocated if the patient is young. In severely comminuted fractures, modified cast brace with pelvic band is used.

Surgery

This is the preferred method of treatment in adults and ORIF is chosen for those fractures, which can be made stable by closed or open reduction. The choice of internal fixation with implants at different levels of the fracture is between interlocking nail, PFN **(Fig. 17.8)**, Zickel's nail, Gamma nail, etc.

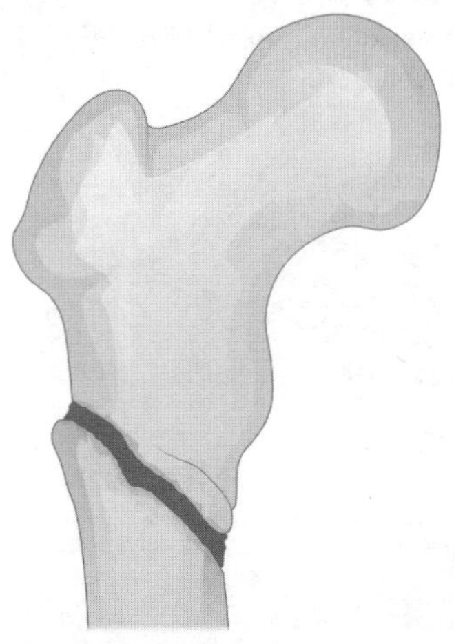

Fig. 17.6: Showing subtrochanteric fracture.

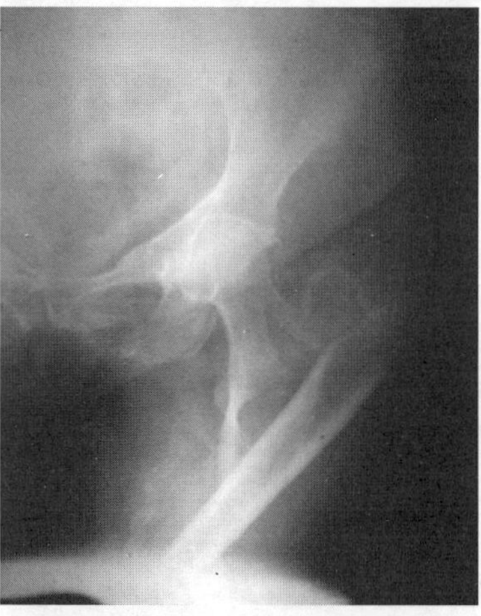

Fig. 17.7: Radiograph showing subtrochanteric fracture femur.

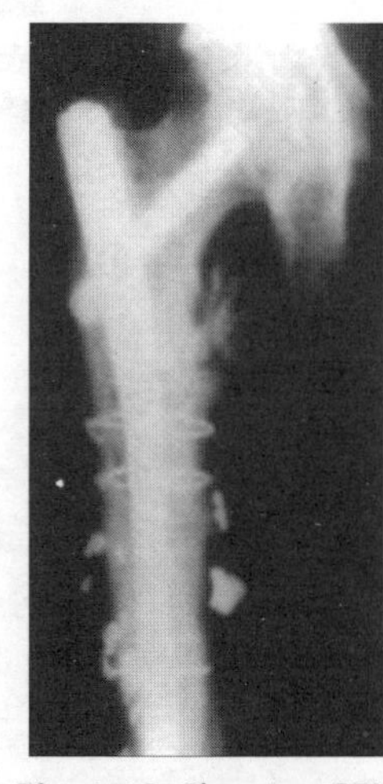

Fig. 17.8: Showing PFN fixation.

INTERTROCHANTERIC FRACTURE

It is seen in elderly patients 10–12 years older than intracapsular fracture neck femur and is more common in females (2.8:1) due to osteoporosis.

Mechanism

Direct trauma as in RTA, fall, etc.

Indirect trauma due to muscle pull, etc.

Clinical Features

The patient will have pain, marked shortening of the lower limb, complete external rotation deformity, swelling, ecchymosis and tenderness over the greater trochanter.

Radiology

A true anteroposterior view in internal rotation and a lateral view helps to study the fracture pattern **(Fig. 17.9)**.

Treatment

Conservative treatment this is indicated in poor medical and surgical risk patients, terminally ill patients and very old patients. Methods commonly employed are:

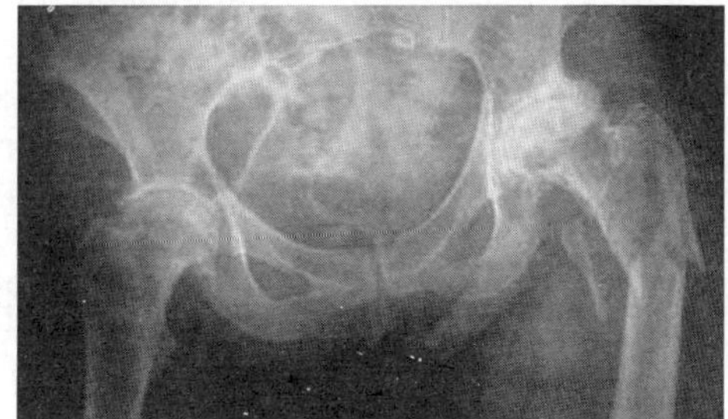

Fig. 17.9: Radiograph showing comminuted trochanteric fracture femur.

❖ Skeletal traction through distal femur or tibia for 10–12 weeks through a BB frame or a Thomas splint.

❖ Russell skin traction is the most widely recommended method of skin traction in this variety of fracture.

Surgical Methods

Goal is to fix a stably reduced fracture either by closed or open methods internally and thus maintain a normal femoral neck shaft angle.

Once stable reduction has been obtained either anatomically or by any one of the non-anatomical means (e.g., by osteotomy, etc.), rigid internal fixation is done preferably by DHS screw and plates **(Fig. 17.10)**.

Complications

Due to the cancellous nature of bone, these fractures unite well unlike fracture neck femur but malunion is quite common. Coxa vara, nonunion is less than 2% (rare) and traumatic osteoarthritis is seen. These fractures also carry a higher incidence of mortality (> 10%). Avascular necrosis is very rare (0.8%)

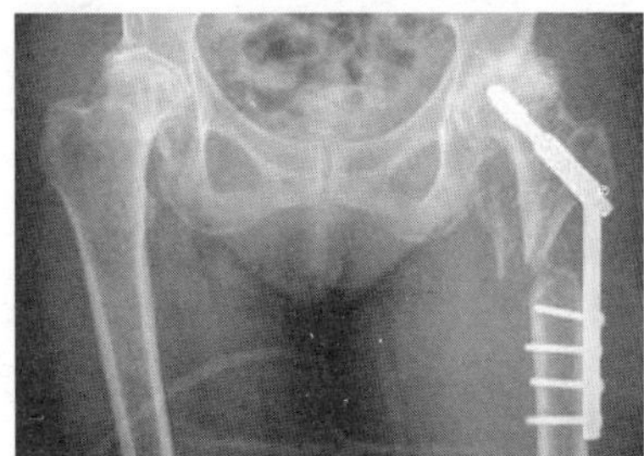

Fig. 17.10: Showing DHS, fixation of choice in intertrochanteric fracture.

DISLOCATIONS OF HIP

POSTERIOR DISLOCATION OF HIP JOINT

It is an interesting observation that if anterior dislocation is common in shoulder joint, it is the posterior dislocation, which is common in the hip joint. Incidence is around 70%.

Mechanism of Injury

It is usually due to a backward directed force along the line of femur in a flexed hip dashboard injury **(Fig. 17.11)**. If the femur is more adducted at the time of impact, pure dislocation results and if the femur is slightly abducted fracture dislocation results.

Clinical Features

There is usually history of trauma and the patient has a flexion, adduction and medial rotation deformity of the affected limb **(Figs. 17.12A to C)**. There is marked shortening and gross restriction of all hip movements. Head of the femur is felt as a hard mass in the glutei region and it moves along with the femur. There could be features of sciatic nerve palsy. It may be difficult to feel the femoral pulse (Vascular sign of Narath is negative).

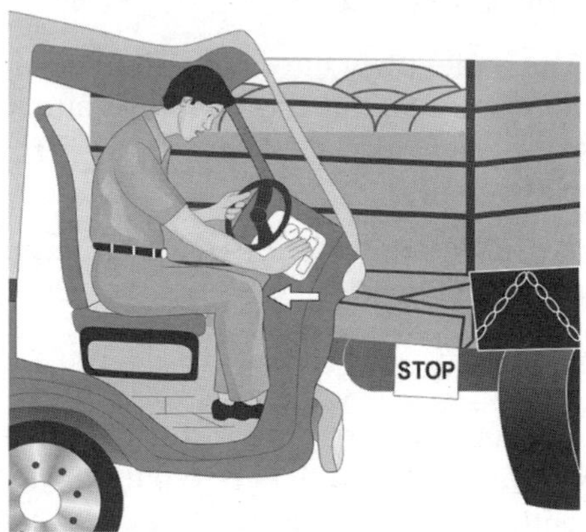

Fig. 17.11: A dashboard injury.

Investigations

Radiography

AP views of the pelvis showing both the hip joints are usually preferred. Lateral view and oblique views of the affected joint gives clue to the fractures of the posterior acetabular rim **(Fig. 17.13)**.

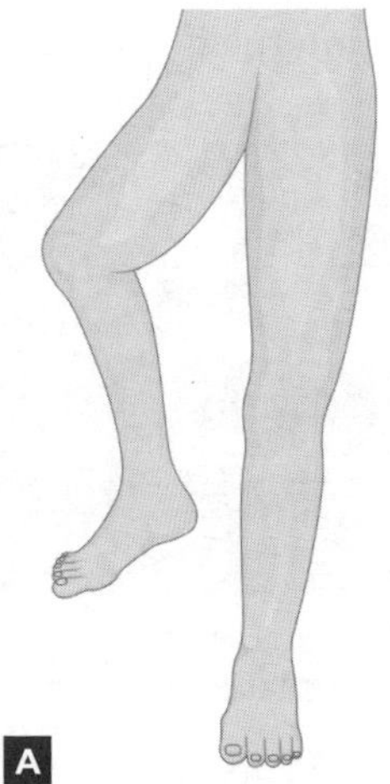

A

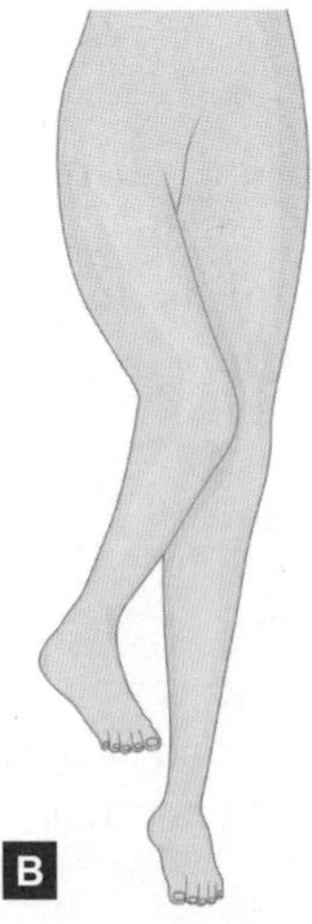

B

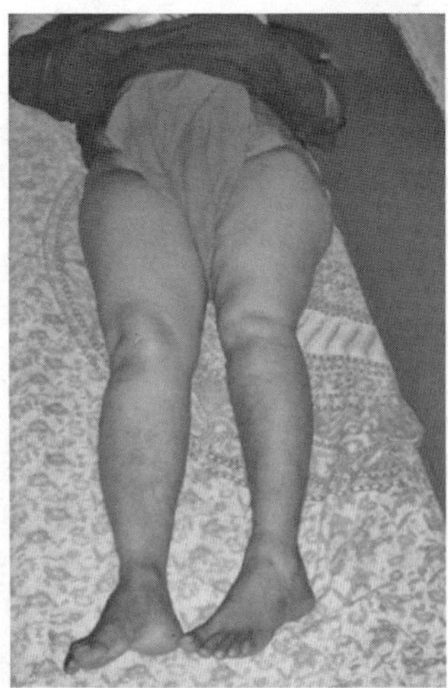

Figs. 17.12A and B: Appearance of classical deformities in dislocation hip: (A) Anterior; (B) Posterior.

Fig. 17.12C: Clinical photograph showing posterior dislocation of the hip.

CT Scan and MRI

CT scan and MRI study of the hip joint is more reliable in assessing the acetabular fractures.

Treatment

In order to prevent early onset of secondary osteoarthritis and to reduce pain, immediate reduction of the hip has to be carried out under general anesthesia.

Techniques of Reduction

There are various methods of reduction of the hip joint but the most commonly employed method is the "classical method" (**Fig. 17.14**). In this method, the patient is supine and is on the floor under general anesthesia. The hip is flexed to 90° and with an assistant stabilizing the pelvis, a longitudinal traction is given in the line of femur. If a reduction is achieved a loud click sound is heard. Immediately after the reduction tests for the stability of hip joint is done by moving it around in all directions. In fracture dislocations, the hip joint redislocates again.

Note: To clinically assess the stability after reduction, flex the hip to 90° and apply a posterior force. If the hip remains reduced, it is considered stable.

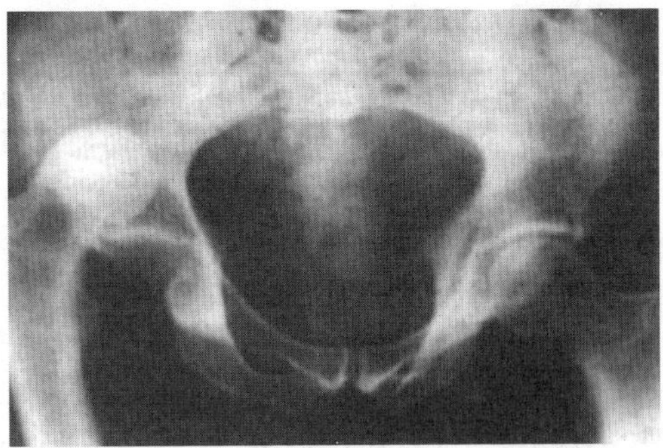

Fig. 17.13: Radiograph showing posterior dislocation of hip.

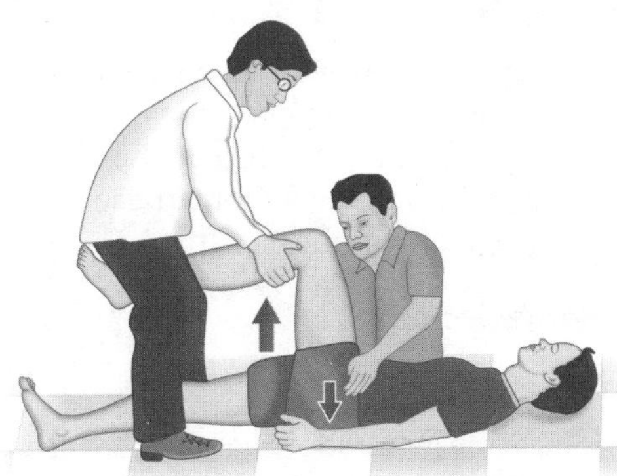

Fig. 17.14: Classical Watson Jones technique for reduction of hip dislocation.

After Treatment

After reduction, the patient is put on skin traction or immobilized in a Thomas splint for 3 weeks. Full weight bearing is permitted after 6 weeks.

Indications for Open Reduction

The following are some of the important indications for open reduction:

❖ **Failure of close reduction:** This could be due to obstruction by bony fragments or by soft tissues, such as acetabular labrum and capsule or locking of fracture surfaces or due to buttonholing of femoral head through the capsule.
❖ Instability after reduction is usually due to large posterior chunk of acetabulum.
❖ Sciatic nerve palsy, etc.

Note: Posterior dislocation of the hip should be reduced early to prevent post-traumatic osteonecrosis and relieve compression on the sciatic nerve.

ANTERIOR DISLOCATION OF HIP JOINT (ADH)

This is relatively less common than the posterior variety and accounts for 10–15% of the cases.

Mechanism of Injury

❖ Dashboard injury as in posterior dislocation but here the thigh is in abduction at the time of impact.

❖ Fall from heights, say a tree, when one of the legs is stuck in the branches and leaves the hip joint widely abducted.

❖ Direct blow to the back as in a RTA **(Fig. 17.15)**.

❖ While standing at the bank of a river, with one foot in the boat and the other on the shore. Now if the boat suddenly moves forwards, the resulting abduction force dislocates the hip anteriorly.

Clinical Features

Patient may complain of severe pain and restriction of the hip movements. The hip is in flexion, abduction and external rotation position. The head may be felt in the groin, and the femoral pulse is readily felt (Vascular sign of Narath is positive).

Investigations

Radiography

AP views of the pelvis showing both the hip joints are usually preferred **(Fig. 17.16)**.

CT scan and MRI

CT scan and MRI study of the hip joint may be required in some situations.

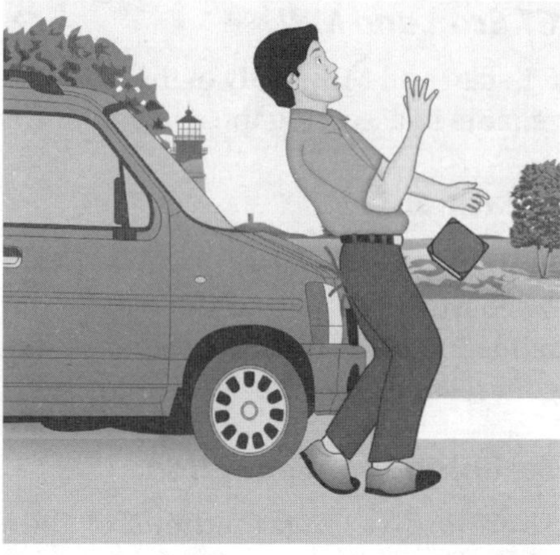

Fig. 17.15: Showing common mechanism of injury of anterior dislocation of the hip.

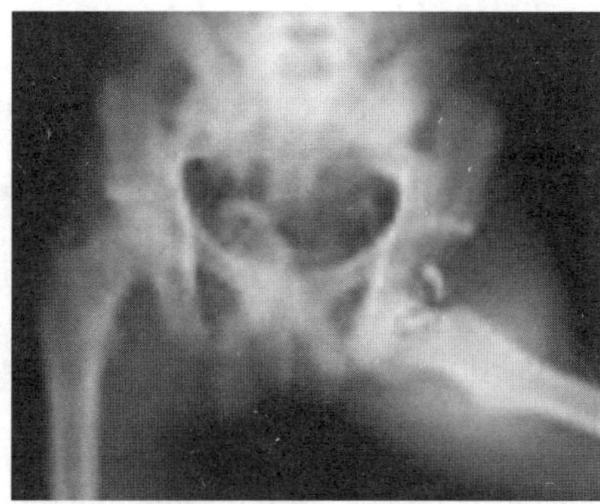

Fig. 17.16: Radiograph showing anterior dislocation of the hip.

Treatment

Consists of prompt closed reduction only and this is similar to the posterior dislocation of hip.

CENTRAL DISLOCATION OF HIP (CDH)

This is the least common and most difficult of all dislocations of the hip joint.

Mechanism of Injury

It could be due to a direct blow on the greater trochanter as in the case of RTA **(Fig. 17.17)** or fall on the sides. It is invariably associated with the fractures of the acetabulum, and this is what makes it a very difficult problem to treat.

Clinical Features

Interestingly none of the features as in ADH or PDH is seen. On the other hand, in CDH there is no limb shortening,

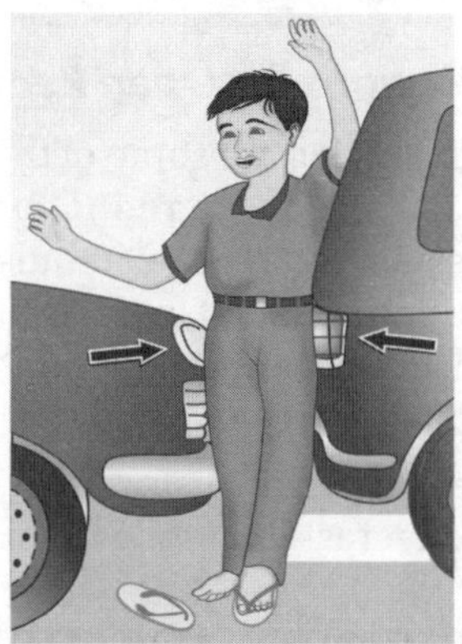

Fig. 17.17: Showing mechanism of injury for central fracture dislocation.

no external rotation deformity, head is not externally palpable. The limb is in neutral position; there is pain, severe restriction of hip movements and a huge bruise over the greater trochanter. Head is felt easily by a per rectal examination typical of CDH.

Investigations

Routine plain X-rays **(Fig. 17.18)**, CT scan are the recommended investigative procedures.

Treatment

Reduction is achieved through skeletal traction over the greater trochanter in line of the neck of femur. Open reduction is reserved for cases of failed closed reduction. The skeletal traction is maintained for 10–12 weeks if the acetabulum is reasonably reconstructed or else open reduction and surgical reconstruction of the acetabulum is recommended.

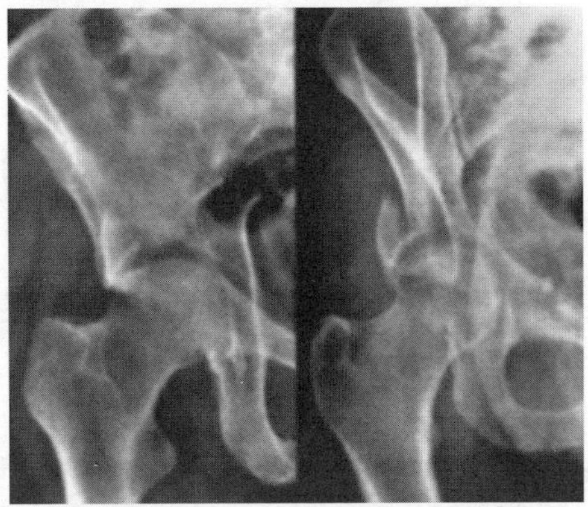

Fig. 17.18: Radiograph showing central fracture dislocation of hip.

Injuries of the Femur

FRACTURE SHAFT FEMUR

Mechanism of Injury

Usually, it is due to direct or indirect forces following a major violence as in RTA **(Fig. 18.1)**, and is common in young adults because the strong metaphyseal areas transmit the forces to the shaft causing fracture. In old age, the metaphyseal areas are brittle and hence the shaft fracture is rare, but fracture of metaphyseal region is common.

Clinical Features

Apart from all the features of fractures there could be shortening of the lower limb and complete external rotation deformity such that the lateral border of the foot touches the bed **(Fig. 18.2)**. Since, the fracture femur is usually due to major violence, the patient may also present with features of shock: (unconsciousness, pallor, cold nose, tachycardia, cold and clammy skin, hypotension, etc.).

Radiography

Routine anteroposterior and lateral views **(Fig. 18.3)** of the femur suffice but care should be taken to include the neighboring joints (hip and knee) to rule out the possibilities of injuries to these joints.

Management

Conservative Methods (Figs. 18.4 to 18.7)

Children: It is mainly conservative in children.

❖ **0–2 years:** Plaster spica in human position or modified Bryant or Gallow's traction **(Fig. 18.4)**.

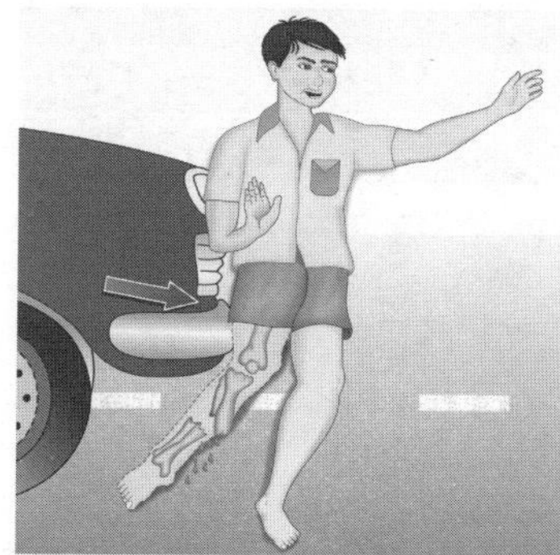

Fig. 18.1: Bumper injuries in RTA commonly cause fracture femur and tibia.

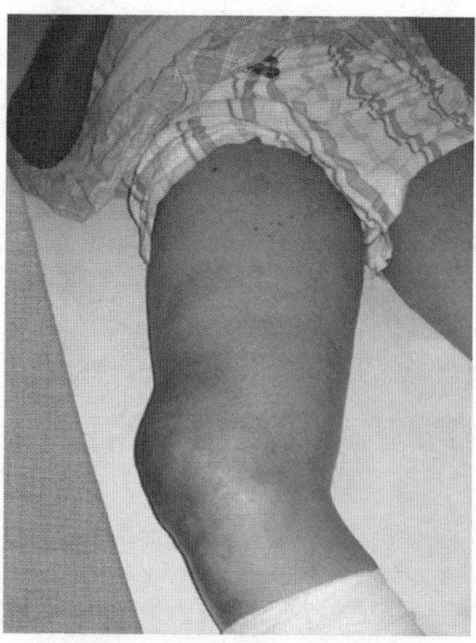

Fig. 18.2: Showing deformity of the thigh in a femur fracture.

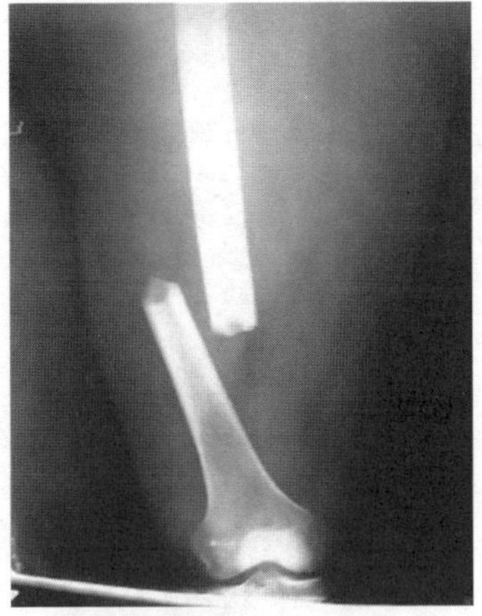

Fig. 18.3: Radiograph showing fracture shaft femur.

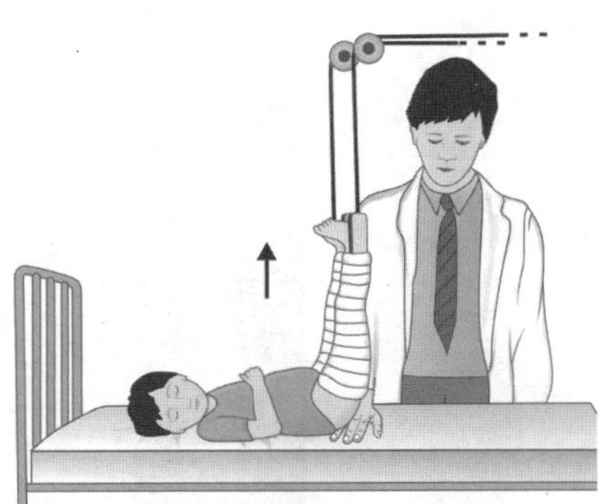

Fig. 18.4: Gallow's traction.

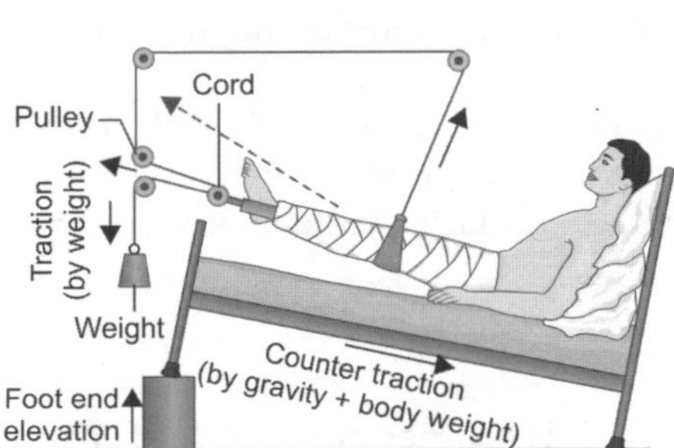

Fig. 18.5: Russell traction.

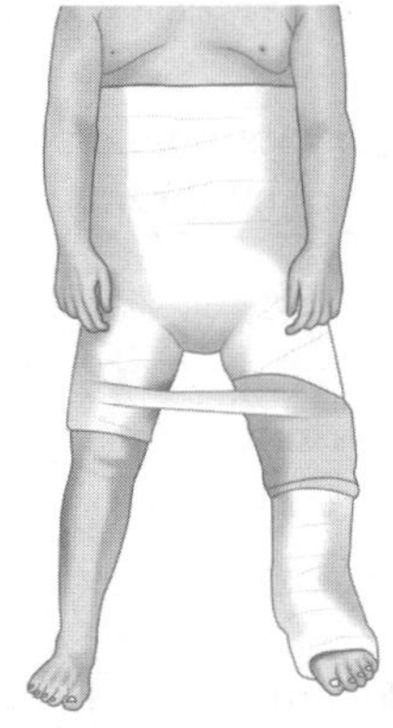

Fig. 18.6: Treatment of fracture shaft femur in children by hip-spice.

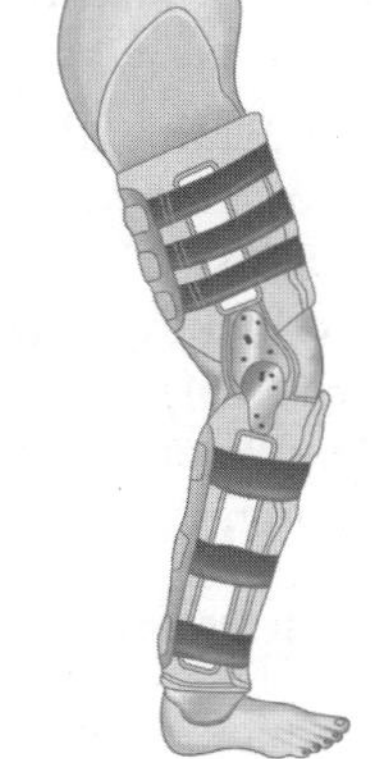

Fig. 18.7: Fracture shaft of femur treated by a functional cast brace.

- ❖ **2–10 years:** Most femoral fractures are seen in this age group. Here split Russell traction **(Fig. 18.5)** is more useful.
- ❖ **10–15 years:** 90–90° femoral skeletal traction or hip spica or both **(Fig. 18.6)**.
- ❖ **>15 years:** Treatment is as in adults.

Note: Human position is 90° of flexion and 45° of external rotation at the hip.

Surgery

The best method of managing a fracture shaft femur in adults is by open reduction and rigid internal fixation with either:
- ❖ **Intramedullary (IM) nails:** This is used for fractures from 2.5 cm below the lesser trochanter to that 8–10 cm above the knee joint. It can be used in simple or comminuted fractures **(Fig. 18.8A)**. It can be done immediately following the trauma or delayed for a few days.

DCP plate and screws: Earlier this was a very popular method of treating fracture shaft femur. Dynamic compression plating is used for proximal and distal one-third fractures where medullary

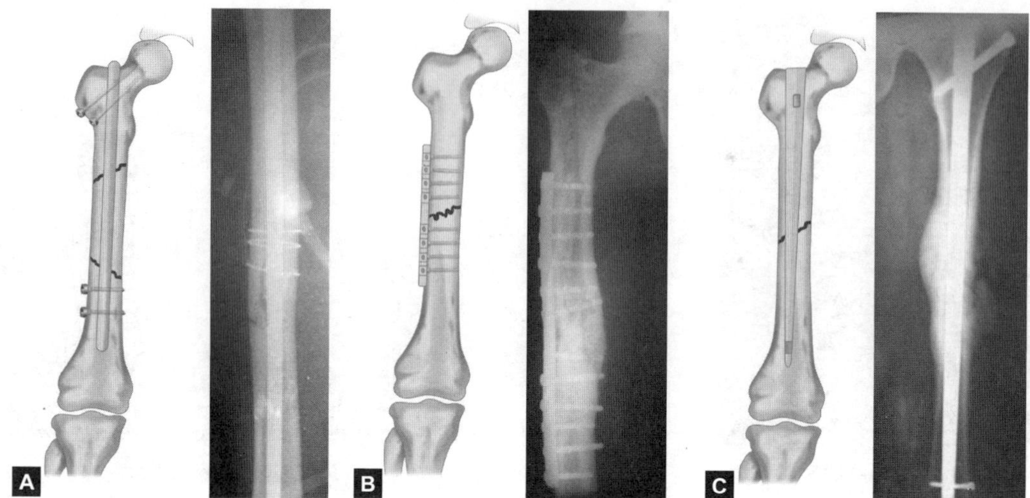

Figs. 18.8A to C: Plain X-ray showing methods of internal fixation for fracture shaft femur: (A) Kuntschner's intermedullary nails; (B) DCP plate and screws; (C) Interlocking nail.

canal is wide and intramedullary nailing is not suitable. However, it is less commonly used nowadays due to the availability of better methods of fixation like the interlocking nailing, etc. **(Fig. 18.8B)**.

❖ **Interlocking nails:** Of late, this is being regarded as the gold standard in the method of internal fixation of fracture shaft femur **(Fig. 18.8C)**. These extend the indications of standard IM nail.

❖ **Flexible medullary nails:** It is like Ender's nail, which is usually passed from below upwards through the distal femur.

DISTAL FEMUR FRACTURE

The distal part of the femur encompasses the lower one-third. It varies between 7.6 cm and 15 cm of distal femur. The supracondylar area is a transition zone between the distal diaphysis and the femoral articular surface. The distal femur is subjected to the quadriceps force anteriorly and the flexion force of the gastrocnemius posteriorly. The fractures of the distal femur could be classified into supracondylar, intercondylar, unicondylar and comminuted fractures **(Figs. 18.9A to C)**. The intercondylar fractures could be wither T, Y or comminuted. The distal femur fracture accounts for 4.7% of all femoral fractures.

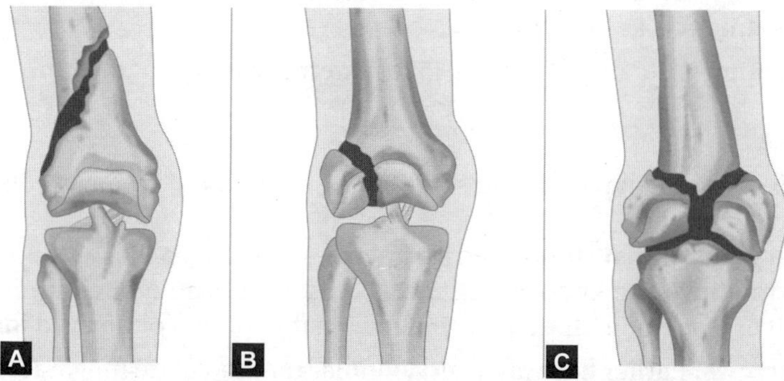

Figs. 18.9A to D: Fractures of distal femur: (A) Supracondylar fracture; (B) Unicondylar fracture; (C) Intercondylar fracture.

Mechanism of Injury

These fractures are usually due to severe valgus or varus forces with axial loading and rotation due to RTA, fall, etc.

Clinical Features

It consists of the usual features of fractures but what is specific to this fracture is the flexion deformity caused by the pull of gastrocnemius. Hemarthrosis is commonly seen especially with fractures extending into the joint.

Radiography

Radiograph helps to study the fracture pattern more accurately **(Fig. 18.10)**.

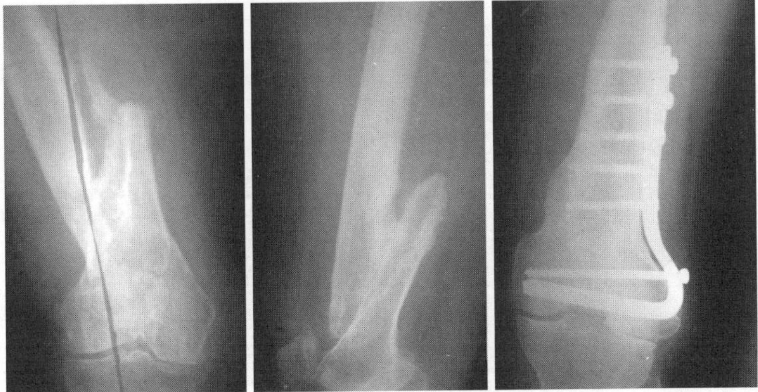

Fig. 18.10: Radiographs showing fracture distal femur and its fixation.

Treatment

The treatment usually consists of conservative methods, traction and operative methods.

Conservative Methods

This has a limited role and is usually useful in impacted and undisplaced fractures. In the former, a long leg or spica cast is sufficient and in the latter a long above knee cast after an initial period of skin or skeletal traction is all that is required.

Traction Methods

The choice is mainly skeletal traction through the upper tibia over the BB frame. This method of treatment is sparingly used is some instances of communited or compound fractures **(Fig. 18.11)**.

Operative methods

This consists of ORIF and is preferred as the closed reduction is associated with troublesome complications, such as limited knee motion, residual varus and internal rotation deformities. The advantages of open reduction are early mobilization of the knee joint due to an accurate reduction and rigid fixation.

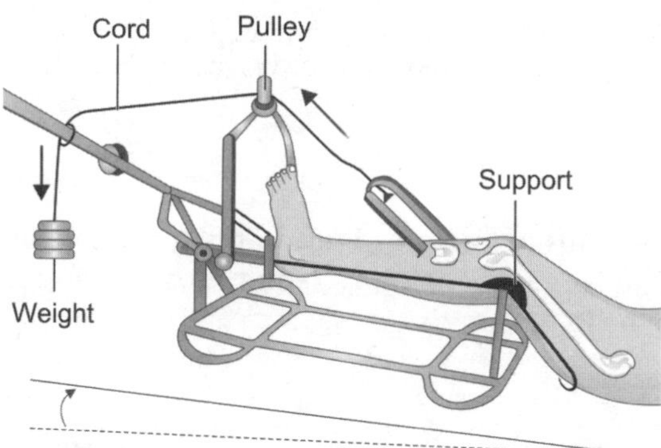

Fig. 18.11: Skeletal traction through Böhler-Braun frame for supracondylar fracture. Note the support is given at the fracture site and not the knee to prevent angulation.

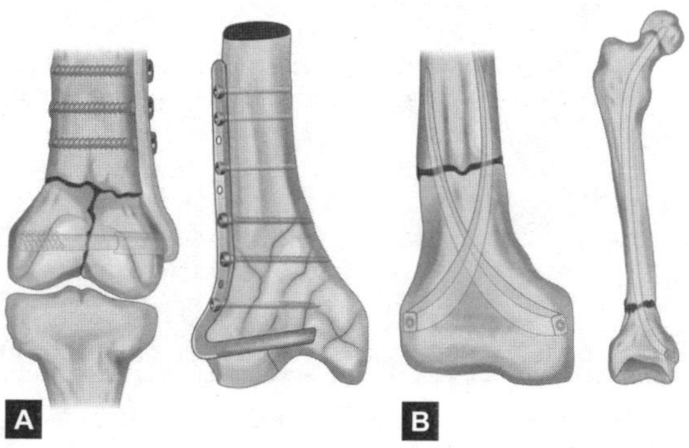

Figs. 18.12A and B: Methods of internal fixation for supracondylar fracture. (A) Blade-plate fixation; (B) Enders nail.

Fixation methods

The choice is between medullary fixation and blade plate fixation. Rush pins, Ender's nail, medullary nails, split nails, etc., are some of the commonly used medullary fixation methods. While AO plates, Elliott or Jewett plates comprise the blade fixation methods **(Figs. 18.12A and B)**.

Injuries of the Leg

PROXIMAL TIBIAL FRACTURE

Proximal tibia consists of the medial and lateral condyles along with the upper tibial articular surface and includes the proximal 10–12 cm of the tibia. These fractures are usually due to bumper injuries, are frequently intra-articular and unite well considering the cancellous nature of the bone (**Figs. 19.1A to F**).

Clinical Features

The patient with proximal tibial fractures presents with pain, swelling, deformity, hemarthrosis, decreased movements of the knee and instability in valgus or varus (**Fig. 19.2**).

Investigations

The routine AP and lateral radiographs of the knee helps to detect a majority of tibial condyle fractures (**Fig. 19.3**). Oblique view may be required to localize the fractures accurately.

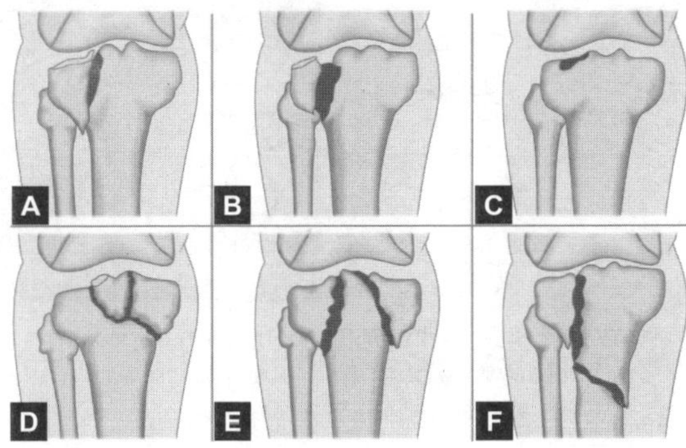

Figs. 19.1A to F: Showing Hohl-Moore's types of proximal tibial fractures.

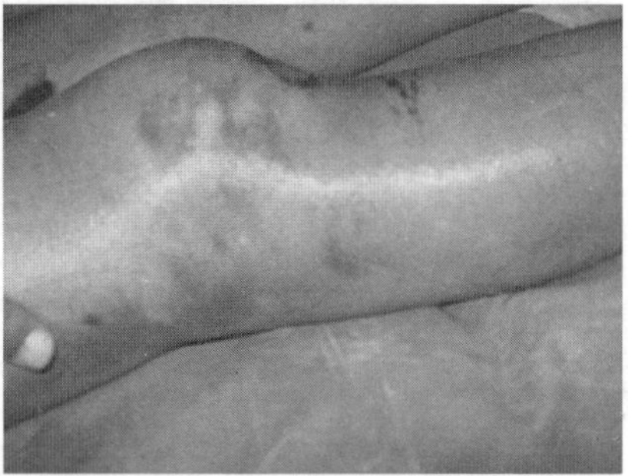

Fig. 19.2: Clinical photograph showing proximal tibial fractures.

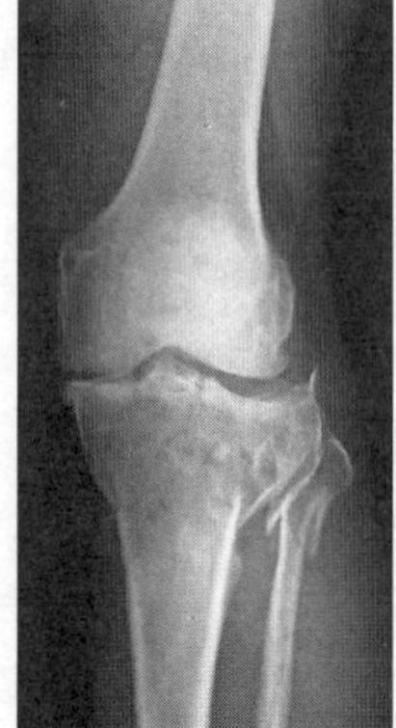

Fig. 19.3: Plain X-ray showing comminuted proximal tibial fractures.

Treatment

Conservative Treatment

It is indicated for fractures with <4 mm depression or displacement and consists of a long cast.

Surgery

Open reduction and rigid internal fixation with cancellous screws, buttress plate, etc., for grossly displaced fractures **(Figs. 19.4 and 19.5)**.

Skeletal Traction

This is reserved for grossly comminuted fractures.

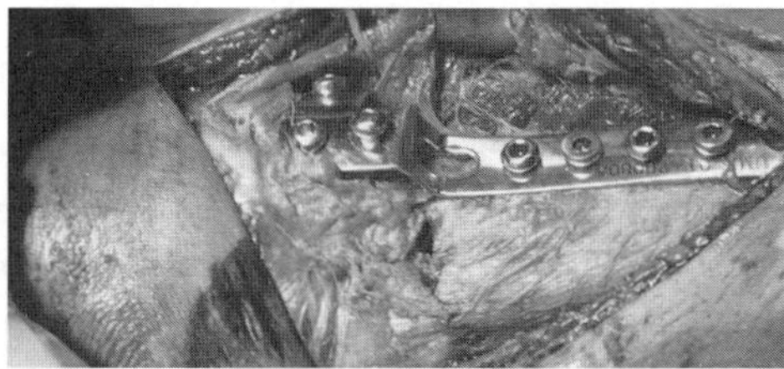

Fig. 19.4: Operative photograph showing fixation of proximal tibial fractures with a buttress plate.

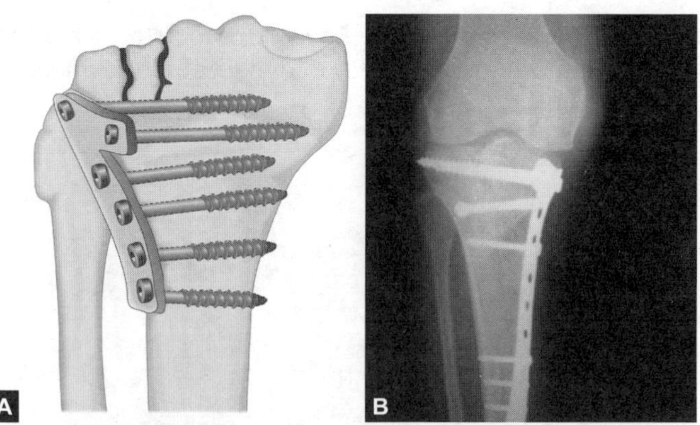

Figs. 19.5A and B: Showing internal fixation of proximal tibial fracture with buttress plate and screws.

FRACTURE OF TIBIA AND FIBULA

Tibia and fibula like their upper limb counterpart's radius and ulna are twin bones residing together and hence more often than not break together. But unlike in the forearm where both radius and ulna play stellar roles in the forearm function, in lower limbs tibia does bulk of the work while fibula is non-functional and is reduced to the role of providing attachment to the bulkier leg muscles.

Mechanism of Injury

Direct Violence

Due to road traffic accident (most common mode of injury), fall, etc. Open fractures are common in this mode of injury.

Indirect Violence

Due to falls, twisting force, usually cause spiral fractures.

The leg fractures could be simple or compound and more often, it is compound due to the subcutaneous location of the tibia. Tibia and fibula may be breaking in isolation or more commonly together.

Clinical Features

In these fractures, the common symptom is pain and the obvious sign is the deformity, apart from other features of fractures **(Fig. 19.6)**. Damage to the blood vessels and nerves is not that common but fibular neck fracture may injure the lateral popliteal nerve and if the posterior tibial vessels are injured, compartmental syndrome may develop.

Radiography

Radiograph for acute cases requires AP and lateral views **(Fig. 19.7)**. For delayed cases AP, lateral and oblique views may be required.

Methods of Treatment

Conservative Management

This consists of closed reduction **(Fig. 19.8)** and a long leg cast application **(Fig. 19.9)**.

Sarmiento's Total Contact below Knee Cast (Fig. 19.10)

After reduction of the fracture and application of a long leg cast for several weeks, a total below knee cast which is moulded around the tibial condyles and patella in the fashion of patellar tendon bearing prosthesis is applied.

Advantages

❖ Allows knee movements.
❖ Sitting can be permitted early.
❖ Ease of ambulation for patients with bilateral fracture.
❖ Decreases the incidence of delayed union and nonunion.

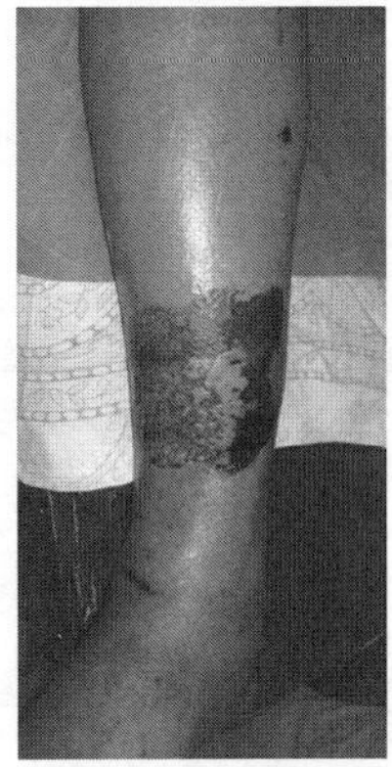

Fig. 19.6: Clinical photograph showing the appearance in fracture both bones leg.

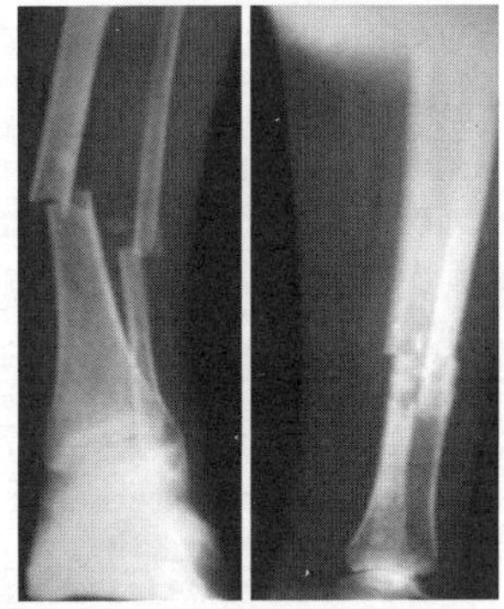

Fig. 19.7: Plain X-ray AP and lateral views showing fracture of shaft tibia and fibula.

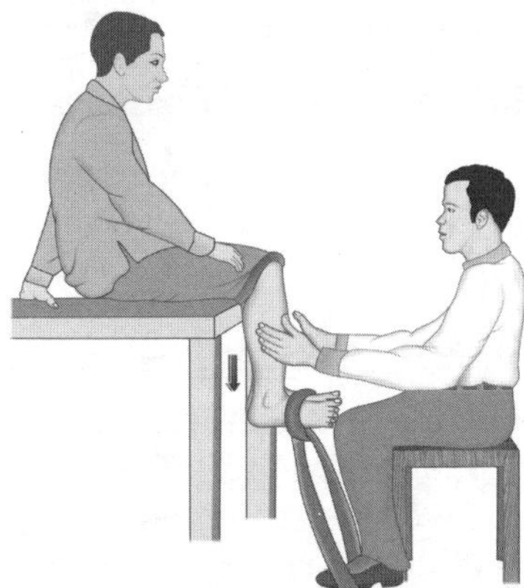

Fig. 19.8: Reduction technique of reduction of fracture tibia by the surgeon himself.

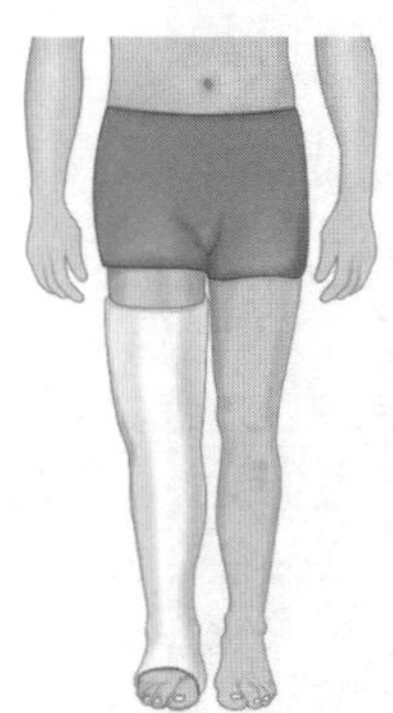

Fig. 19.9: Fracture tibia treated with long leg cast.

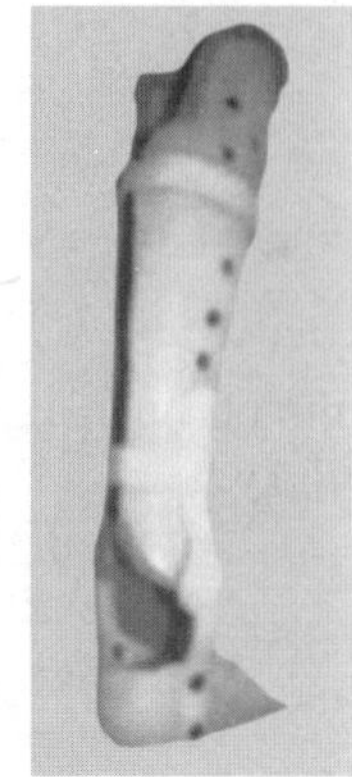

Fig. 19.10: Sarmiento's total contact below knee cast.

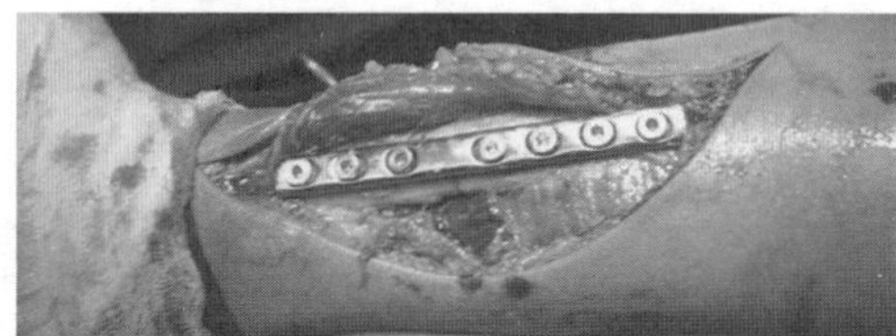

Fig. 19.11: Operative photograph showing fixation of tibial shaft fracture with DCP plate.

Open reduction and internal fixation (ORIF)

As mentioned earlier only 5% of the cases require operative treatment in tibial fractures. After open reduction, the tibial fracture can be fixed internally either by a DCP plate **(Fig. 19.11)**, IM nail or interlocking nail **(Figs. 19.12A and B)**. Luckily most of the times, fibula needs no fixation. Interlocking nail is the current gold standard internal fixation method and is preferred over plating.

OPEN TIBIAL FRACTURE

As mentioned previously, open fractures are frequently seen in tibial fractures due to its subcutaneous location. The principles of treatment, methods of treatment consist of thorough debridement and external fixation or interlocking nailing.

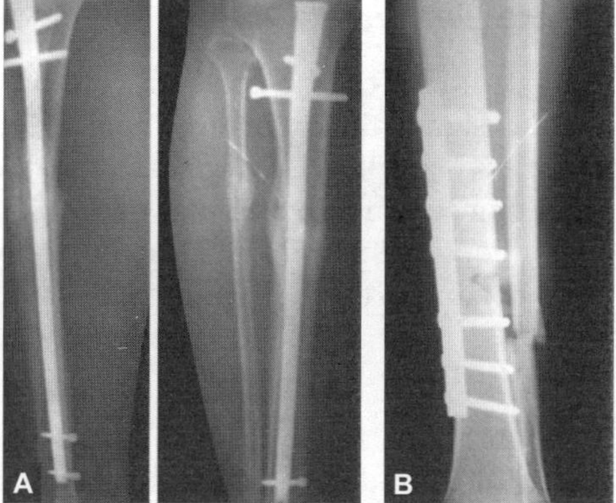

Figs. 19.12A and B: Plain X-ray showing methods of internal fixation in tibial fracture: (A) Interlocking nailing; (B) DCP plate and screws.

Role of External Fixators

This is useful in compound fractures of the tibia as it enables to stabilize the fracture and helps to take care of the wound **(Fig. 19.13)**.

PYLON FRACTURES

These are intra-articular fractures caused by the impaction of the talus on the distal tibial articular surface due to high-energy trauma and fall from a height. These fractures are frequently comminuted and are associated with extensive soft tissue injury. The treatment of choice is open reduction, limited internal fixation and autogenous bone grafting.

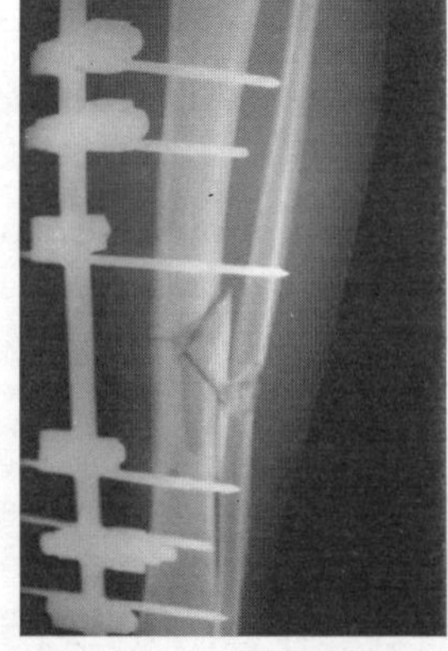

Fig. 19.13: External fixator treatment for compound fracture tibia.

Knee Trauma

KNEE LIGAMENT INJURIES

Etiology

Athletes Knee

Ligament injuries are very common in athletes who are involved both in contact and non-contact sports. The injury could be either direct due to the collision with another athlete or indirect due to rotation and twisting injuries.

Road Traffic Accident (RTA)

Here the mechanism is usually direct and could be due to a dashboard injury.

Fall

From a height with twisting force.

COLLATERAL LIGAMENT INJURIES

Collateral ligament injury is due to direct or indirect violence as described earlier. Medial collateral ligament injury is more common due to the valgus stress caused by striking the lateral aspect of the knee joint during collision in sports **(Fig. 20.1)**. The varus force on the medial side required to cause the lateral collateral ligament injury is less common because of the protection offered by the other leg. The severity of tear ranges from Grade I to III **(Fig. 20.2)**.

Medial Collateral Ligament Tear

This is more common than the lateral collateral ligament injury for reasons mentioned earlier.

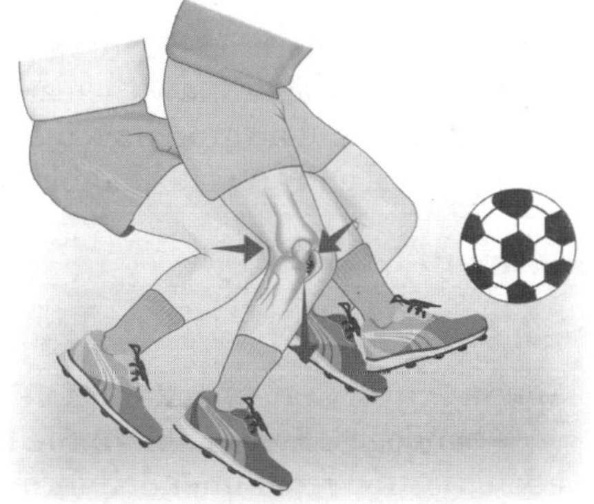

Fig. 20.1: Showing athletic injuries in knee ligament damage.

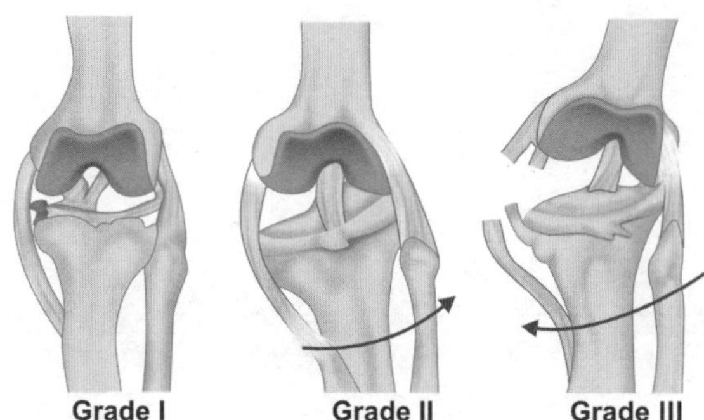

Fig. 20.2: Sprain of medial collateral ligament of the knee.

Mechanism of Injury

Patient gives history of valgus and external rotation force in mild sprains. In severe sprains, patient gives history of valgus stress force due to the direct blow on the lower thigh or upper leg seen commonly in contact sports, such as football, rugby, etc. It may be associated with ACL tear or meniscal injury.

Clinical Features

A patient with medial collateral ligament injury may present with pain, swelling, hemarthrosis, painful and restricted knee movements, instability, etc. On examination, the point of local tenderness could be at the adductor tubercle, joint line or at the insertion of the tibial collateral ligament. About 10–20% of patients have damage to the extensor mechanism of the knee.

Note: MCL more often than not tears at its insertion near the adductor tubercle.

Clinical Tests

These are abduction stress test, which is positive at 30° of flexion **(Figs. 20.3A and B)**. Tests to rule out other knee structures like the anterior drawer test and Lachman's test *should be done.*

Investigations

1. Stress radiographs at 15–20° of valgus.
2. MRI helps to localize the MCL tear.
3. Arthrograms and arthroscopy to evaluate and rule out meniscal and cruciate pathology.

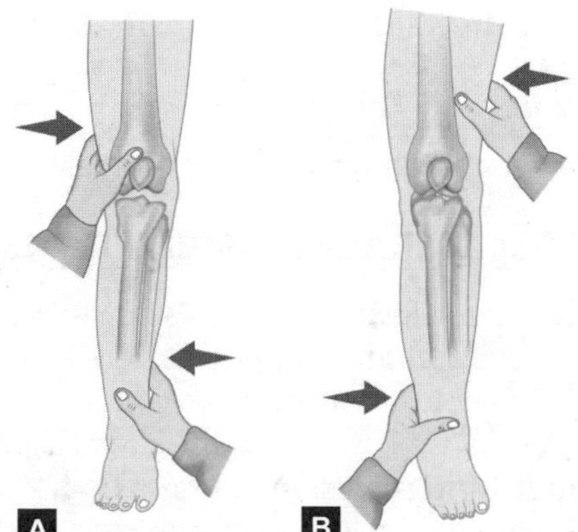

Figs. 20.3A and B: Showing stress tests for collateral ligament injuries: (A) Valgus or abduction stress test; (B) Varus or adduction stress test.

Treatment

Fresh Injury

❖ Sprain I RICE Concept (R-est, I-ce, C-ompression with bandages, E-elevation of the limb to prevent edema) is the recommended form of treatment. Other symptomatic treatment methods include nonsteroidal anti-inflammatory drugs (NSAIDs), etc., to relieve pain, spasm and swelling.

- ❖ Sprain II long leg cast for 4–6 weeks with knee in 30–40° of flexion.
- ❖ Sprain III surgical repair consists of direct repair of the collateral ligament injury using non-absorbable sutures.

Reinforcements

Here along with the repair, additional reinforcement using fascial or tendon graft is done. This is reserved for patients reporting for treatment after 2 or 3 weeks.

Old Cases

Here it is mainly reconstruction. If TCL is intact but lax then distal transfer is done. If ligament is destroyed, reconstruction using hamstrings or semitendinosus is done.

LATERAL COLLATERAL LIGAMENT INJURY

Mercifully, this is not as common as its medial counterpart thanks to the protection provided by the other leg which disallows the varus force, so essential to tear the fibular collateral ligament. Unlike the MCL tear, it more commonly tears at the insertion near the head of the fibula **(Fig. 20.4)**.

Clinical Features

Patient may complain of pain and swelling on the lateral side of the knee. Varus stress test is positive at 30° flexion. Investigations and treatment proceeds on the similar lines as for the MCL injury.

In old cases however, in fibular collateral ligament injury: If the ligament is adequate and thick, distal transfer is recommended. If the ligament is torn badly and destroyed, then reconstruction using fascia lata, biceps tendon, etc., is done.

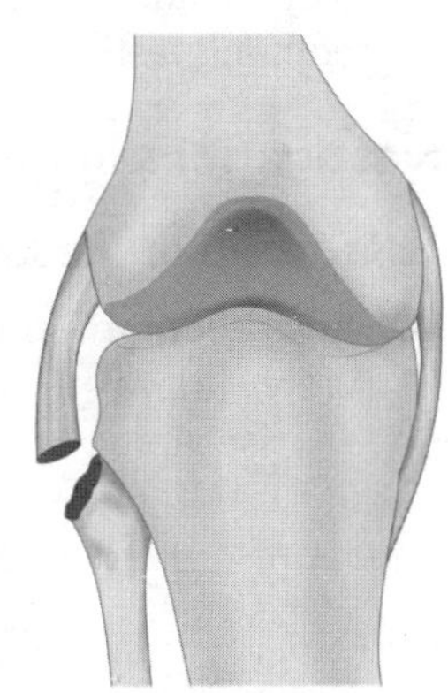

Fig. 20.4: Avulsion of lateral collateral ligament from the head of the fibula.

CRUCIATE LIGAMENT INJURIES

Anterior Cruciate Ligament (ACL) Tear

This is the most common knee ligament injury. Athletes and sportspersons are more prone and are due to the indirect forces, such as flexion, abduction and internal rotation. It rarely tears in isolation and is associated with injuries to medial meniscus and medial collateral ligament (*Popularly known as the Unhappy triad of O'donoghue*).

Mechanism of Injury

The most common mode of injury is external rotation with abduction of the flexed knee or hyperextension of knee in internal rotation **(Fig. 20.5)**.

Clinical Features

This is a disabling injury and the knee may immediately collapse and is painful. Popping sensation felt or heard at the time of injury signifies ligamentous injury (ACL tear). The patient also tells that

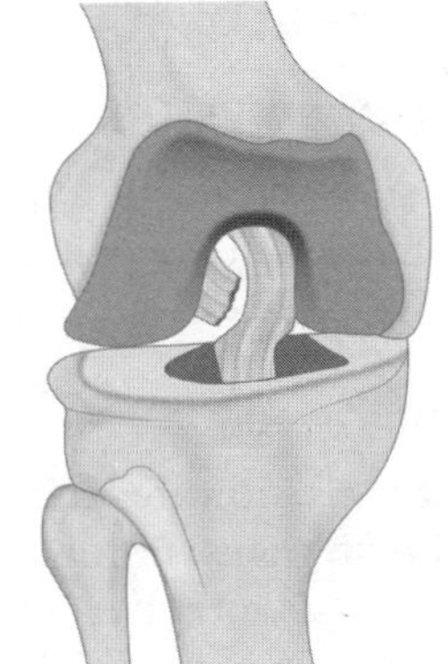

Fig. 20.5: Showing ACL tear.

the knee "gave away" or buckled at the time of injury. Swelling of the knee could develop immediately or over a period and could be due to either hemarthroses or traumatic synovitis. The distended knee is held in partial flexion by the hamstrings.

Clinical Examination

Always examine the normal knee first and form a basis for "comparison." Clinical findings depend on associated ligamentous injury or meniscal injury or bone damage. Depending on the combination, there will be specific instabilities that will allow anterior displacement of tibia on the involved side. Anterior subluxation of >5° suggests lax or disrupted ACL. Isolated injury is rare. This can be elicited by the anterior Drawer test **(Fig. 20.6)** and the Lachman's tests **(Fig. 20.7)**.

Investigations in ACL Tear

Radiograph of the Knee

The views recommended are anteroposterior (AP) view, lateral view, intercondylar notch view, sunrise views, etc. Radiographs are usually normal in ACL tear. Avulsion fracture of tibial spine if present indicates ACL tear.

MRI

This is the best diagnostic tool. It is noninvasive and demonstrates the ACL tear with remarkable accuracy.

Arthroscopy

Diagnostic arthroscopy to detect ACL tear is remarkably accurate. It also helps to rule out damage to meniscus and other internal structures of the knee.

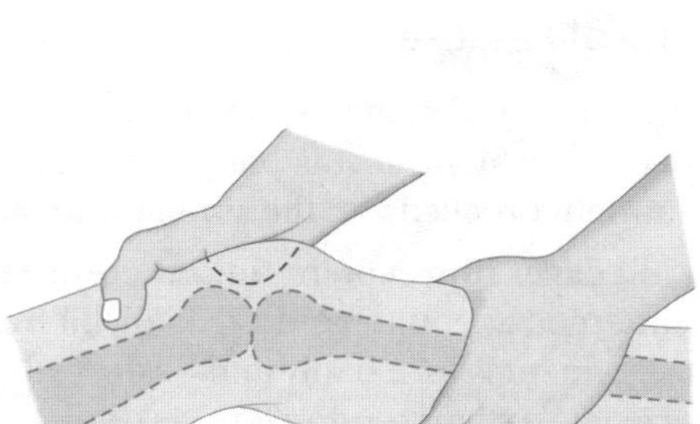

Fig. 20.6: Showing anterior Drawer test.

Fig. 20.7: Showing Lachman's test.

Treatment of ACL Tear

Conservative Treatment

Conservative treatment is indicated for minor ACL tears with no knee instability. Initially, the treatment is as per the RICE regime. In later stages treatment is by rest, long leg casts for 4–6 weeks NSAIDs, physiotherapy, etc.

Surgery

Surgery is indicated in more severe tears and if the knee is unstable.
* **Fresh cases:** Primary repair is indicated in young adults and athletes. Repair is successful, if ACL is torn at its femoral or tibial attachments. It is not successful in mid-position tears. Failure rate is as high as 50%.

❖ **Old cases:** Reinforcement of ACL tear should be augmented except when avulsion is with a fragment of bone, which is fixed with a screw. It could be either intra-articular or extra-articular or both by using iliotibial band, semitendinosus tendon, etc. Reconstruction in chronic ACL insufficiency could be either intra-articular or extra-articular replacement by using quadriceps, tendon, patellar tendon (central 1/3), semitendinosus tendon, etc.

Posterior Cruciate Ligament (PCL) Tear

This is less common than ACL tear. It is ruptured due to severe rotational injury, dashboard injury or complete dislocation of the knee. Isolated PCL tear is rare and is accompanied with other ligament injuries.

Clinical Presentation

Patient complains of pain, swelling and tenderness over the popliteal fossa. Clinically, posterior drawer test and sag sign will be positive **(Fig. 20.8)**.

Investigations

Investigations are similar to ACL injuries.

Treatment

In fresh cases, the treatment is more or less similar to the ones described for fresh ACL tear. However, in old cases surgical re-construction is the treatment method of choice. Reconstruction is done by using medial head of gastrocnemius, etc.

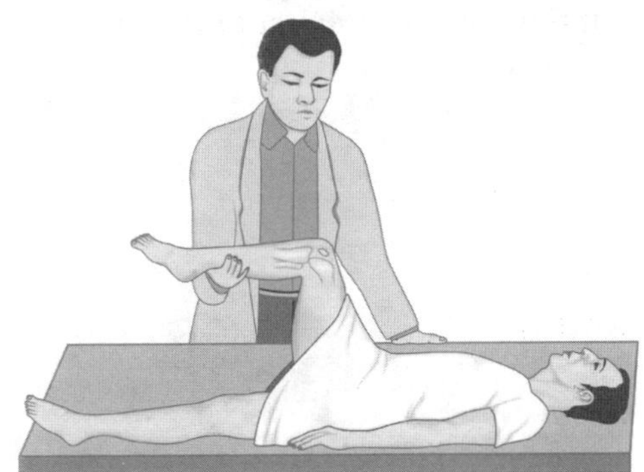

Fig. 20.8: Showing method of eliciting a posterior sag sign.

Rehabilitations
Knee rehabilitation is extremely important the surgery. It consists of mobilization exercise, strengthening exercise, electrotherapy CPM, etc.

MEDIAL MENISCUS INJURIES

Medial meniscus is more commonly injured than the lateral and is usually associated with other ligament injuries of the knee.

Note: Bucket handle tear is the most common variety of medial meniscus injury.

Mechanism of Injury

Mechanism of injury is a rotational force when a flexed knee extends.
❖ In young, it can occur only when weight is being taken, knee is flexed and there is a twisting strain. Young active athletes are more prone.
❖ In middle life, fibrosis has decreased the mobility of meniscus and hence tear occurs with less force.

Predisposing Factors

These could be abnormal meniscal shape, abnormal stress due to chronic ligament laxity, etc.

Clinical Features

A patient with medial meniscal injury complains of local swelling and limbs. There may/may not be history of locking. Joint line tenderness, McMurray's test, Apley's tests are positive **(Figs. 20.9 and 20.10)**. Patient may give history of locking in few instances.

Investigations

❖ Radiograph is usually normal. The views recommended are anteroposterior, lateral, intercondylar notch and sunrise views of the patella.

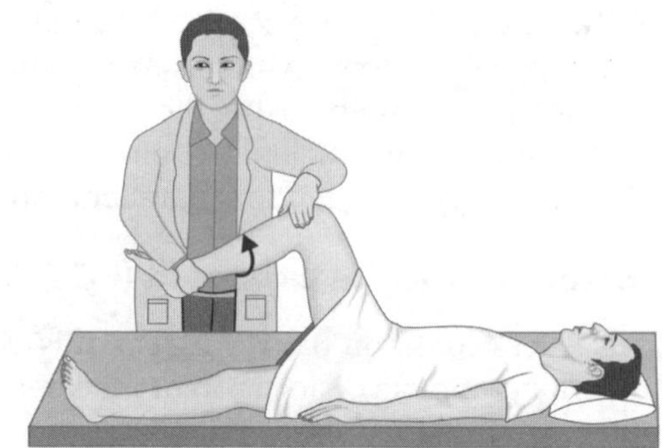

Fig. 20.9: Showing method of McMurray's test.

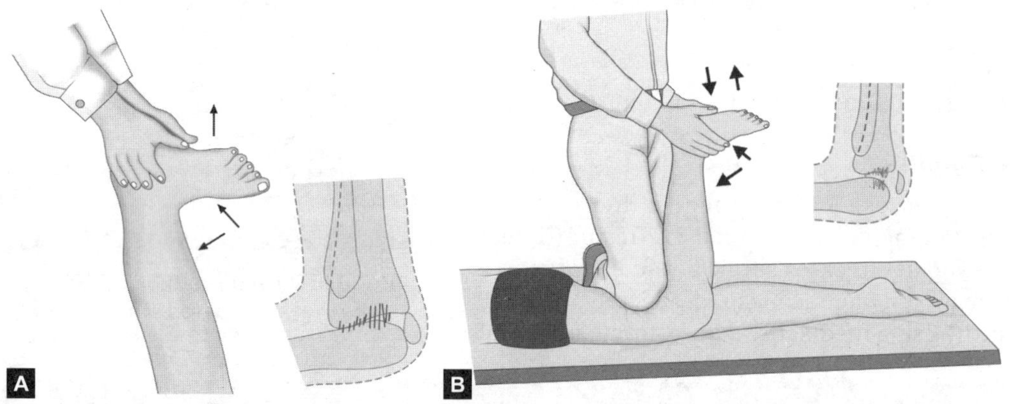

Figs. 20.10A and B: Showing methods of performing Apley's: (A) Distraction test; (B) Compression test.

❖ Arthroscopy helps to identify the torn meniscus more accurately.
❖ Arthrography may reveal the tear. Double contrast arthrography is 95% accurate **(Fig. 20.11)**.
❖ MRI is expensive but useful and is the gold standard investigation.

Treatment Methods

Conservative

This is indicated in patients soon after injury with no locking and with infrequent attacks of pain.

Measures

❖ Abstinence from weight bearing.
❖ Rest, ice packs compressive bandage elevation of the limb (RICE concept).
❖ Buck's skin traction.

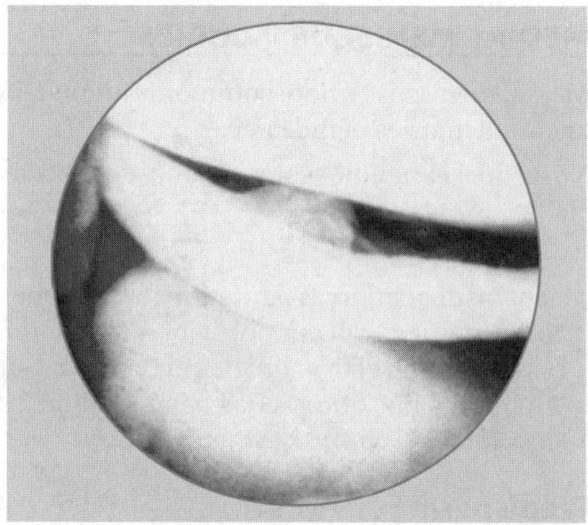

Fig. 20.11: Arthroscopic view of a bucket handles of medial meniscus injury.

❖ Joint aspiration.

❖ Quadriceps exercises.

❖ If symptom persists a cylindrical cast may be considered.

Manipulations Under Anesthesia

If joint is locked due to the torn menisci, manipulation under anesthesia is recommended. This is no longer done.

Surgery

It is indicated, if joint cannot be unlocked and if symptoms are recurrent. Closed partial meniscectomy via an arthroscopy is better than total removal of the menisci by open surgery **(Fig. 20.11)**. Complete removal of the menisci incapacitates the knee; hence, the emphasis is on conservative surgery than radical removal. Suture of a peripheral tear by either open or arthroscopy is also tried.

FRACTURE OF PATELLA

Patella is the largest sesamoid bone in the body. Incidence is around 1%.

Mechanism of Injury

Direct Trauma

This is due to dashboard injuries and due to direct fall over the patella. They usually cause comminuted fractures, and are the common causes.

Indirect Trauma

Indirect trauma (quadriceps contraction) sudden forceful contraction of the quadriceps as in sports person and athletes can cause patellar fractures. Here the fracture is usually transverse and sometimes avulsion fractures of the proximal or distal poles may be seen.

Age: Common in 40–50 years age group.

Male: Female: 2:1

Classification (Fig. 20.12)

1. Undisplaced
2. Displaced
   a. Transverse—involving upper or lower poles (50–85%).
   b. Oblique fracture
   c. Vertical fracture (12–27%).
   d. Comminuted fracture (30–35%).

Clinical Features

Patient gives history of trauma following which there is pain and swelling at the knee joint. Patient is unable to extend the knee and both the active and passive movements are restricted. On examination, there

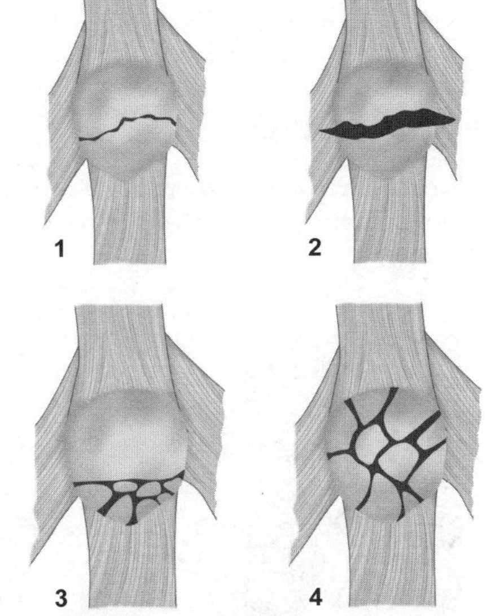

Fig. 20.12: Showing types of patellar fractures: (1) undisplaced fracture, (2) transverse fracture, (3) distal pole fracture, and (4) comminuted fracture.

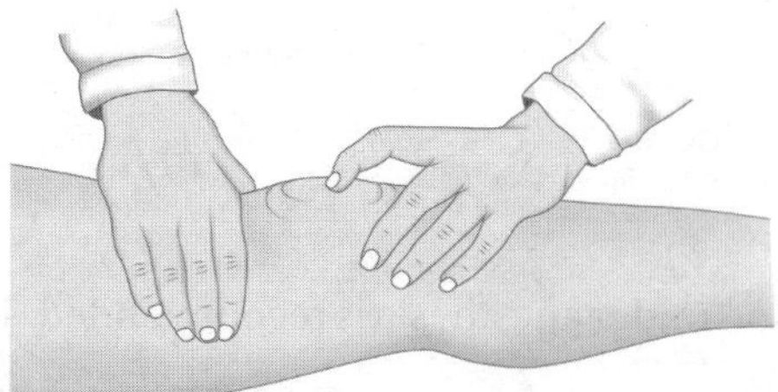

Fig. 20.13: Showing method to eliciting patellar tap.

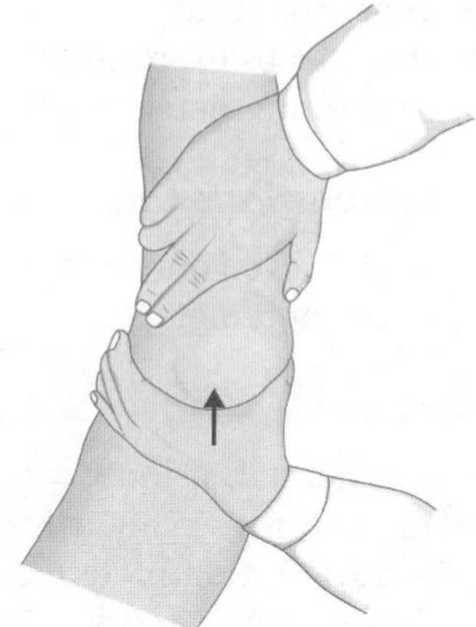

Fig. 20.14: Showing method of eliciting fluctuation test to defect gross knee effusion.

could be a palpable gap, tenderness, signs of effusion and a positive patellar tap **(Fig. 20.13)** test. Cross fluctuation test is frost-free **(Fig. 20.14)**.

Investigations

Radiograph of the knee joint consists of AP view, lateral view **(Fig. 20.15A)** and skyline or axial view (to rule out undisplaced vertical fracture.

Note: Bipartite patella and osteochondral fractures cause confusion in the diagnosis **(Fig. 20.15B)**

Management

Undisplaced Fracture

Nonoperative treatment will produce good results in undisplaced fracture and if displacement is <1 to 2 mm and the methods include compression bandage, ice applications, aspiration of hemarthrosis, cylindrical cast **(Fig. 20.16)**, early weight bearing and quadriceps exercises.

Displaced Fracture

In this variety, surgery is the treatment of choice. Surgery is performed as early as possible preferably within 7 days.

Surgical Methods

Open reduction and internal fixation: This is indicated in transverse fractures of the patella. Internal fixation is done either by the circumferential wiring or by tension band wiring (TBW) **(Fig. 20.17)**.

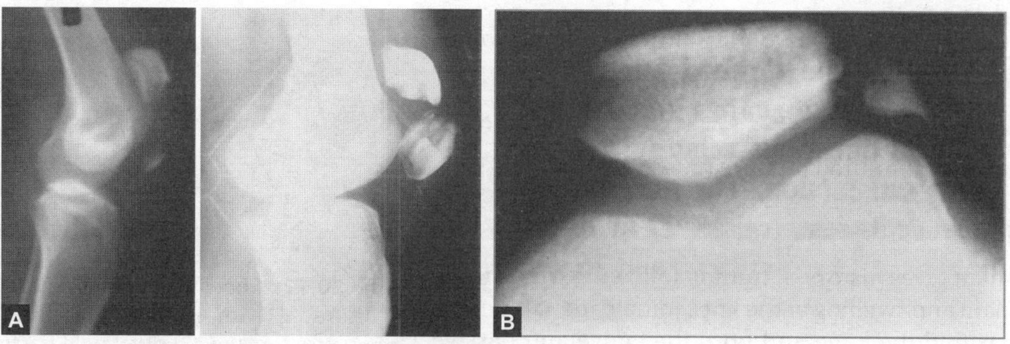

Figs. 20.15A and B: Plain X-ray showing: (A) Transverse fracture of patella; (B) Bipartite patella.

Patellectomy

This could be either partial (for smaller distal or proximal pole fracture) or complete (for comminuted fractures). The emphasis is now on preserving as much patella as possible to prevent the disadvantages of patellectomy.

Acute Dislocation of Patella

Lateral dislocations of patella are very common and are due to lateral force acting on a semi-flexed knee. Patient complains of severe pain, swelling and inability to bend the knee. Patella is seen and felt on the lateral side.

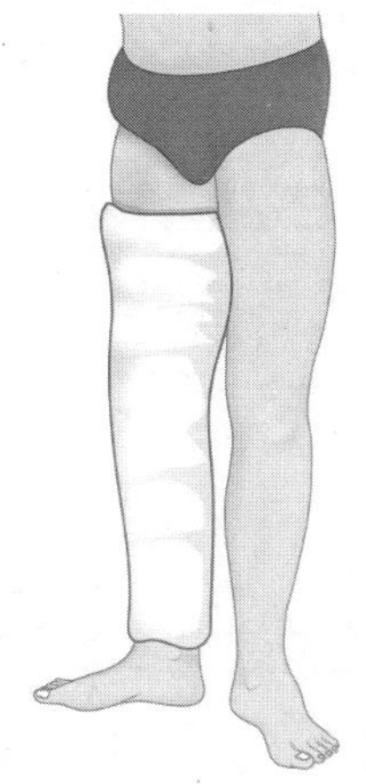

Fig. 20.16: Showing cylindrical cast.

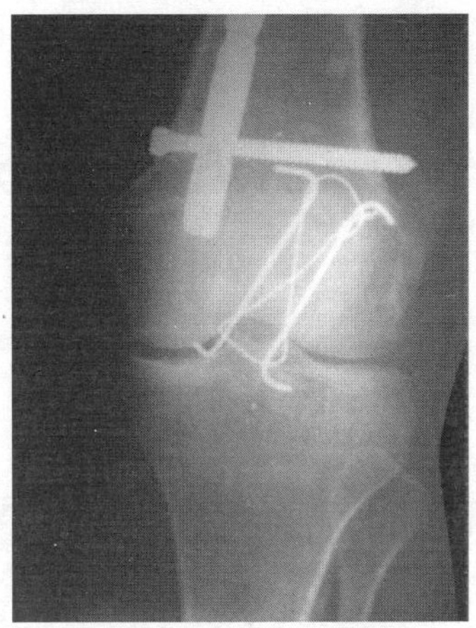

Fig. 20.17: Showing TBW.

Treatment

Closed reduction and above knee POP casting is done under GA. Immobilization in a long leg cast may be required for a period of 4 weeks.

ACUTE DISLOCATION OF KNEE

This is an uncommon injury and is due to severe violence as in RTA, fall, etc. It is usually associated with injuries to collateral, cruciates and meniscus. Patella may also be fractured or dislocated **(Fig. 20.18)**.

Treatment

Conservative

An attempt may be made for closed reduction under GA. A above knee POP cast is applied for 12 weeks.

Surgery

Open reduction may be required if the closed reduction fails or if there are extensive ligament injuries, which may require repair, reconstruction or both. Knee is immobilized in above knee POP cast for 12 weeks.

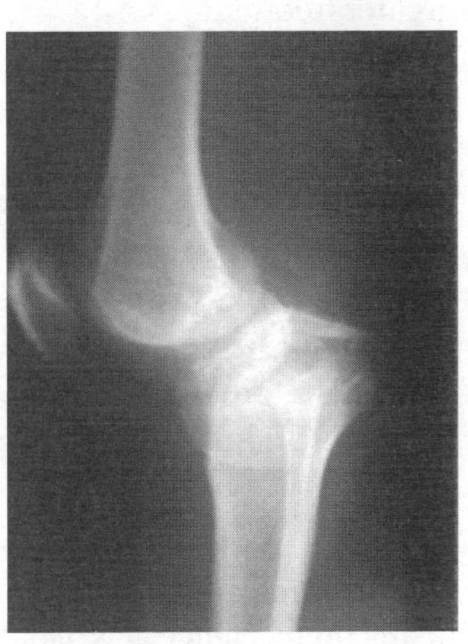

Fig. 20.18: Plain X-ray showing posterior dislocation of the knee.

Injuries Around the Ankle

ANKLE FRACTURES

The ankle mortise is formed by the distal articular surface of the tibia, fibula, the intervening tibiofibular ligament and the inner articular surfaces of the medial and lateral malleoli. The strong ankle mortise and the ligaments make these dislocations a rarity. However, fracture dislocations do occur at a greater frequency.

Pott described ankle injuries for the first time in 1768.

Mechanism of Injury

❖ Twisting injury while walking, running, sports, athletes, etc., are the most common mode of ankle injuries **(Figs. 21.1A to C)**.
❖ **Fall from a height:** These are indirect injuries brought about by the displacing talus.

Classification

Ankle injuries are classified after the mechanism causing them. Hence, it is of paramount importance to understand the movement of the ankle to comprehend the classification.

Clinical Features

Patient usually gives history of inversion, eversion or rotational injury **(Fig. 21.2)**, following which there is pain, swelling, deformity of the ankle **(Fig. 21.3)**. Movements are decreased, Drawer's test, inversion and eversion stress tests may be positive.

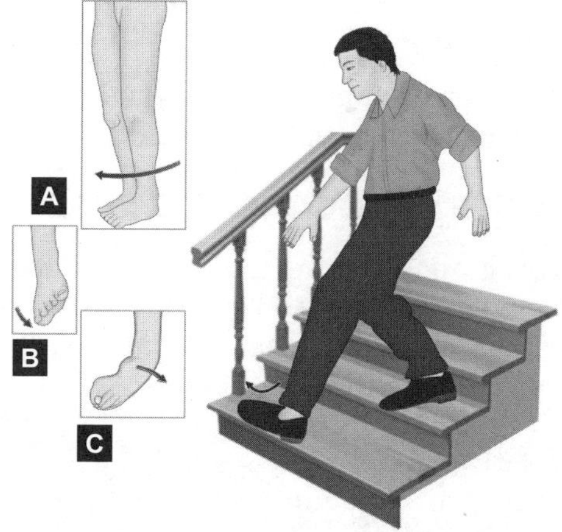

Figs. 21.1A to C: Showing common mechanism of ankle injuries: (A) External rotation force; (B) Abduction force,: (C) Adduction force.

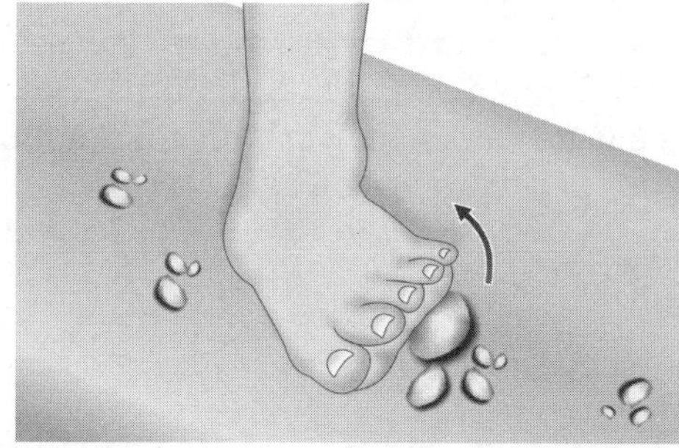

Fig. 21.2: Showing mechanism of eversion injuries.

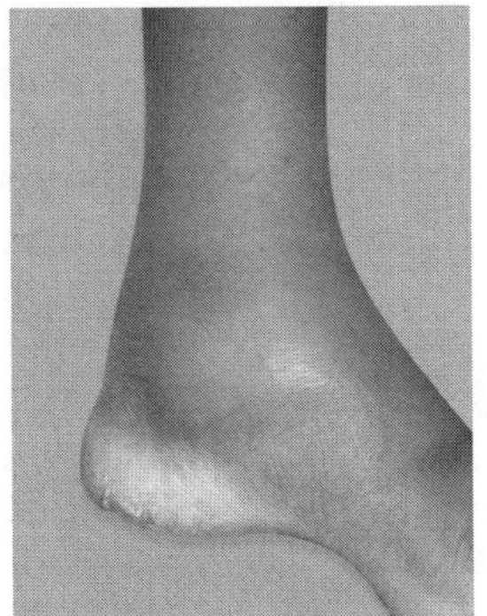

Fig. 21.3: Clinical photograph of ankle injury.

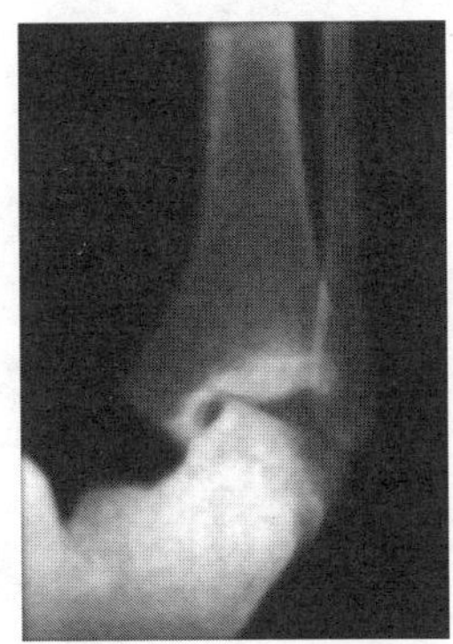

Fig. 21.4: Radiograph showing inversion injury of ankle.

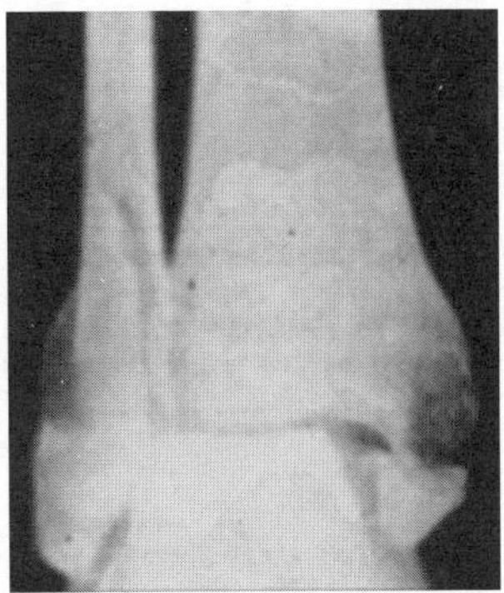

Fig. 21.5: Radiograph showing bimalleolar ankle fracture.

Radiology

Anteroposterior, lateral and mortise views of the ankle are recommended in the radiographs. Radiology in ankle injuries speaks quite eloquently provided one sees it properly **(Fig. 21.4)**. Unlike in other fractures, radiology here helps you to study the fracture anatomy, enables you to guess the nature of injury and plan the line of treatment **(Fig. 21.5)**.

Treatment of Ankle Injuries

Goals of the Treatment

Whatever the ankle fractures, basic principles of treatment remain the same and consist of the following:

- ❖ Anatomical positioning of the talus and restoration of the ankle mortise.
- ❖ To obtain a joint line that is parallel to the ground and the knee joint.
- ❖ Smooth articular surface.

  If these three things are not achieved, post-traumatic osteoarthritis results.

For stable injuries no reduction is required, immobilization with only plaster splints till the swelling decreases and then a below-knee plaster cast is applied with foot in neutral position **(Fig. 21.6)**.

Unstable injuries require reduction and immobilization in plaster casts. The commonly encountered unstable injuries are:

- ❖ **Fracture due to external rotation:** This is more common and can be managed both by conservative and operative methods.
  - ◆ *Conservative method:* This consists of reversal of the injuring forces by closed reduction and a below-knee plaster cast is applied for a period of one month **(Fig. 21.7)**.
  - ◆ *Surgical method:* In these both, the malleoli are fixed, first the lateral malleoli is fixed with pin or screws and later the medial malleolar fracture is fixed with a single screw perpendicular to the fracture line. Below knee splint is given initially and later a cast is applied.

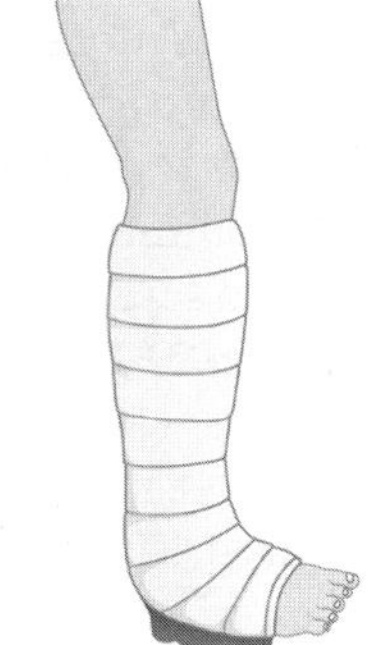

Fig. 21.6: Showing a below knee plaster cast.

- ❖ **Fracture primarily due to abduction:** These are less common than the fractures due to external rotation. Nevertheless, the principles of the treatment remain the same. Adduction force is required to bring about reduction and if closed reduction fails, open reduction is

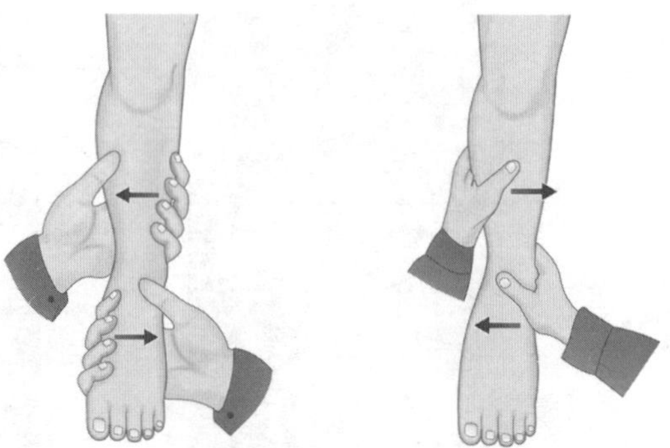

Fig. 21.7: Showing method of closed reduction.

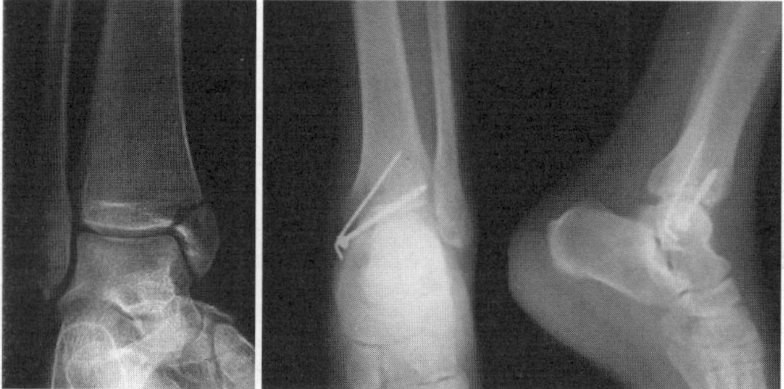

Fig. 21.8: Plain X-ray showing method of fixation of medial malleolar fracture.

preferred. During the open reduction, both the malleoli are fixed with malleolar or cortical screws **(Fig. 21.8)**.

❖ **Fracture primarily due to adduction** unlike external rotation and abduction, adduction violence is more frequently an isolated event. Wedging of small comminuted fragments into the fracture line often prevents closed reduction, so that open reduction and internal fixation (ORIF) is required more frequently.

Medial malleolus is approached first, since it is more unstable, and the fracture is fixed with two screws one at a right angle to tibial cortex and another at right angle to the fracture line **(Fig. 21.8)**. Lateral fibular fracture is stabilized with plate and screws.

❖ **Fracture resulting from primarily vertical compression:** This may be isolated or associated with other forces described above. The anterior and posterior tibial plafond margins are fractured. Two types are described:

1. *Posterior marginal fracture* for undisplaced fracture below knee cast is sufficient. For more than 25% of articular surface involvement, ORIF with 2 screws is preferred.
2. *Anterior marginal fracture (tibial plafond injury)* It may include a crush of the anterior lip or it may include a major fragment. If crushed, calcaneal traction is given and if there is a large fragment, ORIF is required.

Complications of ankle fracture: Include post-traumatic arthritis, reflex sympathetic dystrophy, neurovascular injury (injury to posterior tibial vessels and nerve), nonunion (due to soft tissue interposition), malunion, etc.

ANKLE SPRAIN

These are common injury in sports. If improperly treated, it may result in chronic laxity, pain or delayed recovery.

Lateral Ligament Sprain

This is the most common musculoskeletal injury with an incidence of 1/10,000/day. In 85% of cases, it is due to inversion of supinated plantar flexed foot. The lateral ligament commonly injured is anterior talofibular ligament followed by calcaneofibular ligament **(Fig. 21.9)**. The posterior talofibular ligament is rarely sprained.

Clinical Features

The patient complains of pain, swelling and tenderness over the affected ligament **(Fig. 21.10)**. *Anterior drawer test* is positive and it is performed by stabilizing distal tibia with one hand, then grasps the posterior heel with the opposite hand and applies anterior force. If the displacement of talus is >8 mm anterior, it suggests laxity of the anterior talofibular ligament. Next, the talar tilt test is performed, if the tilt is >5°, it suggests laxity of anterior talofibular and calcaneofibular ligaments.

Radiograph of the Ankle

Plain X-ray of the ankle joint AP, lateral and oblique views. If the talar tilt of the injured ankle is 10° greater than the uninjured ankle, it is considered as significant.

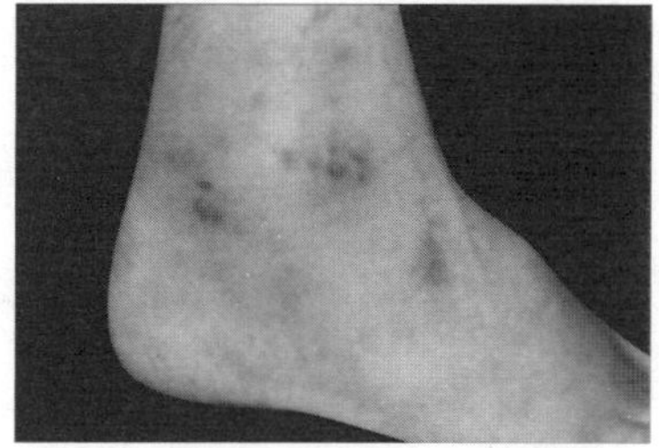

Fig. 21.9: Showing lateral ligament sprain (due to adduction injury).

Fig. 21.10: Showing clinical appearance of an ankle sprain.

Grading of Ankle Sprains

Grade I minimal pain, mild swelling and I no laxity.

Grade II: Mild-to-moderate laxity, soft tissue swelling, anterior drawer and talar tilt is slightly positive.

Grade III: Severe swelling and pain, the anterior drawer and talar tilt tests are highly positive.

Treatment

Grade I sprain: Rest, ice therapy, compression bandage, foot elevation, (RICE), nonsteroidal anti-inflammatory drugs (NSAIDs), crutch walking, etc., are the recommended treatment. Ankle straps helps to provide stability **(Fig. 21.11)**.

Grade II sprain long: Leg cast, range of motion exercises, strengthening exercises, etc., are helpful.

Grade III sprain same: Lines as mentioned above and sometimes may rarely require surgical repair.

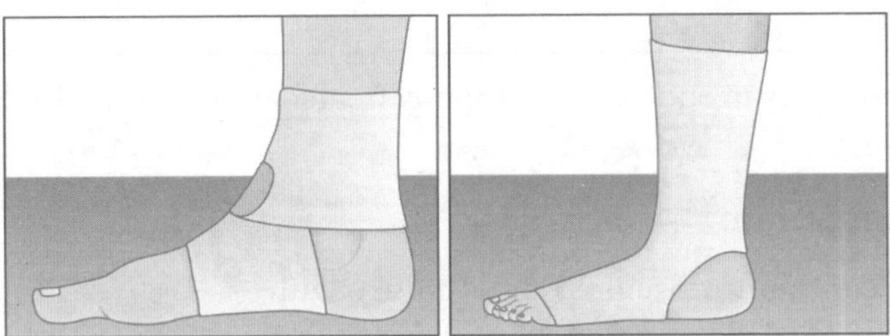

Fig. 21.11: Showing ankle strap.

Medial Ligament Sprain

This is due to pronation eversion injury. In mild sprains, only the superficial part of the deltoid ligament is torn but in severe forms, the deep part of the deltoid ligament is also torn resulting in a lateral talar tilt. If this exceeds >2 mm, significant alteration in the weight-bearing mechanism takes place resulting in post-traumatic arthritis. For mild sprains, conservative treatment is sufficient and for severe sprains, surgical reduction and repair are considered **(Fig. 21.11)**.

Injuries of the Foot

FRACTURE OF THE CALCANEUM

Calcaneus is the most often fractured tarsal bone. No ideal method of treatment has been described yet.

Mechanism of Injury

Twisting forces cause many of the extra-articular fractures.

Fall from height and land on the feet phenomena causes a vast majority of intra-articular fractures **(Fig. 22.1)**.

Fall from height: Lateral process of the talus acts as a wedge and is forced through the Gissane's angle resulting in four fracture patterns:
1. Undisplaced
2. Tongue shaped

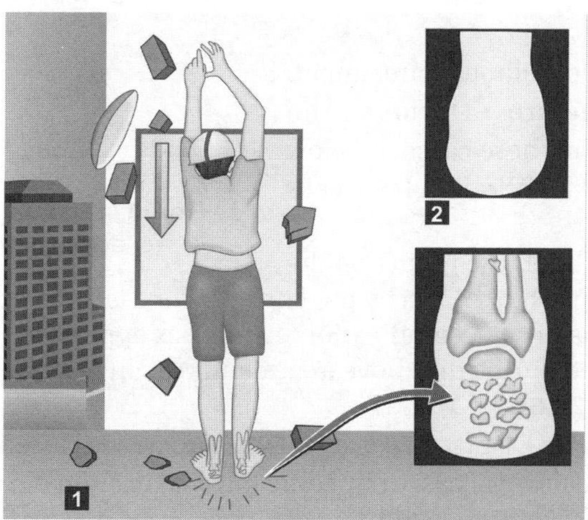

Fig. 22.1: Showing common mechanism of calcaneal fractures of fall and land on heels in worker's (Inset showing comminuted fracture of calcaneal).

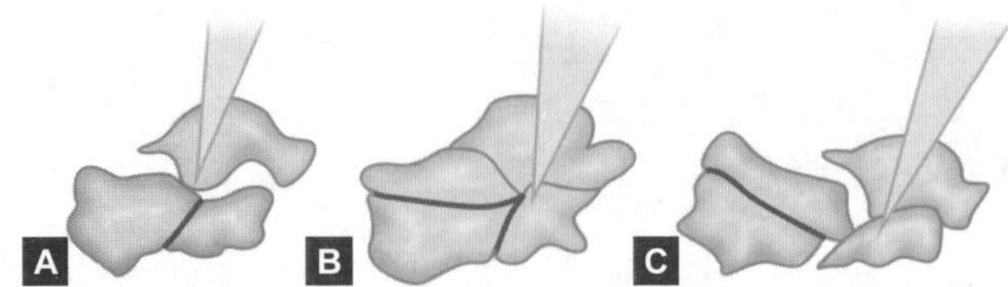

Figs. 22.2A to C: Varieties of Intra-articular fractures: (A) Undisplaced fracture; (B) Tongue-shaped fracture; (C) Comminuted fracture.

3. Joint depression
4. Comminuted **(Figs. 22.2A to C)**

Clinical Features

After the fall, the patient may experience pain, swelling in the heel. Due to the compression, the heel may be broadened **(Fig. 22.1)**. Patient may also complain of inability to bear weight on the heels. There may be ecchymosis around the heels after two days. Inversion and eversion of the foot may be affected but the ankle function remains unaltered. In undisplaced or incomplete fracture eliciting heel tenderness helps clinch the diagnosis **(Figs. 22.3 and 22.4)**.

Radiograph

X-ray of the calcaneum especially the lateral view helps to make an accurate diagnosis **(Fig. 22.5)**. Sometimes, a special view like the axial view may be required.

Treatment

The following are the basic methods of treatment:
1. **For undisplaced fractures:** Obviously, no reduction is required in these cases. A below knee cast applied for a period of 4–6 weeks usually helps.
   Calcaneal cast: Here, after the reduction the leg and the foot are immobilized in a below-knee plaster cast for a period of 4–6 weeks. After the removal of the plaster cast, compression bandage is applied for another 4–6 weeks and the foot is kept elevated during the above treatment. Weight bearing is permitted only at the end of 12 weeks **(Fig. 22.6)**.
2. **For displaced fractures:** Displaced calcaneal fracture needs closed reduction and fixation by either below knee calcaneal cast or by some internal fixation devices.

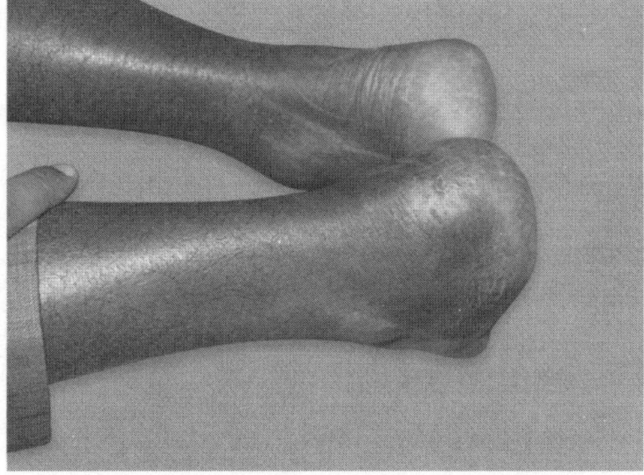

Fig. 22.3: Showing broadened heel in calcaneal fractures.

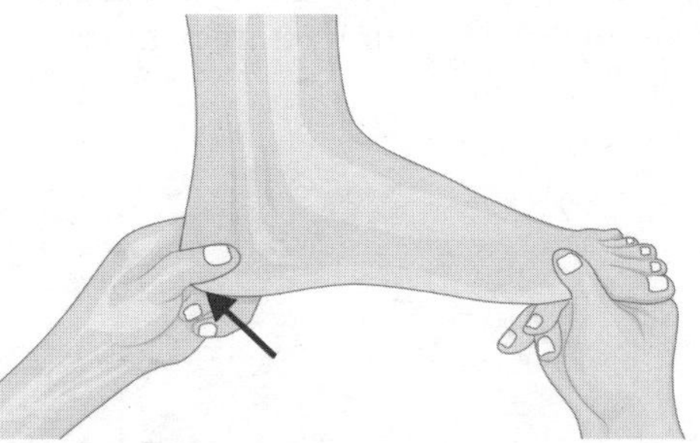

Fig. 22.4: Showing method eliciting heel tenderness in calcaneal fractures.

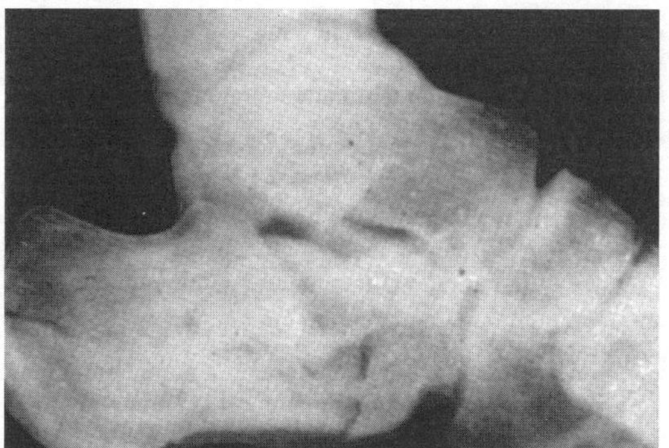

Fig. 22.5: Radiograph showing calcaneum fracture.

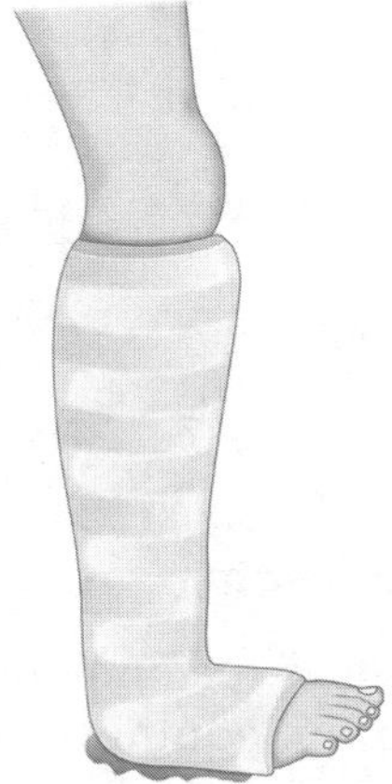

Fig. 22.6: Showing short leg POP cast with walking heel for calcaneal fracture.

3. **Open reduction:** Open reduction and internal fixation with small plate and screws with bone grafting is difficult and is rarely adopted.

FRACTURE OF THE TALUS

Incidence is around 30%. Just as calcaneal fracture is common in people who are more prone for fall from heights, so is fracture neck of talus. It is more commonly seen in people who drive four wheelers and aircraft and get involved in a head on collision accidents.

Mechanism of Injury

The common mode of injury is hyperdorsiflexion of the foot on one leg. It may be associated with fracture of tarsal bones and fracture of the metatarsal bones.

The driver of any four-wheeler, such as car, bus, lorry, etc., or of an aircraft, meets with an accident and has a head on collision with another vehicle, tree or any other object. If his foot is on the brake pedal at the time of impact, then it is forced into hyperdorsiflexion. In this position, the anterior rim of the tibia slices through the weak and unprotected neck of the talus breaking it. It was earlier popularly called the 'aviator's fracture' due to aircraft accidents. Now, it is more commonly seen in automobile accidents **(Fig. 22.7)**. Depending upon the severity of the forces, the fracture could be undisplaced or displaced **(Fig. 22.8)**.

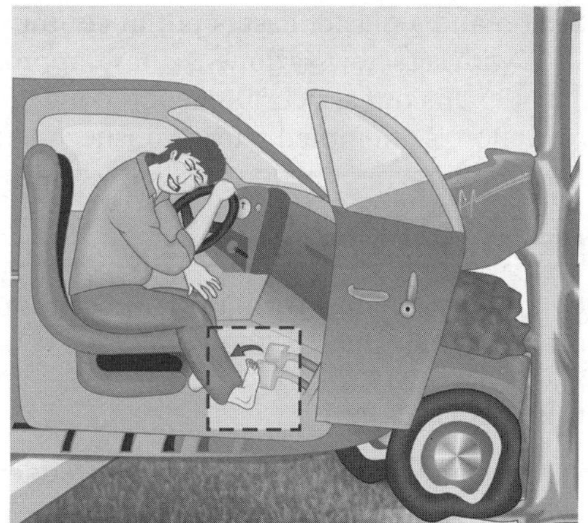

Fig. 22.7: Showing the common mechanism of talus fracture.

Clinical Features

There will be history of pain swelling and inability to bear weight—movements of the ankle and subtalor joints are painfully restricted.

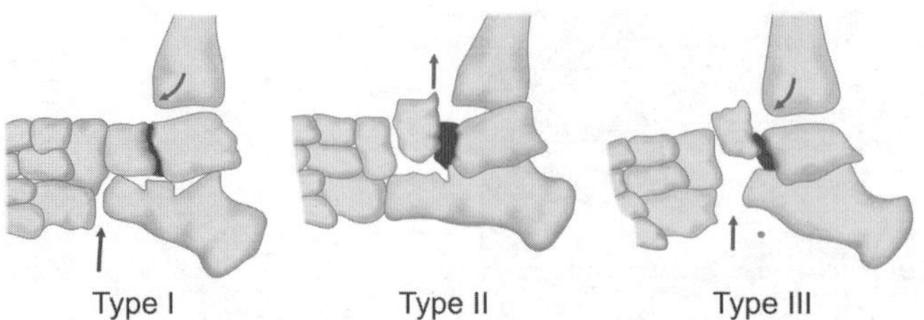

Fig. 22.8: Showing different types of neck of talus fractures.

Radiography

The views recommended are AP view with foot in maximum equinus and 15° pronation, lateral and oblique views of the ankle joint **(Fig. 22.9)**.

Treatment

Undisplaced Fractures

This is best treated by below-knee plaster cast for a period of 8–10 weeks.

Displaced Fractures

In this, closed reduction is done by traction in plantar flexion and a plaster cast is put in equinus. If this fails, ORIF with lag screws is done. In these, approximately 25% are open fractures. Debridement is done first and closed reduction is attempted later. If unsuccessful, ORIF with K-wires or open reduction with lag screws is attempted.

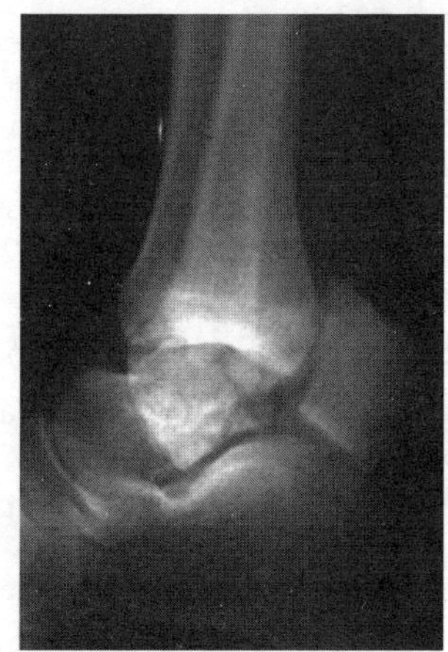

Fig. 22.9: Plain X-ray showing fracture of talus.

METATARSAL FRACTURES

Common mechanism of injury is direct due to fall of a heavy object on the foot.

Clinical Features

Patient complains of pain, swelling and tenderness over the dorsum of the foot **(Fig. 22.10)**. There could be considerable soft tissue swelling. Limp is present. Pain in the foot increases with weight bearing.

Radiology

Plain X-ray with AP, lateral and oblique views help to make the diagnosis **(Fig. 22.11)**.

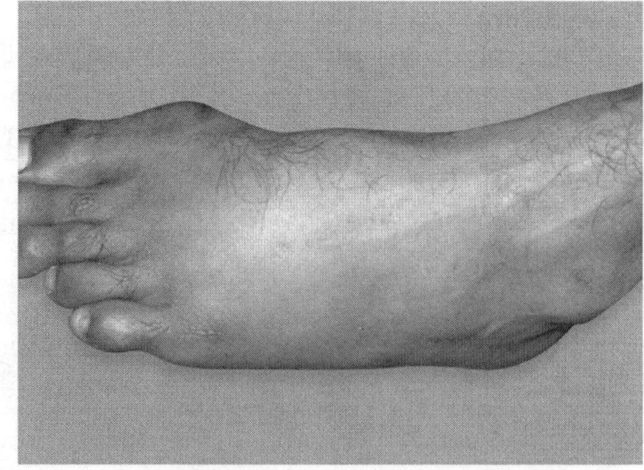

Fig. 22.10: Clinical photograph showing swelling dorsum of the forefoot.

Treatment

Conservative treatment is by NWB below-knee plaster cast for 6 to 8 weeks for stable fractures with no loss of bone length.

Operative treatment is reserved for displaced and unstable fractures by closed reduction and percutaneous fixation with K-wires, screws only or with plate and screws.

JONES FRACTURE

Definition

It is a fracture of the diaphysis of the fifth metatarsal bone approximately 1.5 cm above the tip of the tuberosity.

Mechanism of Injury

It is an avulsion fracture due to the pull of the peroneus brevis muscle.

Clinical Features

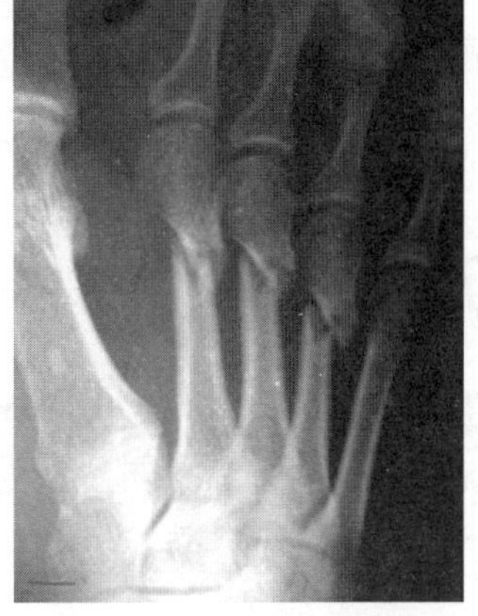

Fig. 22.11: Plain X-ray showing multiple metatarsal fractures.

Patient complains of pain, swelling and limp. On examination, tenderness can be elicited over the base of the fifth metatarsal bone.

Radiology

Radiograph of the foot helps to confirm the diagnosis **(Figs. 22.12A and B)**.

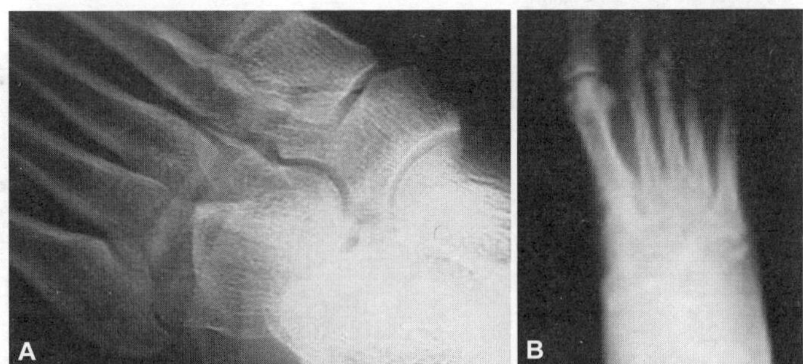

Figs. 22.12A and B: Showing: (A) Jones fracture; (B) Avulsion fractures of the styloid proces.

Treatment

Treatment is essentially conservative and consists of the application of a below knee plaster for a period of 3–4 weeks.

MARCH FRACTURE

This is a stress or fatigue fracture of the metatarsals particularly the second or third metatarsal bone. It is more often encountered in military personnel who indulge in frequent and prolonged marching and hence its name. It is also seen in police officers, dancers, nurses and surgeons who require to dance or stand for a long duration. Pain, tenderness and limp could be the usual complaints. Radiograph helps in the diagnosis **(Fig. 22.13)** and treatment is rest and symptomatic like NSAIDs, splints, elasto crepe bandage application, etc.

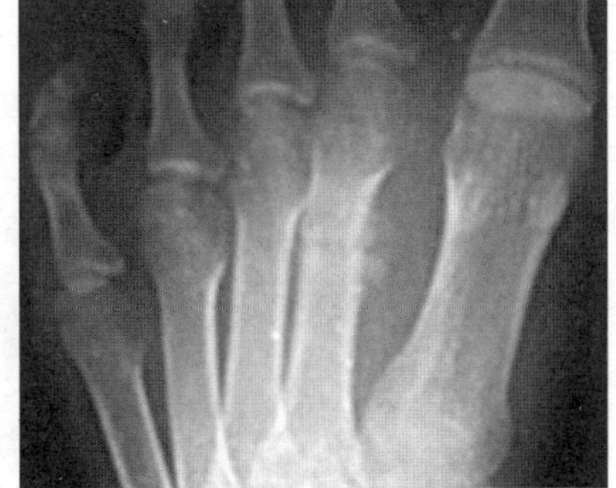

Fig. 22.13: Plain X-ray showing march fracture.

PHALANGEAL FRACTURES

This is the most common injury of the foot. Proximal phalanx is more commonly injured than all other phalanx. Direct blow due to fall of a heavy object on the toes is the common mechanism of injury.

Clinical Features

The patient presents with pain, swelling, limp and difficulty to wear the footwear.

Radiology

Standard AP and lateral films of the forefoot help to make the diagnosis **(Fig. 22.14)**.

Treatment

It consists of buddy taping for undisplaced and slightly displaced fracture **(Fig. 22.15)**. Operative Treatment is indicated for grossly unstable intra-articular fractures. The treatment method of choice is closed reduction and percutaneous K-wire fixation or open reduction, K-wire or screw fixation **(Figs. 22.16A and B)**.

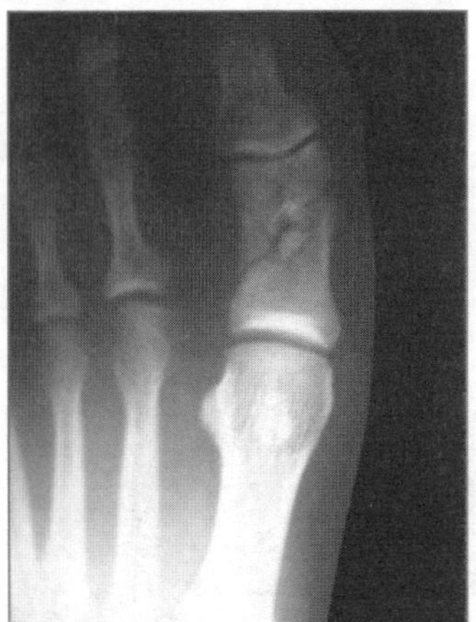

Fig. 22.14: Plain X-ray showing proximal phalangeal fracture of the great toe.

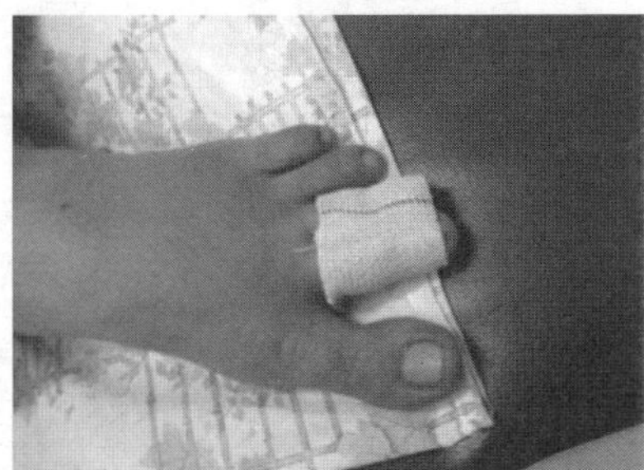

Fig. 22.15: Showing Buddy taping for undisplaced phalangeal fractures of toes.

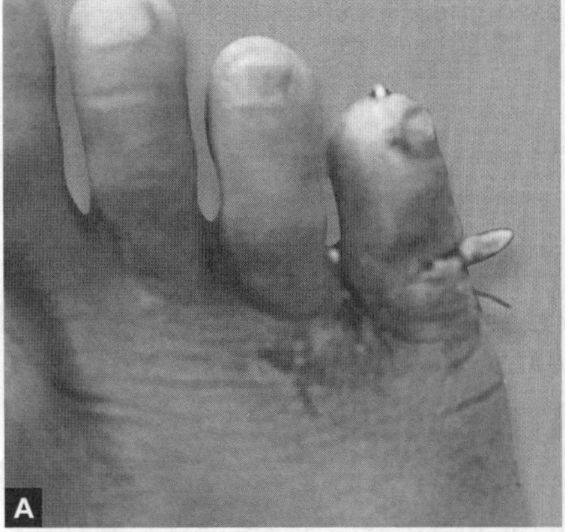

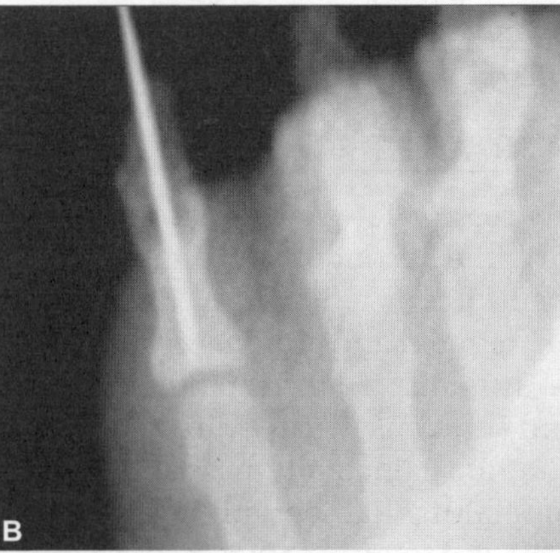

Figs. 22.16A and B: Showing K-wire fixation for displaced phalangeal fracture of the toe.

Non-traumatic

23
CHAPTER

Skeletal Tuberculosis

GENERAL PRINCIPLES OF SKELETAL TUBERCULOSIS

Skeletal tuberculosis is always *secondary,* the primary foci being either in the lungs, lymph nodes or gastrointestinal tract. The incidence of bone and joint tuberculosis is 2–3%. About 50% of these cases are found in the vertebral column. The other major areas affected in order of predilection are hip, knee, foot, elbow, hand, shoulder, and others. *Skeletal tuberculosis occurs mostly in the first three decades of life but no age is immune.*

Etiology

- ❖ **TB bacillus:**
  - ◆ Human variety, *Mycobacterium tuberculosis* (more common)
  - ◆ Bovine (rare)
- ❖ **Route:** Always secondary, may spread to the bone through
  - ◆ Blood, e.g., through Batson's plexus in tuberculosis of spine
  - ◆ Lymphatic spread
  - ◆ Direct
- ❖ **Precipitating factors:**
  - ◆ General factors, such as anemia, debility, etc., help precipitate the infection.
  - ◆ Local factors, such as trauma, etc., localize the problem to the bone.
- ❖ **Local trauma** causes vascular stasis and intraosseous hemorrhage.

Pathology

Pathology following a minor skeletal injury, the vessels ruptures and there is hemorrhage. The tubercle bacilli present in the circulation settle and proliferate in the blood clot so formed. A tubercle follicle is formed and it consists of lymphocytes, giant cells and endothelial cells. Small such tubercle follicles coalesce to form a larger follicle which undergoes caseation at the center and fibrosis at the periphery. The caseation at the center of the affected bone breaks down forming pus. It spreads towards the subperiosteal region, breaks the periosteum and tracks along the lines of least resistance. It reaches the skin and forms the cold abscess (not warm). Later on, it breaches the skin forming the sinus.

Changes in the Marrow

In the early stages, there is increase in the polymorphs. In the later stages, it is replaced by lymphocytes. The marrow is slowly surrounded by fat cells and is replaced by fibrous tissue.

Lamellae

There may be osteoporosis due to the action of osteoclasts or due to metaplasia. Osteosclerosis may also be seen.

Periosteum

Increased vascularity in the periosteum leads to new bone formation and the consequent subperiosteal thickening.

Joint Involvement

Joints may be affected due to direct spread from the vicinity of a tubercular bone infection or more commonly from a synovitis. Unlike a septic arthritis, synovitis is low grade here. The pannus causes a slow destruction of the cartilage and other structures of the joints. This slow destruction mostly leads to fibrous ankylosis and very rarely a bony ankylosis. Eventually various deformities may develop and the pus so formed may burst open the skin forming a cold abscess.

Note: In skeletal tuberculosis, healing is usually by fibrous ankylosis except in spine where bony ankylosis is more common.

Clinical features

The diagnostic triad **(Fig. 23.1)** best sums up clinical features.

Insidious Onset

Skeletal tuberculosis does not happen suddenly. It takes months and sometime year to develop wreaking have with the effected bones. Slow to affect and even slower to regress is the hallmark of the disease.

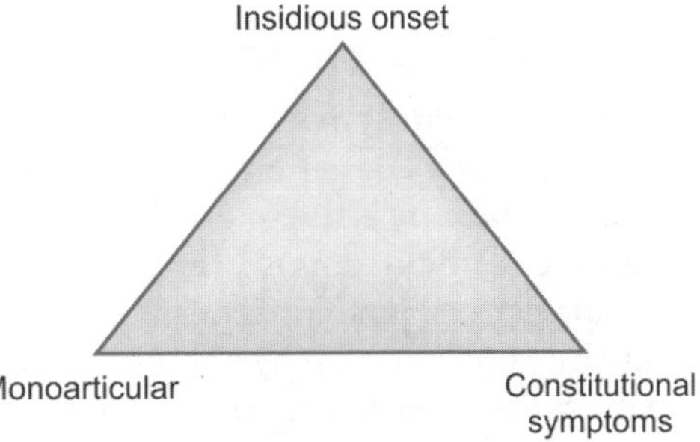

Fig. 23.1: Diagnostic triad of skeletal tuberculosis.

Monoarticular

The patient usually complains of pain in one joint, which is dull aching and chronic in nature. He or she may give history of night cries which is due to the rubbing of inflamed articular surfaces against each other due to the release of muscular spasm at rest. The joint movements are decreased in all directions, initially due to muscle spasm and later due to arthritis. *The wasting of the limb muscles is gross and is out of proportion.* Regional lymph nodes may be enlarged.

Constitutional Symptoms

This is present in approximately 20% of the cases. It consists of low-grade fever, lassitude in the afternoon, loss of appetite and weight, night sweats, anemia, tachycardia and evening rise of temperature.

Laboratory Investigations

These consists of hemoglobin estimation, total and differential count, raised ESR, urine routine tests, etc.

Other Investigations

- **Positive evidence of the disease:**
  - Identification of organism on culture from the joint, histology, etc.
  - Reproduction of disease by inoculating guinea pigs.
- **ZN stains** for acid-fast bacilli in aspirate or excised tissue.
- **Guinea pig test**
- **Mantoux test:** It is significant only in the first 3–4 years of life, adults are usually positive. Negative test does not rule out tuberculosis.
- **X-ray:**
  - No typical finding for tuberculosis.
  - Earliest sign is decalcification of bones (rarefaction).
  - Late signs are joint destruction.
- **Biopsy** of regional lymph nodes may show "tubercles".
- **Exploratory arthrotomy:** It is the certain way of ascertaining diagnosis. The tissue may be cultured or may be injected into a guinea pig.
- **Serum ELISA test:** This helps to detect the antibodies against *Mycobacterium* bacteria.

Note: Do not forget to take a chest X-ray in skeletal tuberculosis.

Treatment

Principles of Treatment

- **General treatment:** This includes rich protein diet, hematinics, adequate exposure to sunshine, etc. The general treatment aims at building up the general resistance of the patient.
- **Chemotherapy** is the mainstay of treatment and is discussed in detail below.
- **Local treatment aims** to prevent, correct, or decrease the deformities. By positioning the joints in appropriate functional position by proper splints. If the disease is osseous, aim at ankylosis in functional position by immobilization. If the disease is synovial aim at mobility by traction.
- **Operative treatment** consists of biopsy partial capsulectomy, synovectomy, osteotomy, curettage, joint debridement arthrodesis, etc., depending on the stage of tuberculosis.
- **Treatment of tubercular abscess:** Conservative treatment is recommended in most of the cases. Aspiration is done, if the abscess is tense.

Chemotherapy

Drugs used for the treatment of tuberculosis are grouped as follows:

First-line of drugs

These have the greatest level of efficiency and have an acceptable degree of toxicity.

The following are the first-line of drugs used in tuberculosis (mnemonic **PRISE**).

P—Pyrazinamide
R—Rifampicin
I—INH
S—Streptomycin
E—Ethambutol

Second line of drugs

These are useful if the patient develops resistance to the first-line of drugs (mnemonic **CAKECA**).

C—Capreomycin

A—Amikacin

K—Kanamycin

E—Ethionamide

C—Cycloserine

A—Aminosalicylic acid (PAS)

Second-line of drugs are used only for treatment of diseases caused by resistant microorganisms or by non-TB *Mycobacterium*. All drugs are given parenterally and are potentially ototoxic and nephrotoxic. Hence, no two drugs from this group should be used simultaneously. These are not used with streptomycin for the same reasons.

Chemotherapy regimes

- ❖ **Nine-month regime:** Nine months of rifampicin and INH are effective for all forms of disease.
- ❖ **Six-month regime:**
  - ◆ First two months, INH + Rifampicin + Pyrazinamide
  - ◆ Next four months, INH + Rifampicin
  - ◆ When the primary resistance to INH is high, therapy is usually initiated with four first-line drugs.
- ❖ **Third regime:** Here three to four drugs are used in the first four months, two to three drugs in the second four months, one or two drugs in the third four months and one drug (i.e., INH) in the last three to four months of treatment.

TUBERCULOSIS SPINE (KNOWN AFTER SIR PERCIVALL POTT)

This is the most common form of skeletal tuberculosis constituting about 50% of all cases.

As is evident from the above table spinal tuberculosis commonly affects the lower thoracic and lumbar vertebra accounting for nearly 80% of the cases. The reasons cited for this area of predilection are:

- ❖ Large amount of spongy tissue within the vertebral body.
- ❖ Degree of weight bearing which is comparatively more.
- ❖ More vertebral mobility is seen here.

Regional distribution
◀◀ Cervical—12%
◀◀ Cervicodorsal—5%
◀◀ Dorsal—42%
◀◀ Dorsolumbar—12%
◀◀ Lumbar—26%
◀◀ Lumbosacral—3%

Clinical Features

Tuberculosis of spine is usually insidious in onset although sometimes it may present acutely. The constitutional symptoms almost always antedate local spinal involvement. Weakness, anorexia, night sweats and cries, evening or afternoon rise of temperature, loss of appetite and weight are some of those.

Patient may complain of back pain, which is localized over the site of vertebral involvement or is referred depending on the specific nerve root irritation. Thus if cervical roots are involved pain radiates to the arm, if dorsal roots are involved patient complains of girdle pain, if lumbar nerve roots are involved patient complains of radiating pain to the groin, and if sacral roots are involved patient complains of sciatica.

Back stiffness is another common earliest complaint given by the patient. Patient is unable to bend and pick up the objects on the ground. Patient may give history of night cries. If the patient complains of stiffness, weakness, awkwardness of lower extremities, it heralds the onset of paraplegia. In more severe cases, patient may present with cold abscess or paraplegia.

Physical Findings

The patient has a very protective attitude and has a very cautious and careful gait. The muscle spasm straightens out the spine. The spinous process of the involved vertebra is tender to percuss and when an attempt is made to rotate the vertebra. Back movements are decreased in all directions especially forward, flexion. There is pronounced wasting of the back muscles. The clinical attitude of the patient varies according to the region involved. Cold abscess may be seen as paravertebral swelling or in areas already described. Patient may develop or present with neurological complications, such as spastic or flaccid paraplegia. Of the various deformities of spine due to tuberculosis, *kyphotic* deformity is the most common and is seen in over 95% of the cases **(Fig. 23.2)**.

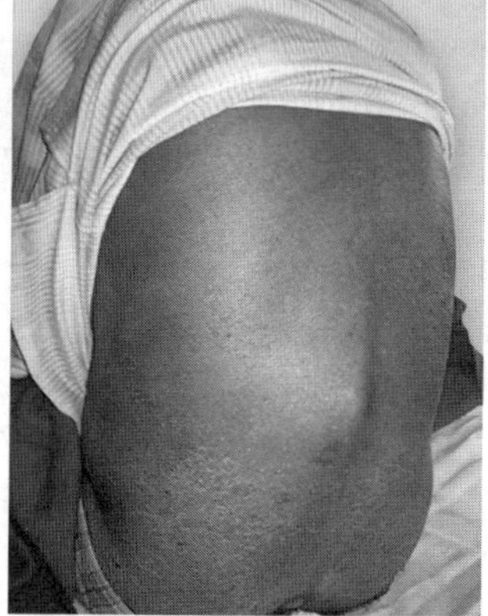

Fig. 23.2: Clinical photograph showing kyphotic deformity in tuberculosis of spine.

General Examination

Reveals signs of anemia, debility, involvement of lungs, lymph nodes, etc.

Investigations

Laboratory Tests

These tests show anemia, lymphocytes, hypoproteinemia, mild increase in ESR, etc. Mantoux test is helpful especially in children below 2–3 years but is not diagnostic. The importance of general tests lies in indicating chronic disease.

Radiographs

X-ray of the affected vertebrae is a very important diagnostic test and it is observed that the average number of affected vertebra is usually three. The following changes are seen on the X-ray:

Early Changes

This consists of disc space narrowing and subsequent loss of disc space in the common paradiscal lesions. The bones look rarefied and osteopenic (about 40% of calcium loss must take place to show a radiolucent sign on the X-ray).

Late Changes

This includes anterior wedge compression in anterior vertebral involvement, central vertebral body collapse also called as "concertina collapse" **(Fig. 23.3)** in central involvement, destruction of the posterior elements in the posterior affection, destruction of the body and the intervertebral spaces **(Fig. 23.4)**.

Soft tissue swelling and its calcification are highly predictable of tuberculosis. In the healing stages,

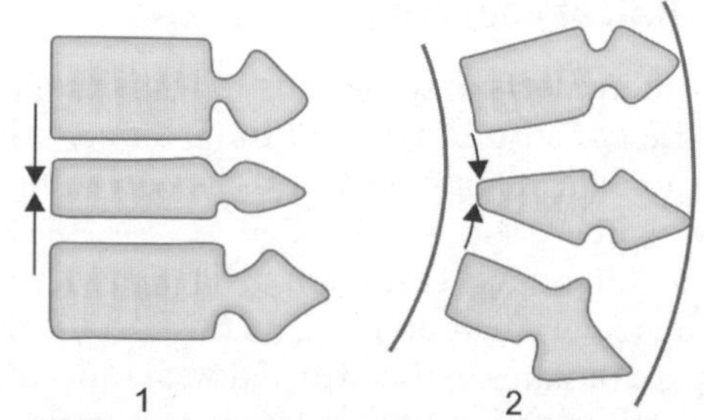

Fig. 23.3: (1) Concertina collapse, and (2) Anterior wedge compression.

the vertebral body and the posterior elements may appear denser due to sclerosis.

Paravertebral shadow

If seen on the X-ray indicates cold abscess **(Fig. 23.5)**:
- Cervical region; it is seen in between the vertebral bodies and pharynx (retropharyngeal).
- Upper thoracic V-shaped shadow and widened mediastinum.
- Below fourth thoracic vertebra shows a fusiform or bird nest shadow appearance.
- Psoas abscess shows unilateral or bilateral widening of psoas shadows in the lumbar region.
- Aneurysmal phenomenon is seen as a tense thoracic vertebral abscess showing a scalloping effect.
- Sclerosis and bony ankylosis indicate healing.

Note: The most common is paradiscal, rarest is appendiceal involvement in spinal tuberculosis.

CT Scans

Identifies paravertebral soft tissue swelling more readily than X-rays. It helps to assess the degree of neural compromise and helps in better evaluation of the pathologic process. Some prefer CT to X-ray to determine the clinical progress. Findings are similar to X-rays.

Note: The only detectable abnormality on plain X-ray and CT scan specifically related to tuberculosis is fine calcification in the paravertebral soft tissue shadow.

MRI

It helps in further delineation of the disease and helps to detect the cord compression. It does not eliminate the need for biopsy. It is 94% accurate **(Fig. 23.6)**. Small calcifications seen on X-rays are not seen on MRI.

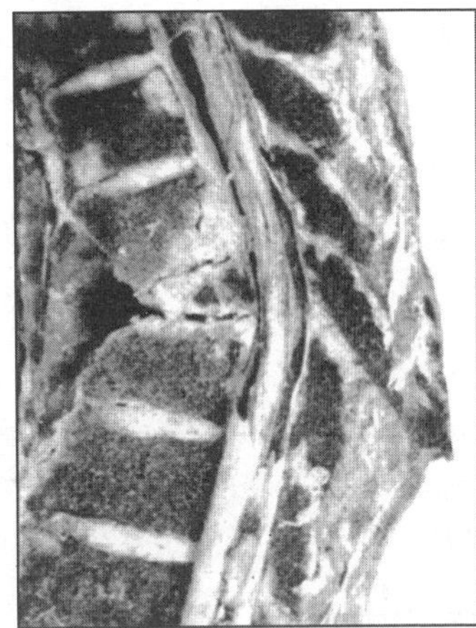

Fig. 23.4: Specimen of tuberculosis spine showing destruction of the intervertebral space and body.

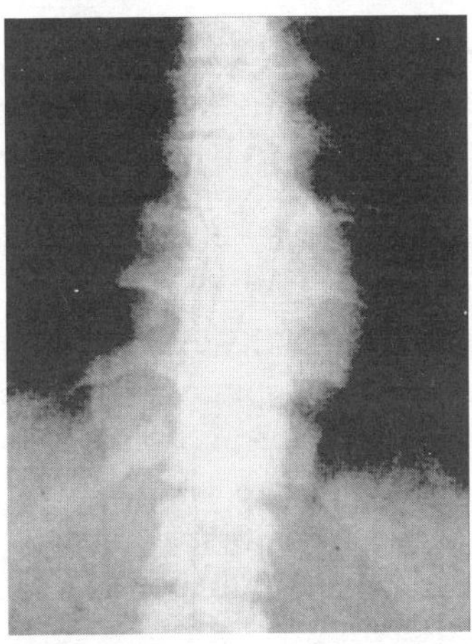

Fig. 23.5: Tense paravertebral abscess of tuberculosis of lower dorsal spine.

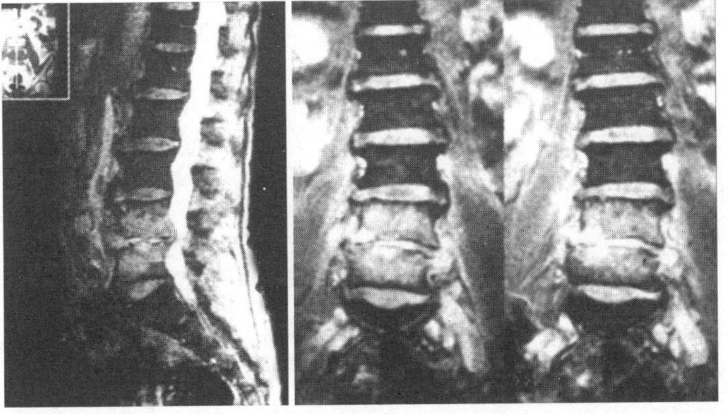

Fig. 23.6: MRI of lumbar spine showing tubercular lesion of L5 vertebra.

Gallium Scanning

It is useful in disseminated TB.

Biopsy

No one diagnostic test is 100% accurate for definitive diagnosis. Hence, diagnosis is dependent on culture of the organism and requires biopsy by percutaneous technique with CT control.

Ultrasound

It is useful to detect size of cold abscess in lumbar vertebral disease.

Note: *CT scan and MRI* are also helpful in detecting tubercular affection of posterior spinal elements, craniovertebral and craniodorsal region, sacrum and sacroiliac region.

Treatment

General Measures

This form of treatment is has already seen discussed.

Local Measures

Rest and immobilization: Bed rest helps considerably in the initial stages. A plaster of Paris body cast helps to immobilize the spine. Collar and Minerva Jacket helps to immobilize the cervical spine.

Mobilization: As the disease subsides, patient may be mobilized with a brace. Collar for cervical spine, ASH brace for the thoracolumbar vertebra are the preferred braces and they need to be worn at least for 2 years **(Fig. 23.7)**.

Chemotherapy: Definitive diagnosis by biopsy and culture is necessary before starting the treatment, because of the toxicity of the chemotherapeutic regime and length of the treatment required.

Surgery

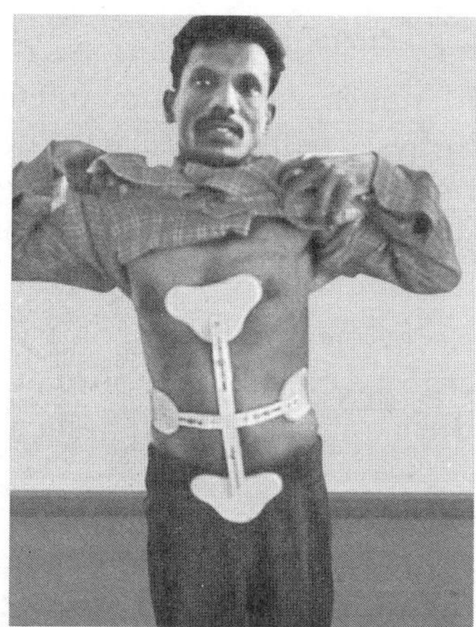

Fig. 23.7: clinical photograph showing Anterior hyperextension brace.

Indications for Surgery

❖ Neurological symptoms
❖ Kyphosis with several vertebral involvement, severe kyphosis, progressive kyphosis, etc.
❖ Resistance to chemotherapy
❖ Recurrence of disease
❖ Cord compression
❖ Progressive impairment of pulmonary function
❖ Spinal instability

Surgical Procedures

The following surgical procedures are described:
Aspiration: This technique is useful to aspirate the contents of a cold abscess through a thick bored needle. The needle should be inserted below the abscess to enable the gravity to help drain the contents.

Minimal debridement: This consists of evaluating the cold abscess through costotransversectomy or decompression. Here the contents are evacuated, the walls thoroughly curetted and bone grafting is done, if necessary. Recently evacuation and debridement of a thoracic cold abscess through a thoracoscope has been successfully tried.

Radical debridement: This is done through the anterior approach and is invariably followed by spinal fusion with a strut graft involving rib or fibula after a thorough debridement.

Objectives of Surgery

Surgery helps to excise the infected tissue, decompress the intraspinal neural elements, reduce the spinal instability and provide stability by spine fusion techniques.

Middle Path Regime

Tuli and Kumar advocated triple drug therapy without surgery. In their series, operative treatment was reserved for patients:

Complications of tuberculosis spine

- Paraplegia
- Cold abscess
- Sinuses
- Secondary infection
- Amyloid disease
- Fatality

- ❖ Not responding favorably to drug therapy after six months of treatment
- ❖ Recrudescence of the disease
- ❖ Patient with neural complications

Operative treatment is combined with 6–12 months of bed rest, followed by 18–24 months of spinal bracing.

TUBERCULOSIS SPINE WITH PARAPLEGIA

The incidence of this complication is 10–30% and it is most often associated with tuberculosis of the dorsal spine.

The following are the reasons cited for paraplegia

- TB is more common in dorsal spine.
- Spinal cord terminates below L1.
- Spinal cord is smallest in this region.
- Normal curve of the thoracic spine encourages marked kyphosis.
- Anterior longitudinal ligament in the dorsal region loosely confines the abscess.

Pathology

Paraplegia could result due to inflammatory causes, mechanical causes, and intrinsic causes and due to spinal tumor disease.

Classification

Seddon's Classification

Early onset paraplegia is associated with the active disease. It is seen within two years of onset of the disease.

Late onset paraplegia is associated with healed disease. It is seen after two years after the onset of disease.

Clinical Features

Rarely paraplegia may be the presenting symptom. Late onset paraplegia may be associated with clumsiness, twitching, increased reflexes, clonus, positive Babinski sign, etc. Motor functions are usually affected first. The paralysis usually follows the following stages in order of severity, muscle weakness, spasticity, in coordination, paraplegia in extension, flexor spasms, paraplegia in flexion (severe form), and flaccid paraplegia lastly **(Figs. 23.8A to D)**.

Investigations

These are the same as described for TB spine. MRI is the gold standard among the investigations for paraplegia due to TB spine.

Principles of Treatment

Three schools of thought are described for management of paraplegia due to tuberculosis.
- ❖ **Bosworth:** Immobilization and early posterior arthrodesis.
- ❖ **Hodgson radical:** Anterior decompression and arthrodesis.
- ❖ **Tuli and Kumar's:** Middle path regime.

<table>
<tr><td>What is middle path regime?</td></tr>
</table>

- ◄◄ Admission, rest in bed or Plaster of Paris cast.
- ◄◄ Chemotherapy.
- ◄◄ X-ray and ESR once in three months.
- ◄◄ Gradual mobilization in the absence of neurological complications.
- ◄◄ Spinal braces—18 months to 2 years.
- ◄◄ Abscesses are aspirated or drained.
- ◄◄ Sinuses heal within 6–12 weeks.
- ◄◄ If no neural complications develop, if response is obtained within 3–4 weeks of triple drug therapy, surgery is unnecessary.
- ◄◄ Excision surgery for posterior spinal disease.
- ◄◄ Operative debridement for patients who do not show arrest of disease after 3–6 months of chemotherapy.

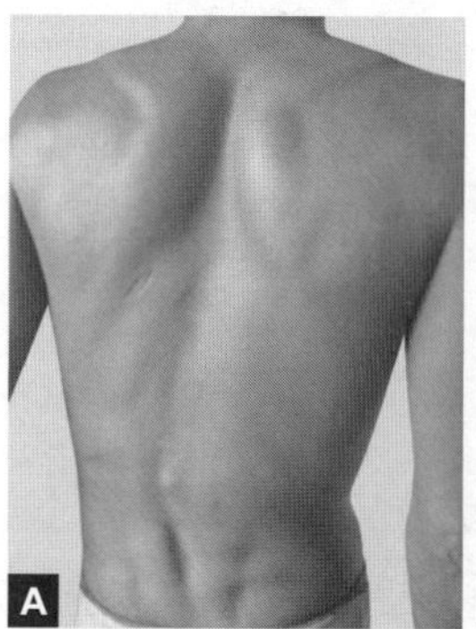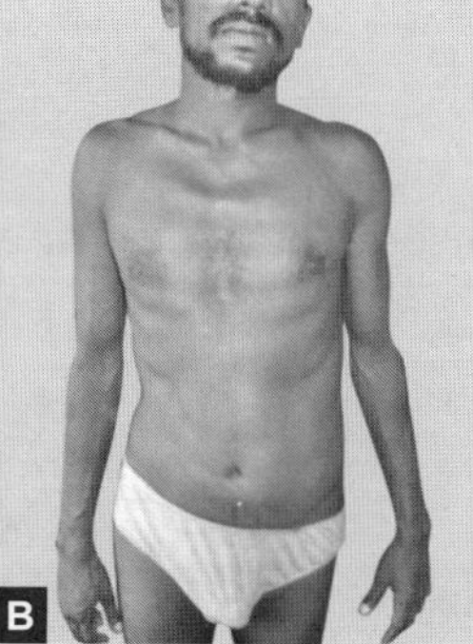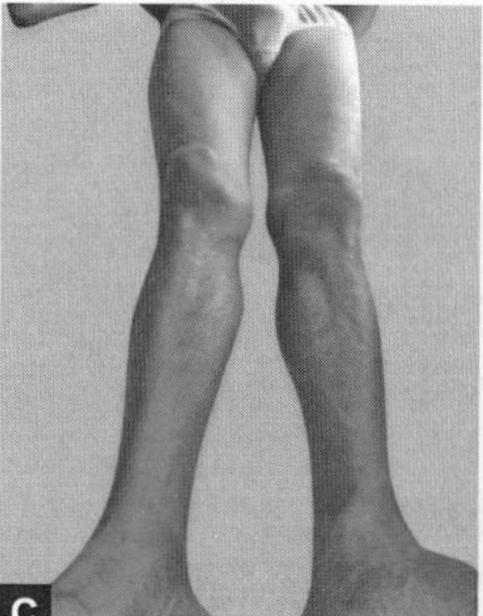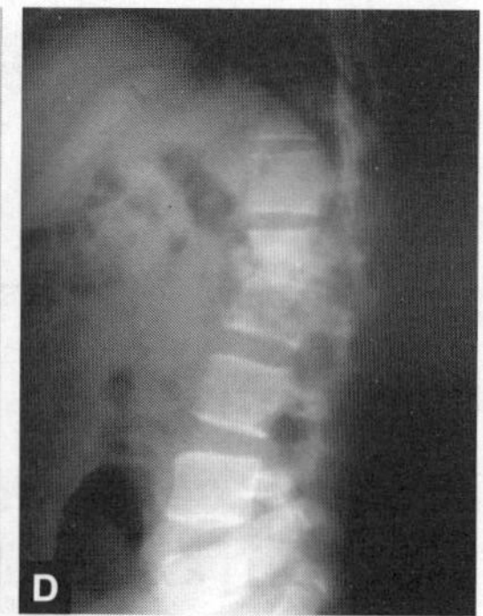

Figs. 23.8A to D: Clinical photograph showing tubercular paraparesis: (A) Knuckle gibbus; (B) Postural abnormalities; (C) Limbs showing paraparesis; (D) Showing destruction of lumbar vertebra on plain X-ray.

Treatment of Pott's Paraplegia

The following measures are adopted in the treatment of Pott's paraplegia.

Conservative Treatment

Chemotherapy is the mainstay of this method and has already been described. Immobilization of the spine to provide rest and thereby promote healing is done by traction (in cervical region) plaster cast or brace (in dorsal region), etc. Management of bedsores, bladder and bowel management is done as already discussed in the management of spinal injury. Physiotherapy and occupational therapy helps in the treatment of the paralyzed lower limbs.

Surgical Treatment

The incidence of surgery has considerably decreased as chemotherapy is found to be successful in treating Pott's paraplegia. Only 5% of the cases require surgery in uncomplicated cases and 60% of the cases with neurological deficits require surgery.

Main Indications for Surgery

- **Failed conservative treatment:** If the patient does not respond to conservative treatment even after 3–6 months.
- In doubtful diagnosis.
- Fusion for mechanical instability by some grafts, implants, etc., either by the anterior or posterior approach.
- Recurrence of the disease after treatment.
- In rapid onset paraplegia.
- In disease secondary to cervical disease and cauda equina paralysis.

Other Indications

- Recurrent paraplegia
- Painful paraplegia due to root compression, etc.
- Posterior spinal disease involving the posterior elements of the vertebra
- Spinal tumor syndrome resulting in cord compression
- Rapid onset paraplegia due to thrombosis, trauma, etc.
- Severe paraplegia
- Secondary to cervical disease and cauda equina paralysis.

Surgical Techniques

Costotransversectomy

This is indicated for a tense paravertebral abscess. As the name suggests excision of the transverse process of the affected vertebra and about an inch of the adjacent rib to facilitate the drainage of abscess is done. If pus is yielded under pressure, one has to wait up to six weeks for improvement. If no improvement occurs anterolateral, decompression is done.

Anterolateral Decompression (ALD)

The structures removed in this procedure is posterior part of the rib, transverse process, pedicle and part of the vertebral body anterior to the cord (**Figs. 23.9 and 23.10**). This is the surgery of choice for Pott's paraplegia. It helps to effectively remove the solid and liquid debris. ALD is done through an extrapleural mediastinal approach. Bone graft may be inserted if needed.

Anterior Decompression

This is technically more demanding. Here the affected vertebra is approached through a transpleural or transperitoneal route, diseased tissue is curetted and a bone graft is inserted.

Laminectomy

In Pott's paraplegia, anterior part of the cord is predominantly affected and laminectomy does not decompress this part of the cord. Moreover, it makes the spine unstable as it removes the healthy areas of the vertebrae. Hence, this procedure is not commonly recommended.

If arthrodesis of the spine is required after the above procedures, anterior arthrodesis is normally preferred. Posterior spinal arthrodesis has limited value and is usually done to stabilize the craniovertebral region. Paralysis secondary to cervical disease is treated by either laminectomy and posterior arthrodesis or radical debridement and anterior arthrodesis. Severe cauda equina paralysis requires lumbar transversectomy.

Cold abscess is another complication.

It can present as one of the three **P's**
- **P**alpable tumor in neck, back, thigh, etc.
- **P**ressure symptoms on the cord.
- **P**resent on radiographs of spine.

Treatment Methods

Early aseptic evacuation is indicated.
- Aspiration of the contents are very fluid.
- Majority require open surgery for evacuation, e.g., costotransversectomy for tense paravertebral abscess.
- ALD for less than tense paravertebral abscess.

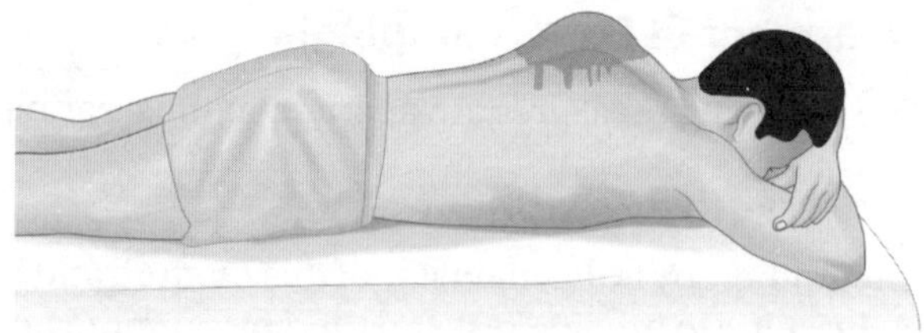

Fig. 23.9: Approach for ALD and costotransversectomy.

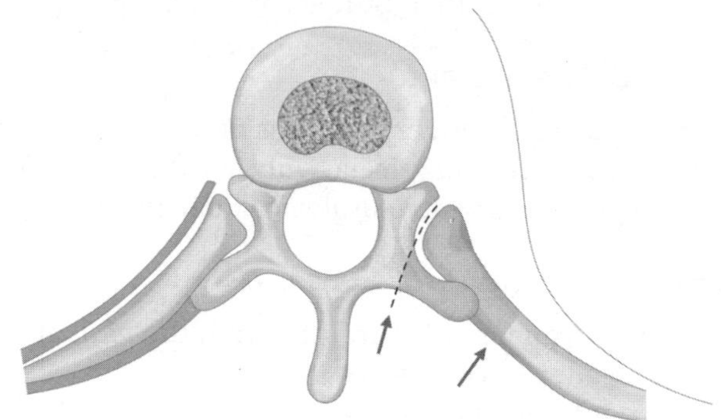

Fig. 23.10: Structures removed in ALD.

Disorders of Joints

ARTHRITIS

It is a non-specific term denoting acute or chronic inflammation of the joint. Clinically, arthritis falls into the following groups:

1. **Osteoarthritis**
   - Primary
   - Secondary
2. **Rheumatoid arthritis**
   - Adult
   - Juvenile
3. **Infective arthritis**
   - Acute
   - Chronic
4. **Metabolic arthritis**
   - Gout
   - Pseudogout
5. **Nonspecific monoarthritis**
6. Neuropathic joint disorders, e.g., Charcot's
7. **Special forms:**
   - Hemophiliac arthritis
   - Psoriatic arthritis
   - Psychogenic arthritis

Nearly 10% of the population suffers from one form of the arthritis or the other.

INFECTIVE ARTHRITIS

PYOGENIC INFECTION OF JOINT OR SEPTIC ARTHRITIS

Definition

Septic arthritis is defined as a bacterial infection of the joint, which causes an intense inflammatory reaction with migration of polymorph nuclear leucokytes, and subsequent release of proteolytic enzymes. This could lead to destruction of the articular cartilage and later the joint.

Causative Organisms

The most common offending organisms are *Staphylococcus aureus* (50%), *Streptococcus* (20%), *Pneumococcus* (10%), *Gonococcus, E. coli,* etc. *H. Influenzae* is very common in children <2 years. *Blood culture is positive only in 60% of cases.*

Predisposing Factors

The predisposing factors are trauma, diabetes, steroid therapy, malignancy, etc. It is more common in children and males.

Sites of Involvement of the Joint

In adults

- ❖ Knee (53%)
- ❖ Hip (20%)
- ❖ Elbow (17%)
- ❖ Shoulder (10%)

In children

- ❖ Knee (39%)
- ❖ Hip (32%)

Routes of entry for organisms: 5 P's
◀◀ **P**rimary focus is in RS, GIT, etc.
◀◀ **P**yogenic osteomyelitis
◀◀ **P**unctured wounds
◀◀ **P**neumonia, typhoid, etc.
◀◀ **P**rimary focus within the joint, absent in few
◀◀ **P**hysician-latrogenic, following intra-articular injections, etc.

Remember

About 90% of cases of septic arthritis are monoarticular and 10% are polyarticular.

Pathology

The organism, which gains entry through one of the above routes, reaches the synovium. Synovitis this develops and leads to the following pathological changes:
- ❖ **Exudation into joint:** This could be serous, serofibrinous or purulent depending upon the severity of infection.
- ❖ **Destruction of articular cartilage** by plasmin, cathepsin, prostaglandins, etc.
- ❖ Capsules, ligaments are destroyed by pus.

Stages

The stages of infective although are stage of synovitis, stage of arthritis and stage of recovery or stage of bony ankylosis **(Fig. 24.1)**.

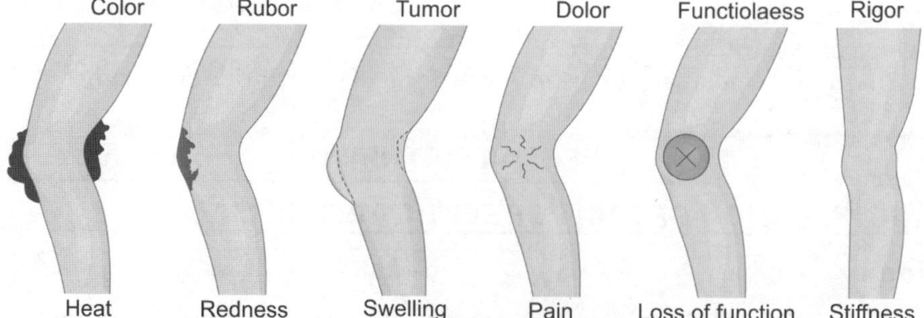

Fig. 24.1: Showing the cardinal signs of inflammation.

Clinical Features

Septic arthritis usually presents as monoarticular affection in 90% and polyarticular in 10% of cases and fever is seen in only 50% of the cases. Limp is a common complaint. The severity of clinical manifestation depends upon the severity of disease **(Fig. 24.2)**.

Investigations

Joint aspirate and synovial fluid analysis: This is the most accurate diagnostic tool for septic arthritis. The synovial fluid is tested for cells, sugars and proteins. Gram-staining is positive in 60% of the cases for gram-positive cocci.

Laboratory investigations: WBCs (polymorphs) are raised to 50,000–1,00,000 (80% of cases), ESR increased >20 mm/hour (in 50% of cases), Hb percentage decreases. Blood culture is positive in 35–50% of the cases.

Radiology

Early Stages

It may be normal in some cases. In others earliest findings in the radiographs are soft tissue swelling and periarticular osteoporosis **(Fig. 24.3)**.

Late Stages

In the later stages, cartilage destruction, loss of joint space, necrosis of bone, epiphyseal disturbances, fibrous ankylosis, and bony ankylosis **(Figs. 24.4A to C)** may be seen.

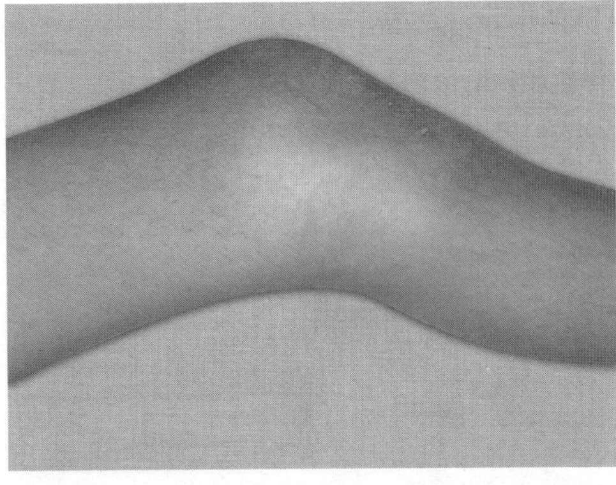

Fig. 24.2: Showing septic arthritis of the knee joint.

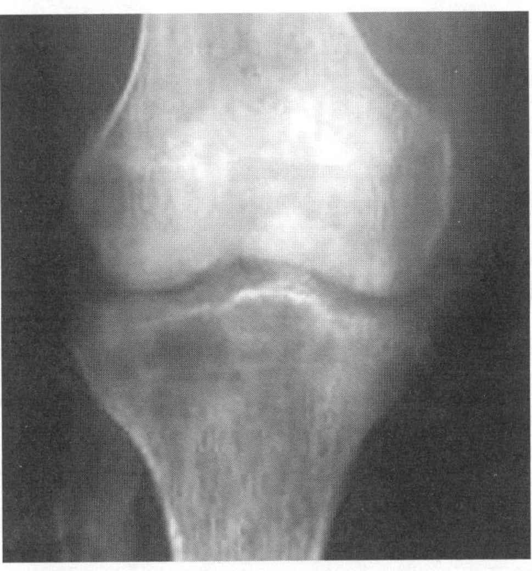

Fig. 24.3: Showing radiological features of the knee joint.

Treatment

1. **Arthrotomy or joint drainage:** The joint is aspirated first, if pus is present, open arthrotomy is indicated. The pus is cultured and is subjected to Gram-staining. Appropriate antibiotics are then chosen and are given intravenously before surgical drainage. Antibiotics are used for a minimum period of 2–4 weeks. IV Amikacin (15 mg/kg) and Cefotaxime (100–150 mg/kg) are the drugs of choice in the initial stages.
2. **Immobilization** of the joints by using plaster of Paris splints in functional position reduces pain and prevents deformities.
3. **Radical treatment:** It is reserved for all except, very early cases, which do not respond rapidly within 24 hours to antibiotics and immobilization.
4. If cartilage is destroyed, aim for ankylosis in functional position by plaster casts.

Complications

- ❖ Joint destruction
- ❖ Pathological dislocation
- ❖ Osteoarthritis in later years
- ❖ Ankylosis—fibrous or bony
- ❖ Acute osteomyelitis
- ❖ Amyloidosis very rarely develops
- ❖ Septicemia, pyemia, etc.

> **Remember**
>
> Tom Smith arthritis is a septic arthritis of the hip joint seen in infants. It is often confused with CDH. Arthroscopic joint drainage is the treatment of choice.

Differential Diagnosis

- ❖ TB arthritis
- ❖ Hemophilia
- ❖ Rheumatic arthritis
- ❖ Acute osteomyelitis

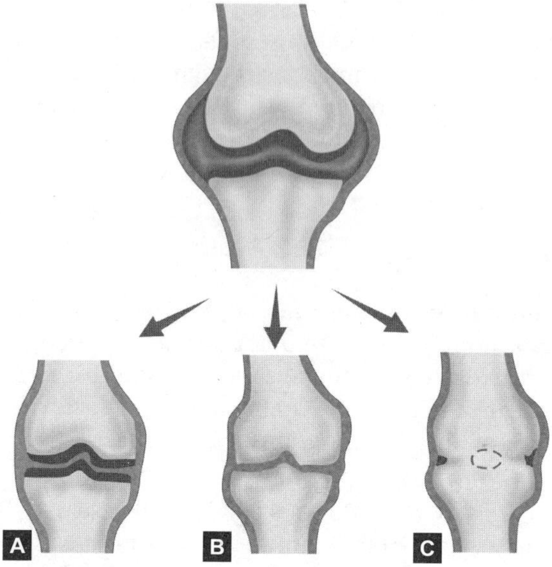

Figs. 24.4A to C: Showing sequelae in infective arthritis: (A) No residual effect leaving back a normal joint; (B) Features suggestive of fibrous ankylosis; (C) Bony ankylosis.

GONOCOCCAL ARTHRITIS

The incidence of gonococcal arthritis is <1% and it is familiarly known as a three weeks infection. The male is to female ratio is 5:1 and the age of predilection is between 20 and 30 years. It usually results due to lack of treatment for gonorrhea. About 40% of the cases are monoarticular, knee being the most common.

Pathology

Gonococcal arthritis can present as acute, subacute and chronic. The important pathological features are synovitis, effusion, cartilage erosion, and destruction of cartilage.

Clinical Features

Gonococcal arthritis is usually sudden in onset. Patient presents with chills, fever, pain and swelling of the joint. On examination, there is raised temperature and tenderness. There may be history of urethral discharge. The disease may become chronic due to inadequate and improper treatment.

Treatment

The treatment methods consist of local measures, such as splints, chemotherapy by intravenous penicillin G, and rest to the part, aspiration with a thick bored needle and arthrotomy to clear the joint debris.

SYPHILIS OF JOINTS

The incidence of syphilis of the joints is definitely on the decline due to the early use of antibiotics. Syphilitic arthritis is caused by *Treponema pallidum* and is classified as congenital or acquired.

Investigations

1. Wassermann's test is positive.
2. *Treponema pallidum* immobilization test is positive.
3. Joint fluid aspiration and synovial fluid analysis for cell, sugar, protein, etc.

Treatment

Antisyphilitic treatment is done but it is often not successful. Penicillin is the drug of choice.

NEUROPATHIC JOINTS (CHARCOT'S)

This causes extensive destruction of the joint as it is painless. The following are some of the important causes of neuropathic joints:

- Syringomyelia (25%)
- Tabes dorsalis (4–10%)
- Syphilis
- Rheumatoid arthritis
- Intra-articular steroids
- Traumatic division of sciatic nerve
- Chronic liver disease
- Prolonged administration of drugs, such as indomethacin, etc.

Sites

Knee, ankle, hip, elbow, shoulder, wrist and intervertebral joints in that order. It is rare before 40 years.

Pathology

The pathological changes seen in the joint are gross destruction of the joint, the capsules are thickened, osteophyte formation is seen, joint cavity is distorted and the loose bodies are present.

Clinical Features

In this condition, premonitory signs are rare; onset is usually sudden and unexpected. Gross swelling and lax joint are commonly seen **(Fig. 24.5)**. In the later stages of the disease, the following features are seen—lax joints, striking absence of pain, joint becomes flail and there is a diffuse erythema around the joints.
X-rays may show gross destruction of the joints in the advanced stages **(Fig. 24.6)**.

Treatment

The treatment of choice is Charnley's compression arthrodesis but efficient bracing still has a major role to play **(Figs. 24.7 and 24.8)**.

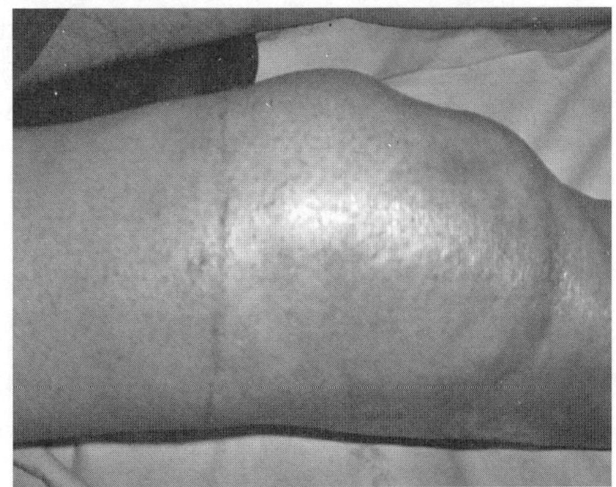

Fig. 24.5: Showing Neuropathic knee joint.

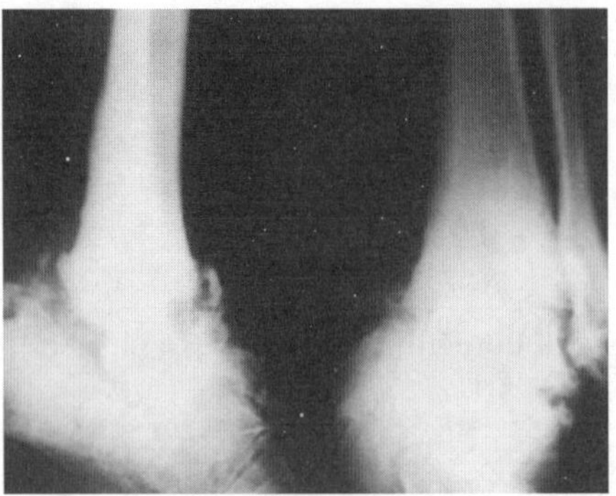

Fig. 24.6: Showing a radiological features of a neuropathic ankle joint.

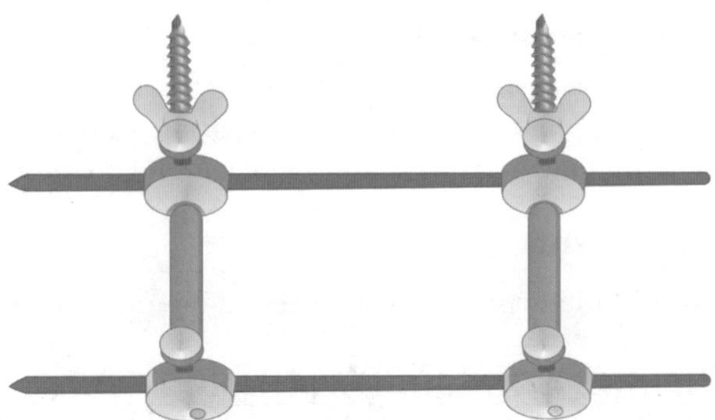

Fig. 24.7: Charnley's compression clamp with 2 pins.

HEMOPHILIC ARTHRITIS (BLEEDER'S JOINTS)

Definition

It is a hereditary coagulative disorder characterized by hemorrhages, which is spontaneous and is due to trivial trauma. It is X-linked, carried by female, manifest in male, cause being *prolonged clotting time. Incidence* is 3–4 per one lakh population.

Pathology

The defective blood interacts with the synovial fluid and causes irritation to the synovial membrane. Due to the proliferation of the macrophages, there is synovial hyperplasia and pannus formation which ultimately causes destruction of the articular cartilage of the joint.

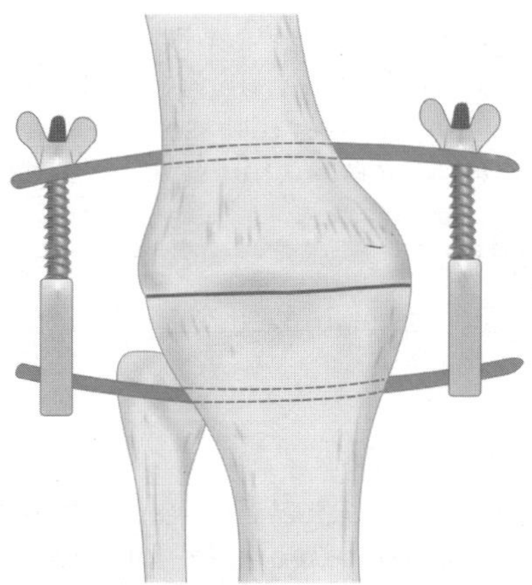

Fig. 24.8: Showing Charnley's compression arthrodesis.

Clinical Features

Bleeding is spontaneous and is usually due to trivial trauma. Acute hemarthrosis occurs within hours. The joint is warm, tender and flexion attitude develops. Acute phase lasts for few weeks. With each attack joint movement decreases, fixed flexion deformity occurs, degenerative arthritis sets in and results in fibrous ankylosis. There is gross muscle atrophy **(Fig. 24.9)**.

Laboratory Investigations

The classical feature of this disease is, bleeding time is normal but the clotting time is prolonged.

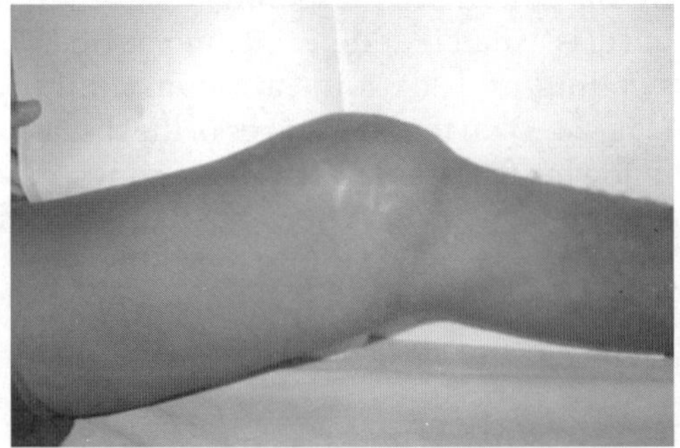

Fig. 24.9: Showing hemophilic knee joint.

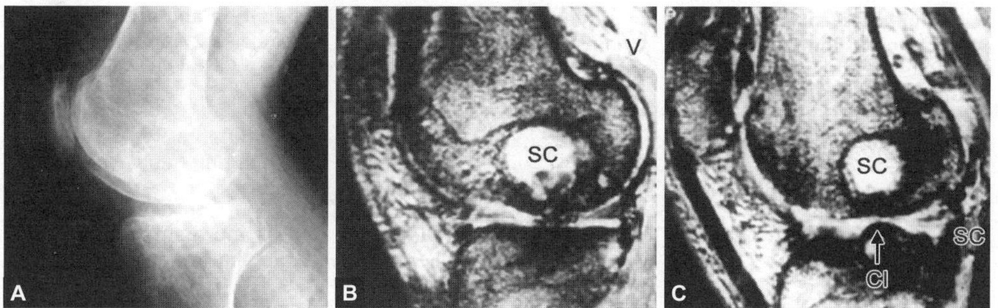

Figs. 24.10A to C: Showing radiological features and MRI features of hemophilic knee joint.

Radiology

This shows soft tissue swelling, juxta epiphyseal osteoporosis, squaring of the patella, widening of the intercondylar notch of the femur, subchondral cysts and features of ankylosis **(Figs. 24.10A to C)**.

Treatment

This varies according to the stages of the disease.

Acute Stage

For injuries of less than four hours, the patient is treated on OPD basis. Factor VIII is replaced and is discharged home on the same day.

Late Cases

Treated as in-patient, trial aspiration prolonged immobilization, factor VIII replacement and later mobilization with calipers and splints are recommended.

Chronic Hemarthropathy

1. **For recent contractures:** Plaster immobilization, dynamic traction and physiotherapy.
2. **For post-subluxation of tibia:** Dynamic traction
3. **For painful unstable joints:** Orthotic splintage
4. Surgery is indicated for painful, stiff joints, stiff contractures and recurrent bleeding into the joint.

Surgical Methods

These include synovectomy, internal fixations for fracture nonunion. Supracondylar osteotomy for severe flexion contractures of knee, arthrodesis for severely disorganized joints, total hip replacement for pain in the hip in advanced stages and tendoachilles lengthening for tendoachilles contractures, etc.

Rheumatoid Arthritis

RHEUMATOID ARTHRITIS

Rheumatoid arthritis is the ***most common*** inflammatory disease of the joints. It is a systemic disease of young and middle-aged adults characterized by proliferative and destructive changes in synovial membrane, periarticular structures, skeletal muscles and perineural sheaths. Eventually joints are destroyed, fibrosed or ankylosed. It is a widespread vasculitis of the small arterioles.

- ❖ **Incidence:** It is 3%.
- ❖ **Sex:** About 80% affected are women; Male:Female ratio is 1:3
- ❖ **Age:** No age is exempted, mean age is 40 years.

Etiology

The exact cause is unknown but genetics and malfunction of the cellular and humoral arms of the immune system are cited as the probable cause.

Genetics

The presence of HLA-drw-4 and HLA-DR 1, strongly suggests the role of genetics in the causation of rheumatoid arthritis.

Current Hypothesis

An initiating antigen triggers an aberrant response, which becomes self-perpetuating long after the offending antigen has been cleared.

Antigenic Agents

Which probably act as predisposing factors are viruses—rubella, Epstein–Barr, etc., genetic (common in people with HLA DR_4 60%), psychological stress, allergic factors, endocrine factors and metabolic factors.

Clinical Features

Rheumatoid arthritis usually presents in three forms:

Classical Presentation

In this group, patient is usually a woman in her mid 30s. Pain, swelling, stiffness of the small joints of hands and feet are the common presenting complaints. Other joints are also affected with varying frequency. Patient also gives history of weight loss, lethargy and depression. Joint swelling could be symmetrical and the patient presents with deformities of bones and joints in the late stages. *The patient gives history of remissions and exacerbation of symptoms with seasonal variations.* This is a very classical complaint in the absence of which diagnosis of rheumatoid arthritis should be carefully made. Symptoms fluctuate from day to day.

Other Presentations

This consists of palindromic presentation involving one or two joints, systemic presentation and is usually seen in middle-aged men presenting with pleurisy, pericarditis, etc. It mimics malignancy. It may present as polymyalgia particularly in elderly patients. It may present as monoarthritic swelling. Sometimes, the presentation may be very explosive unlike the usual chronic presentation. In some cases, it may present as PUO (pyrexia of unknown origin).

Extra-articular Features

Two or more features are present in 75% of the cases. Rheumatoid factor is invariably present and indicates a bad prognosis.

- Subcutaneous nodules are present in 25% of the cases. It is seen over the elbow, sacrum and occiput. Nodules may also be present in lungs, eye, hearts, etc. When present over flexor tendon, it may cause trigger finger.
- Widespread vasculitis leading of Raynaud's phenomenon, digital arteritis, necrotizing arteritis, peripheral neuritis, etc.
- Blood abnormalities commonly encountered in rheumatoid arthritis are chronic anemia, iron deficiency anemia, vitamin B_{12} and folate deficiency, leukocytopenia, thrombocytosis and marrow hypoplasia.
- Osteoporosis could be generalized or localized in bones around the joints.
- Eye changes seen in rheumatoid arthritis are keratoconjunctivitis sicca or Sjögren's syndrome, episcleritis (common), scleritis (serious problem), secondary glaucoma and scleromalacia perforans.
- Lung affections in rheumatoid arthritis are pleurisy, pleural effusion, Caplan's syndrome (RA + pneumoconiosis involving the upper lobes) and fibrosing alveolitis in 2%.
- Heart affections in rheumatoid arthritis are pericardial friction (10%), pericardial effusion (30%), arrhythmias and heart block.
- Neuromuscular system involvement includes carpal tunnel syndrome, mononeuritis multiplex, muscle wasting, subluxation of C_1 and C_2, etc.
- Reticuloendothelial system affections include splenomegaly (5%), Felty's syndrome in 1% (RA+ splenomegaly + neutropenia), generalized lymphadenopathy and painless pitting edema of the feet and ankles.

Orthopedic Deformities in Rheumatoid Arthritis

Rheumatoid arthritis can affect any joint in the body. *It involves the peripheral joints more often and very rarely affects the larger joints.* Of particular importance are the affection of the temporomandibular joint and atlantoaxial joint, which can prove lethal due to the cord compression **(Fig. 25.1)**.

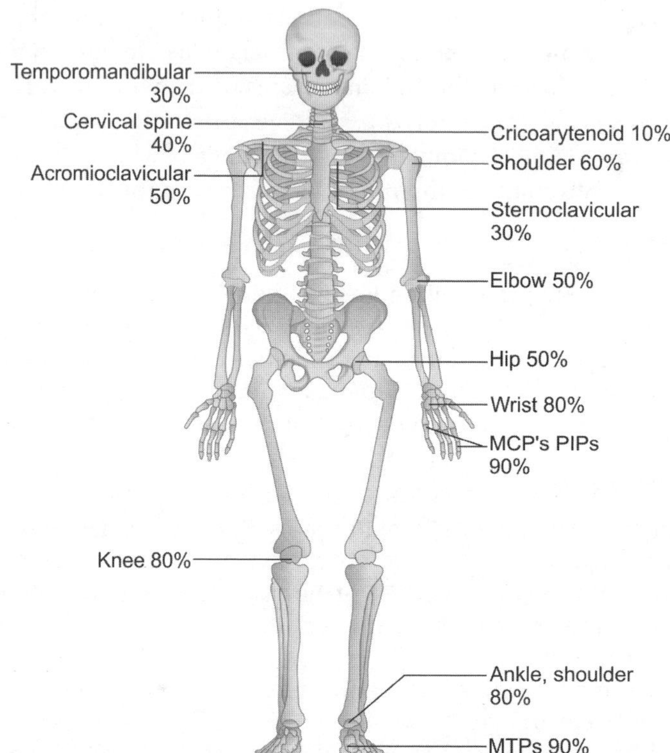

Fig. 25.1: Showing frequency of involvement of different joint sites in established RA.

Orthopedic deformities of the hand (rheumatoid hand) the following are some of the very common deformities seen in the hand **(Figs. 25.2A to D)**.

❖ **Symmetrical peripheral joint swelling** of metacarpophalangeal and interphalangeal joints.
❖ **Ulnar deviation** of the hand is due to rupture of the collateral ligaments at the metacarpophalangeal joints, which enables the extensor tendons to slip from their grooves towards the ulnar side.
❖ **Boutonnière's deformity** is due to the rupture of central extensor expansion of the fingers resulting in flexion at the PIP joint.
❖ **Swan neck deformity** is due to the rupture of the volar plate of the PIP joints which enables the tendons to slip towards the dorsal side. This is also known as *intrinsic plus deformity*. Here there is hyperextension of the PIP joint and flexion of the DIP joints.
❖ **Trigger fingers and trigger thumb** *are* due to nodules over the tendons.

Rheumatoid Foot

It affects the forefoot, midfoot and hindfoot. In the forefoot, patient may develop hallux valgus deformity of the great toe, claw toes, callosity over the dorsum and the sole, widening of the forefoot, etc. The heel may show valgus deformity.

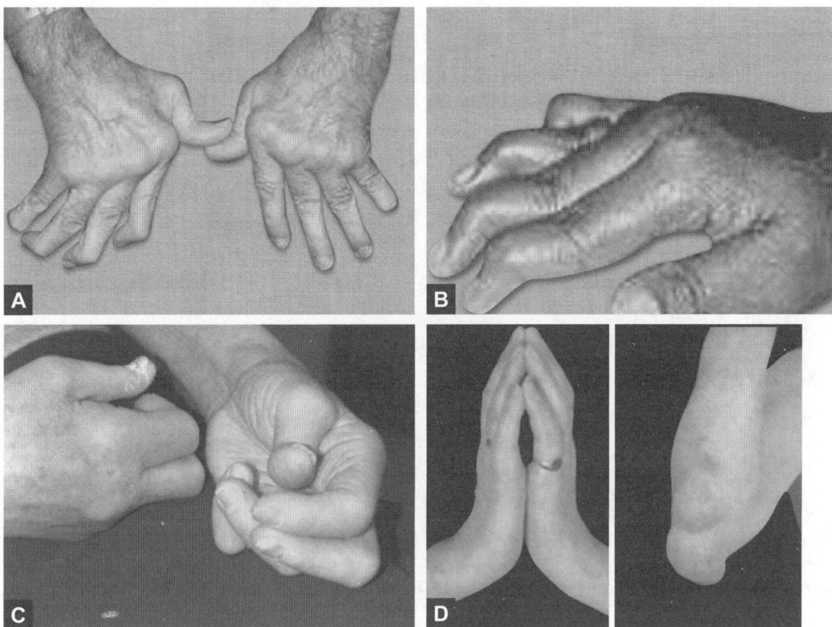

Figs. 25.2A to D: Various orthopedic deformities of the hand in rheumatoid arthritis: (A) Symmetrical swelling of peripheral joints, ulnar deviation of the fingers; (B) Swan neck deformity; (C) Swan neck deformity thumb and Boutonnière deformity of the fingers; (D) Subcutaneous nodules over the elbow.

Other Joints

In the knee, initially, there is a gross soft tissue swelling due to synovitis and in the later stages, the patient may develop fibrous ankylosis or bony ankylosis due to widespread destruction of the articular cartilage by the pannus. Similarly, other major joints of the body, such as the hip, ankle, shoulder, and elbow could be involved.

Laboratory Investigations

Hb percentage is low and shows normochromic, hypochromic anemia. WBCS are decreased or normal, There are increased lymphocytes and the ESR is raised.

Serological Tests

Usually detects only IgM type of rheumatoid factor.

Radiological Features (Fig. 25.3)

X-rays of the hand and feet and other joints slow the following changes:
- ❖ Soft tissue swelling
- ❖ Juxta-articular osteoporosis
- ❖ Erosion of joint margins
- ❖ Joint spaces are decreased
- ❖ Deformities
- ❖ Atlantoaxial subluxation
- ❖ Subchondral erosions and cyst formation
- ❖ Fibrous and bony ankylosis develops in the late stages.

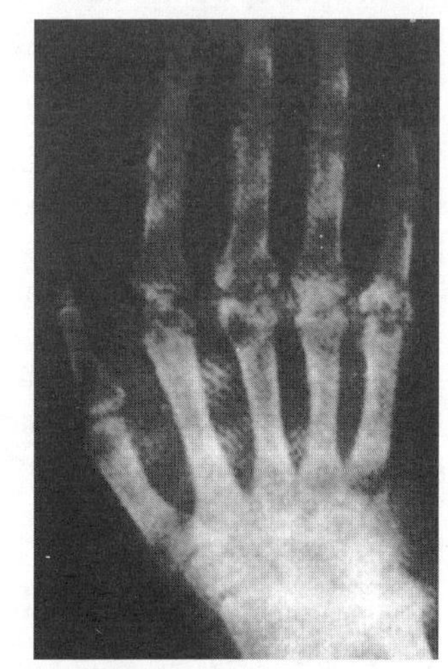

Fig. 25.3 : Radiological features of rheumatoid arthritis.

Other Common Abnormalities

These include increased C-reactive protein (CRP), increased alkaline phosphatase, increased platelets, and decreased serum albumin.

Synovial Fluid Analysis

This is not performed routinely for diagnostic purposes but performed to exclude other causes of inflammation, such as infection.

Synovial fluid in RA is typically yellow, watery and turbid due to high WBC and has low sugar content.

Management (Fig. 25.4)

Aims of Treatment

❖ To keep inflammatory process at a minimum, thereby, preserving joint motion, maintaining healthy muscles and preventing secondary joint stiffness and deformity.
❖ To keep constitutional symptoms at a minimum.
❖ The possible deformities are anticipated and prevented by appropriate splinting.
❖ Finally surgical measures to correct the deformities, eliminate pain and provide stability are undertaken.

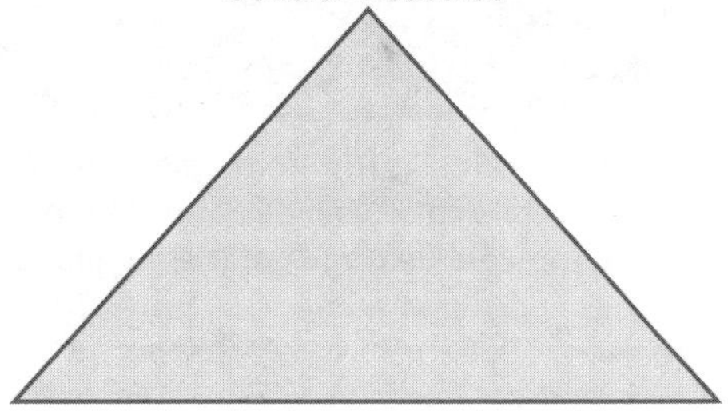

General Measures

It aims at improving the general condition of the patient and to keep the joints properly splinted in functional position to guard against the ensuing ankylosis.

❖ Rest in bed
❖ Good diet, rich in proteins and minerals
❖ Transfusion and hematinics to correct the anemia
❖ Hormones combination of estrogen and androgen to improve the bone stock
❖ Removal of infective foci

Fig. 25.4: Treatment triad for rheumatoid arthritis.

Splints

These are known to serve three main functions:
1. Rest and relief of pain *(rest splints)*
2. Prevention and correction of deformity *(corrective splints)*
3. Fixation of damaged joint in a good functional position *(fixation splints)*

Splinting in the functional position helps in the event that ankylosis ensues. The splint is removed daily. Hot packs are given or patient is placed in Hubbard tank at (92.6–102°F) and the joints are put into full range of motion. While the joints are immobilized, muscle-setting exercises are advocated. After removal of the splints, resistance exercises are begun.

Drug Therapy

It is the mainstay of treatment in rheumatoid arthritis. Three classes of drugs are used regularly.
❖ Analgesics
❖ Anti-inflammatory drugs

❖ Disease modifying antirheumatic drugs (DMARD).
❖ Steroids especially intra-articular injections have an important role.

Physiotherapy Measures in Rheumatoid Arthritis

❖ **Measures to prevent deformities:** Splintages
❖ **Measures to relieve pain:** Heat therapy, tens, etc.
❖ **Measures to mobilize the joints:** Active and passive exercises
❖ **Measures to strengthen the muscles:** Various active, resistive, isometric exercises
❖ Walking aids

Surgery

Aim of surgery in rheumatoid arthritis is to:
❖ Relieve pain
❖ Correct the deformity of the joints
❖ Reduce joint instability
❖ Improve the range of movements of the joints

Surgical Methods

Synovectomy

It may be indicated in patients with rheumatoid arthritis if joint destruction is minimal and if the main cause of pain and swelling is synovitis, which is resistant to medication and physiotherapy. Synovectomy is usually carried out over the knee, ankle, elbow and wrist.

Osteotomy

This should be considered in patients under the age of 60 years with osteoarthritis of the hip or knee due to rheumatoid arthritis. *Osteotomy has the advantage of relieving pain without sacrificing the joint surfaces which have only been partially damaged* **(Fig. 25.5)**.

At the hip, intertrochanteric osteotomy, which contains the femoral head within the acetabulum, is preferred. At the knee, abduction osteotomy is preferred.

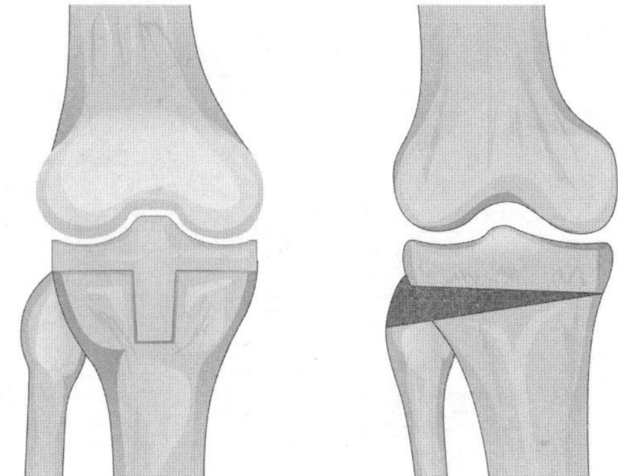

Fig. 25.5: Showing osteotomy.

Arthrodesis of the joint gives excellent long-term pain relief. It is reserved for peripheral joints, such as the wrist, ankle, and IP joints of the hands and feet where the functional loss is less disabling and arthroplasty is less reliable.

Arthroplasties of the hip, knee **(Figs. 25.6 and 25.7)**, ankle, shoulder, elbow, wrist, and hand is indicated in advanced diseases causing severe pain and incapacitating disability due to stiffness and instability.

Self-management Techniques for Rheumatoid and Other Forms of Arthritis: This is the most important aspect of the treatment of rheumatoid and other forms of arthritis. People practicing self-management techniques tend to experience less pain and are more active than those who do not practice self-management. In this management, the patient is made aware of the disease and the rationale behind the treatment. They are made to realize that the success of the treatment is their ultimate responsibility **(Figs. 25.8A to J)**.

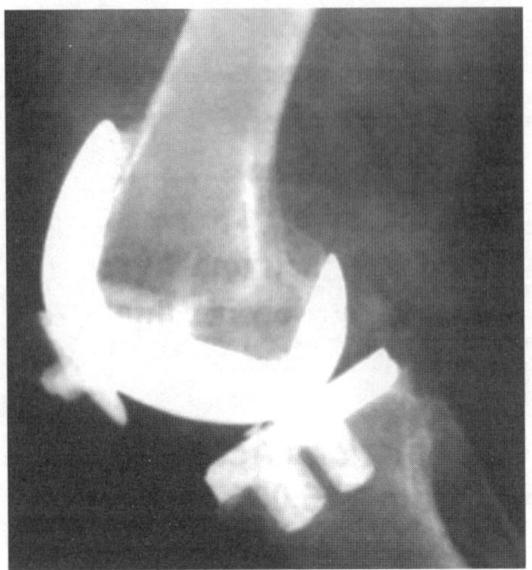

Fig. 25.6: Showing total knee replacement for OA knee.

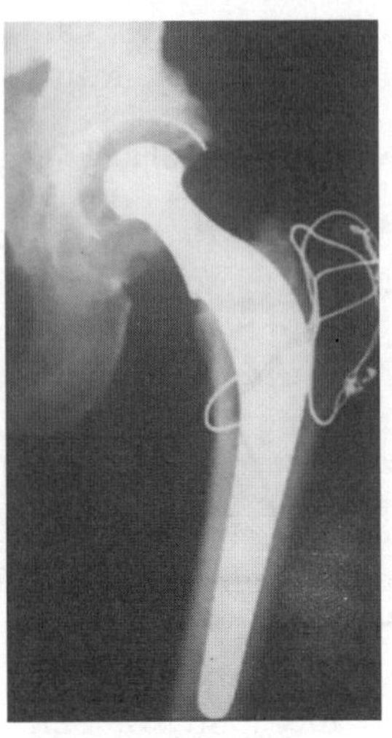

Fig. 25.7: Total hip replacement for osteoarthritis of hip.

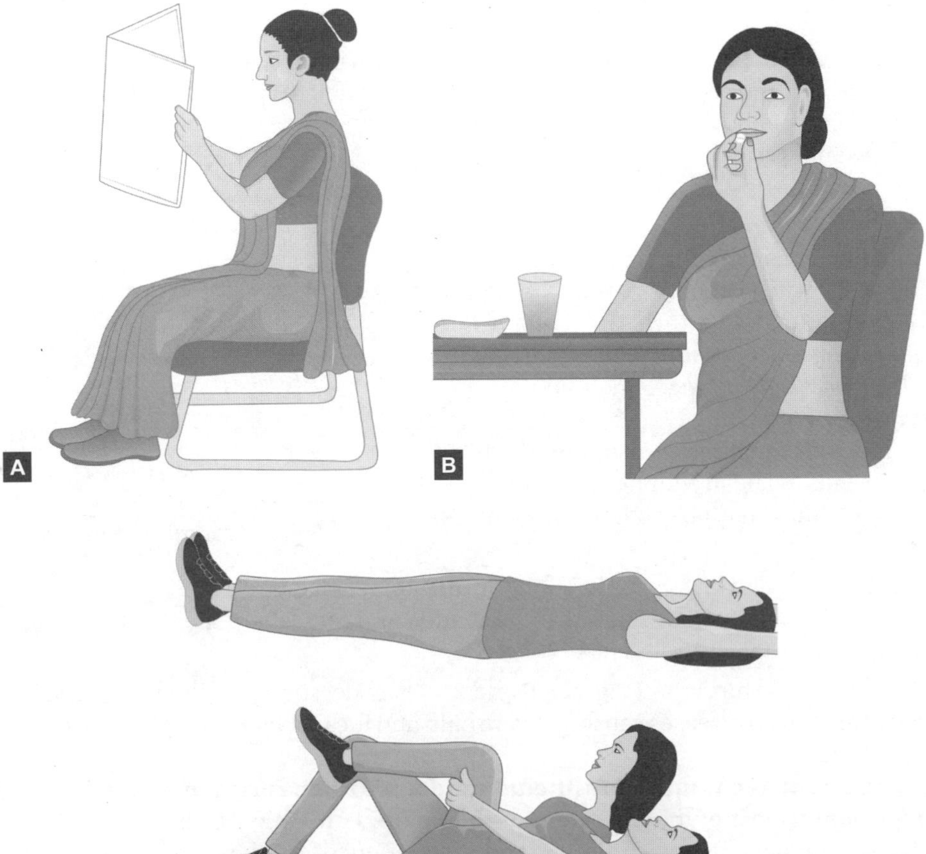

Figs. 25.8A to J: *Contd.....*

Contd.....

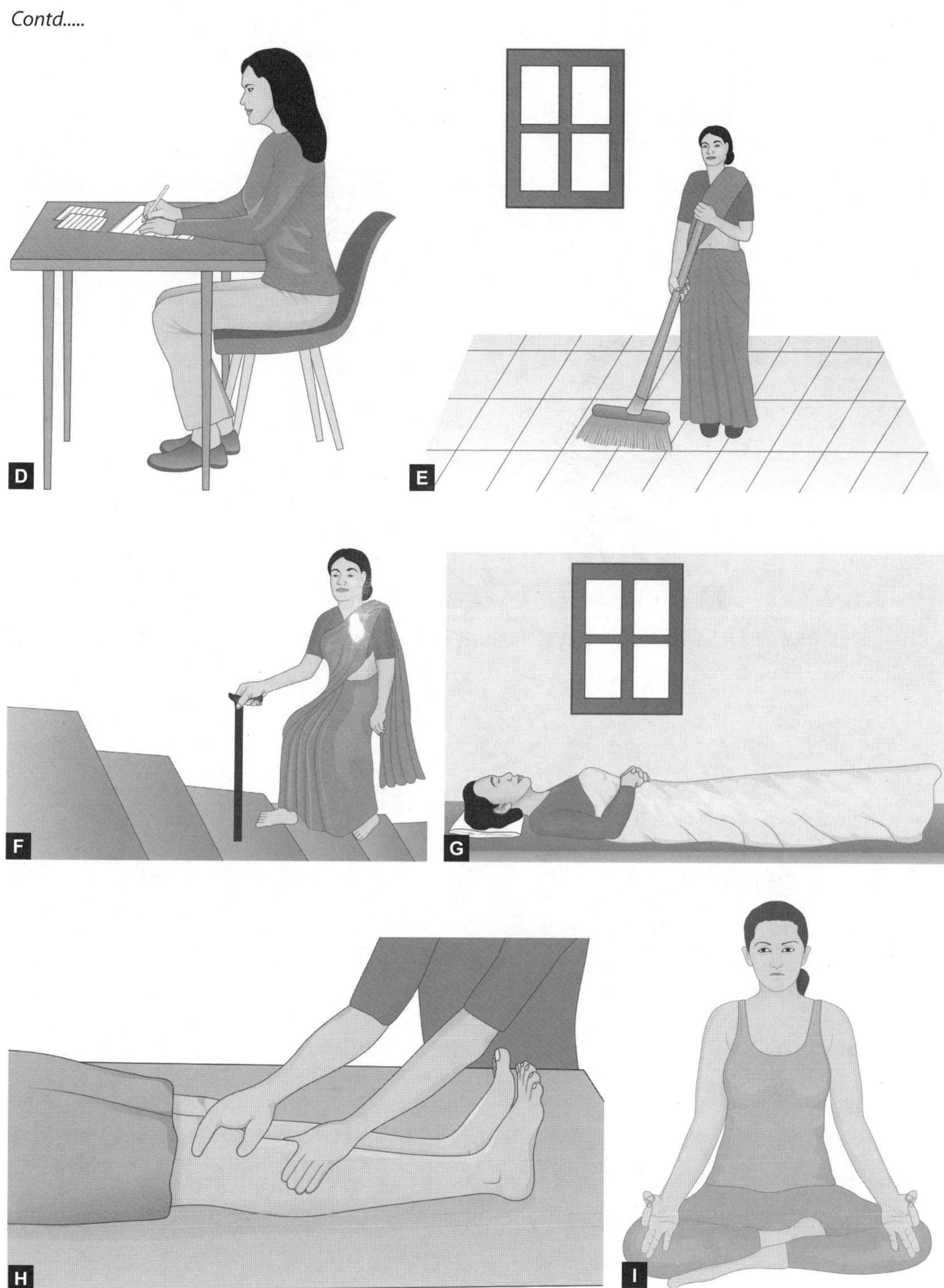

Figs. 25.8A to J: *Contd.....*

Contd.....

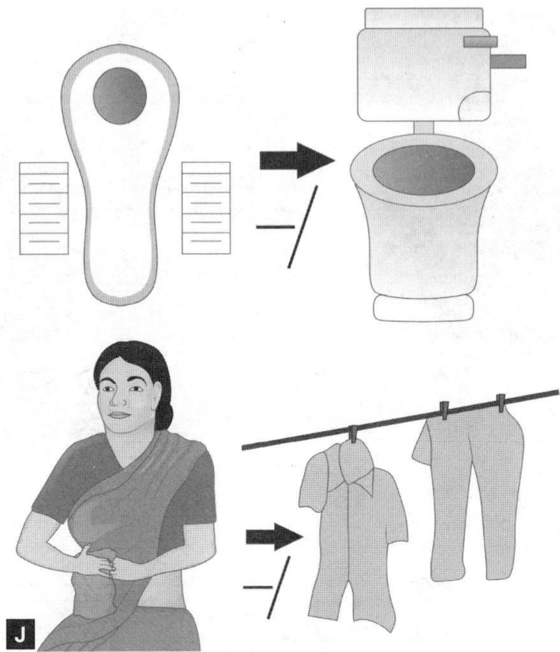

Figs. 25.8A to J: Self-management techniques in the treatment of rheumatoid arthritis.

Degenerative Disorders

OSTEOARTHRITIS

Definition

It is defined as a degenerative, non-inflammatory joint disease characterized by destruction of articular cartilage and formation of new bone at the joint surfaces and margins. There are two varieties—primary and secondary. The former is more common. Knee joint is affected more often than any other joint and is hence discussed first.

Primary Osteoarthritis of the Knee

Etiological Causes for Primary Osteoarthritis

Though exact cause is not known, the following factors are suspected to play an important role in the causation of primary osteoarthritis—obesity, genetics and heredity, occupation involving prolonged standing, sports, endocrinal and metabolic disorders.

Important Predisposing Factors in the Indians

Use of Indian toilets and squatting cross legged on the ground places the knee joints in extreme flexion and this over the years causes enormous stress on the knees and hastens its degeneration (**Figs. 26.1 and 26.2**).

Features

❖ It commonly affects the knee joint.
❖ All races are susceptible.
❖ Common in older age groups.
❖ 80% of people are affected by 40 years, but only 40% show symptoms.
❖ It causes varus deformity of the knee in the late stages.

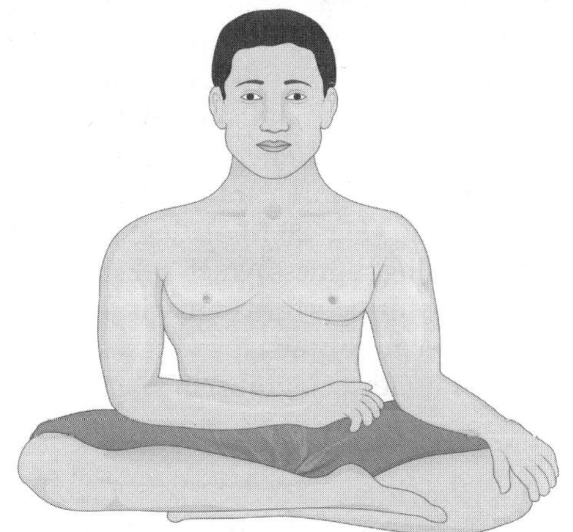

Fig. 26.1: Showing the habit of squatting in the contains that places abnormal stress on the body.

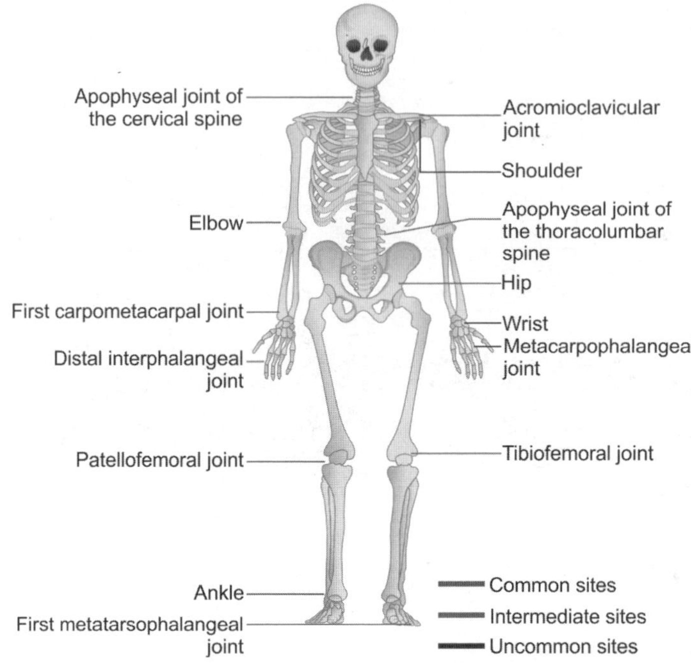

Fig. 26.2: Showing common sites of osteoarthritis.

Sequence of pathological events in osteoarthritis leads to destruction of the articular cartilage **(Fig. 26.3)** which later affects all structures of the joint secondarily **(Fig. 26.4)**.

Clinical Features

Predominant symptom is pain which decreases on walking. The pain is poorly localized and is dull aching in nature. Patient has mild swelling of the knee joint and complains of early morning stiffness. Minimal tenderness and coarse crepitus can be elicited. If there are loose bodies in a joint, patient gives history of locking or giving way. Terminal movements of the knee are restricted **(Fig. 26.5)**. Patient complains of early morning stiffness which subsides over the day after some activity. Genu varum deformity may be seen in very advanced cases **(Fig. 26.6)**. Minimal quadriceps muscle wasting may be seen.

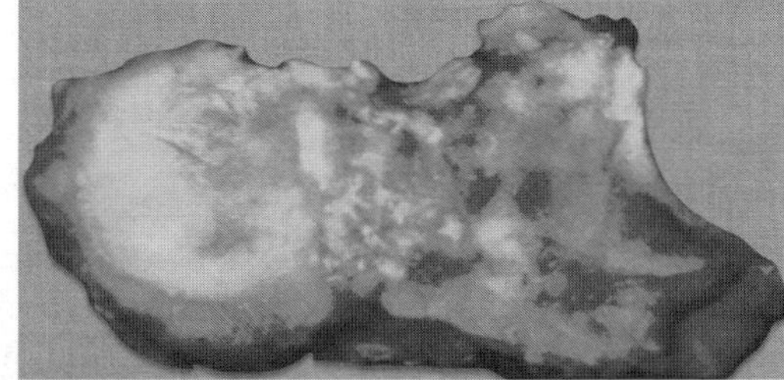

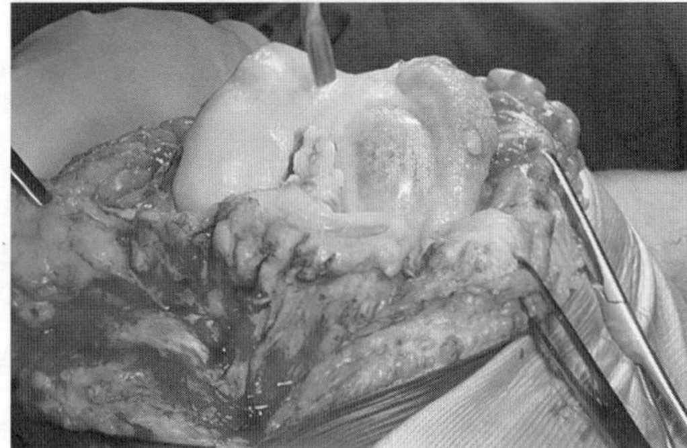

Fig. 26.3: Pathological features of the osteoarthritis knee.

Investigations

Laboratory investigations are usually within normal limits. Radiological examination of the knee joint is the most important diagnostic tool. The radiological features seen in osteoarthritis of the knee **(Fig. 26.7)**.

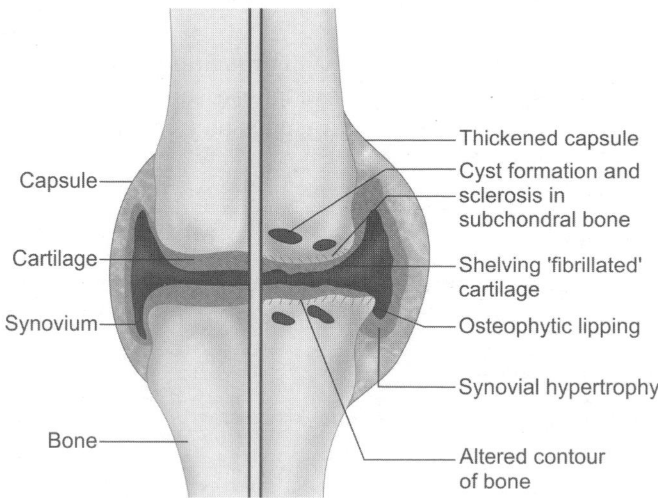

Fig. 26.4: Structures affected in OA Knees.

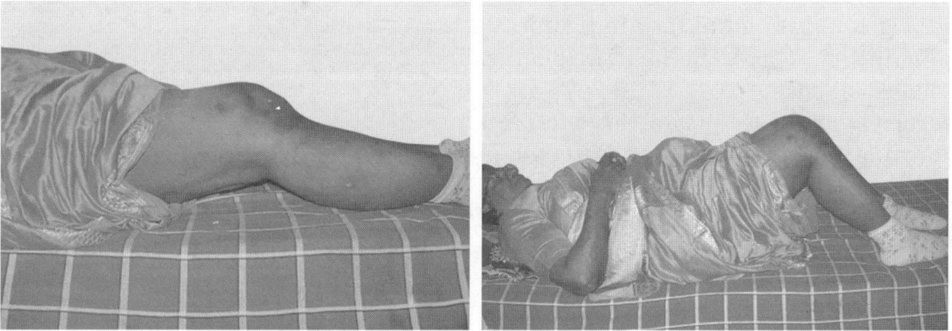

Fig. 26.5: Loss of terminal flexion in osteoarthritis knee.

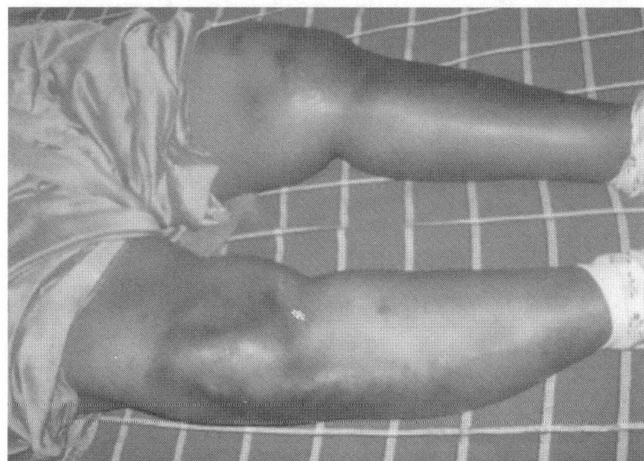

Fig. 26.6: Genu varum deformity in osteoarthritis of knee.

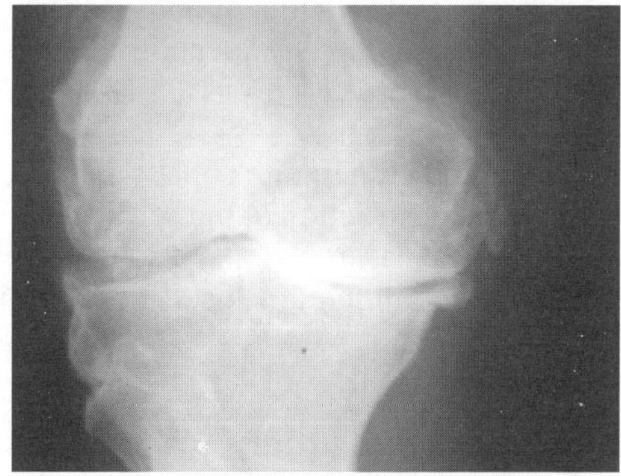

Fig. 26.7: Radiograph of the knee joint: Showing loss of joint space, osteophytes, subchondral sclerosis and varus deformity.

Other Investigations

Synovial fluid analysis shows non-inflammatory picture. Bone scan shows increased uptake of technetium-99m, MRI and CT scan also helps to diagnose, subchondral cysts, osteophytes, etc., but are rarely employed. Arthroscopic procedure helps both in diagrams and therapy.

Treatment

Conservative Treatment

This forms the mainstay of management in osteoarthritis of the knee. About 50% of patients respond to conservative treatment, which consists of the following measures:

Nonpharmocological Therapy

According to the American College of Rheumatology guidelines, this is the most important part of the treatment.

❖ Patient education
❖ Reduction of weight.
❖ Isometric quadriceps exercises **(Fig. 26.8)**.
❖ **Physiotherapy:** This consists of heat therapy and is given through ultrasound, short wave diathermy, TENS, etc. This helps to relieve pain and muscle spasm.
❖ **Exercises:** Exercises play a very vital role in improving the joint mobility and strengthening the muscles of the hip, knee and legs.

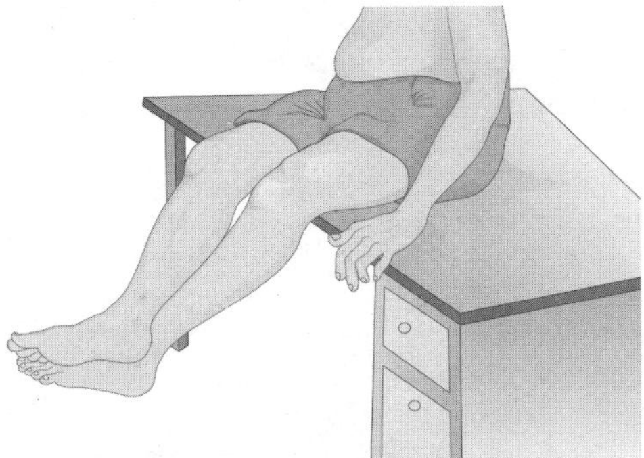

Fig. 26.8: Showing method of quadriceps exercises.

❖ **Modifications of daily living activities:** This is the most important aspect of the management of knee joint osteoarthritis and the patients themselves have practiced this.

Pharmacological Therapy

❖ Acetaminophen (Paracetamol) is an analgesic and is the first line of drug as OA is not an inflammatory condition. It is a least toxic drug and can be given upto 4 g/day.
❖ Nonsteroidal anti-inflammatory drugs (NSAIDs) are indicated if the patient fails to respond to Paracetamol. They are known for the GI side effects.
❖ Cartilage protective drugs like Glucosamine, Chondroitin sulfate are being tried with varied success.
❖ Viscosupplementation consist of injecting hyaluronidase drug into the joint. It is known to slow the destruction of the cartilages.
❖ Intra-articular injections of steroids if the patient fails to respond to the drugs (not more than 3 recommended, local anesthetic is avoided for fear of developing neuropathic joint).

Surgery

Indications for Surgery

❖ Pain that is refractory to conservative measures.
❖ History of frequent locking episodes.
❖ Hemarthrosis due to loose bodies or osteochondral fractures.

❖ Deformity usually genu varum.
❖ Joint instability.
❖ Progressive limitation of knee motion.

Surgical Methods

❖ Excision of osteophytes is rarely done alone.
❖ **Arthroscopic treatment:** Excision of loose bodies, meniscectomy, synovectomy, joint lavage and reconstruction or joint debridement are best done by arthroscopy.
❖ **Proximal tibial osteotomy (Slocum's):** It is indicated for unicompartmental osteoarthritis of knee with pain and also to correct varus (less than 15°) or valgus deformity (less than 12°). Pain is decreased in 80% of the cases following surgery as osteotomy changes the line of weight bearing and brings the more normal surface to carry out the function of load transmission **(Figs. 26.9A and B)**.
❖ **Distal femoral osteotomy:** It is indicated when varus or valgus deformity of the knee is more than 12–15°.
❖ **Total knee arthroplasty:** This is indicated when both the compartments of the knee joint are destroyed or if valgus or varus deformity is more than 15°. It is also indicated in failed conservative treatment **(Fig. 26.10)**.
❖ **Arthrodesis:** It is indicated less commonly than arthroplasty. If the patient is young and involved in heavy occupations, arthrodesis is indicated to give him a stable and strong knee. However, arthrodesis results in a stiff knee which is a severe disability.
❖ **Patellectomy:** It is rarely done except as a last resort. Contemplated in osteoarthritis present for several years.

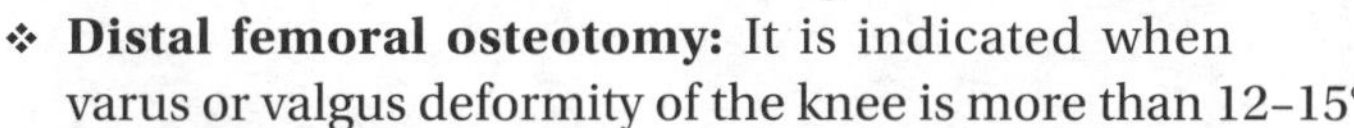

Figs. 26.9A and B: High tibial osteotomy in osteoarthritis: (A) Before operation; (B) After operation.

Fig. 26.10: Showing total knee replacement.

SECONDARY OSTEOARTHRITIS OF KNEE

The causes for secondary osteoarthritis of the knee are as follows:
❖ Obesity, valgus and varus deformities of the knee.
❖ Intra-articular fractures of the knee, etc.
❖ Rheumatoid arthritis, infection, trauma, TB, etc.
❖ Hyperparathyroidism.
❖ Hemophilia.
❖ Syringomyelia.
❖ Neurological diseases like diabetes.
❖ Overuse of intra-articular steroid therapy.

It is generally observed that secondary osteoarthritis occurs in the younger age groups and is more severe than the primary. Apart from all the features of osteoarthritis, secondary osteoarthritis has the features of the corresponding etiological condition.

OSTEOARTHRITIS IN OTHER REGIONS

Osteoarthritis spine (lumbar spondylosis): It is usually seen in the elderly age group and the patient presents with low backache. Osteophytes may compress the nerve roots at their exit at the intervertebral foramen and may cause neurological disturbances **(Fig. 26.11)**. Conservative treatment usually helps but surgery may be required for prolonged pain and neurological deficits.

Osteoarthritis of the small joints: Osteoarthritis may affect the peripheral joints of the hand and foot **(Fig. 26.12)**. It may cause ankylosis at an increased rate in these joints **(Fig. 26.13)**.

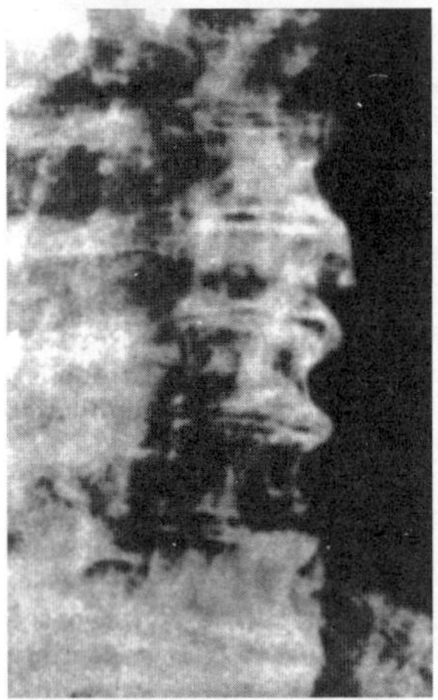

Fig. 26.11: Lumbar spine: Narrowing of disc space and osteophyte formation.

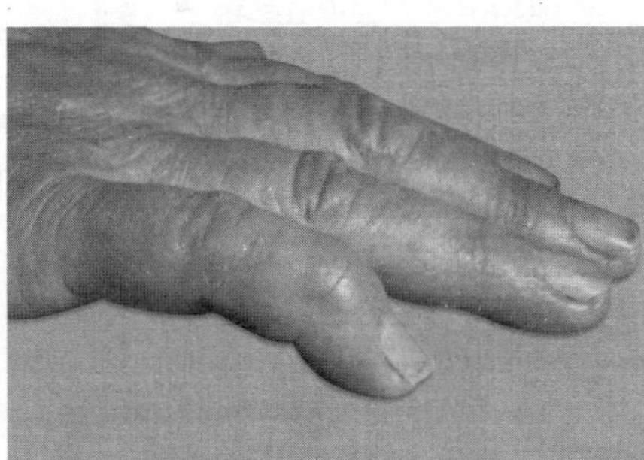

Fig. 26.12: Showing finger OA.

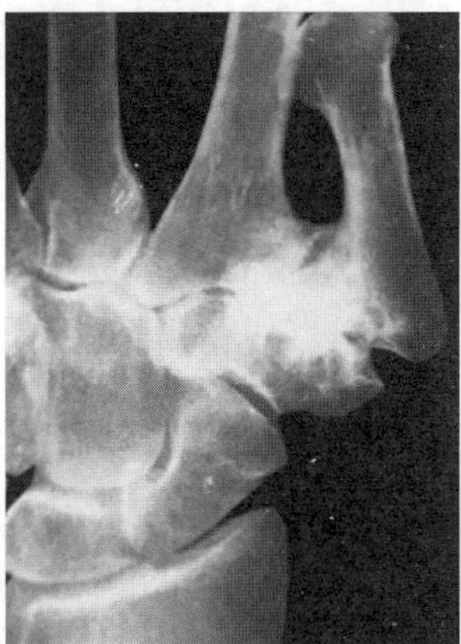

Fig. 26.13: Osteoarthritis of the carpometacarpal joint of the thumb: loss of joint space and sclerosis.

Cervical Disc Syndromes

Cervical spondylosis has been discussed at depth in the chapter as regional disorders of the neck. Students are requested to go through it.

Neuromuscular Disorders

CEREBRAL PALSY (CP)

Definition

This is a disorder of movement and posture caused by a nonprogressive lesion in the immature brain.

Lesions

In cerebral palsy, the lesion could be either in the brain or the upper cervical cord.

Incidence is 0.6–5.9/1,000 live birth.

Lesions in the Brain

In cerebral palsy, the lesions in the brain can occur in the following four areas:
1. Cerebral cortex (spastic type)
2. Midbrain (dyskinesia)
3. Cerebellum (ataxic)
4. Widespread brain involvement (rigidity and mixed)

Causes

In cerebral palsy, the causes are different in prenatal, natal, postnatal and perinatal period.

Note: Birth asphyxia is the commonest cause of CP.

Clinical Features

Clinical features could be mild, moderate or severe. This depends on the location of lesions in the brain. Single muscle involvement is rare as in polio and entire portion of the body supplied by that area of brain is involved. Patients show delayed milestones and primitive reflexes are usually preserved.

Other clinical features depend on the geographic distribution of cerebral palsy and the associated handicapping situations. Involvement of pyramidal tract (65%) causes spasticity, increased reflexes, clonus, etc. This may involve one or more limbs. The most common lower limb deformities are flexion and adduction of the hip, flexion of the knee and equinus of the ankle **(Figs. 27.1 and 27.2)**. In the upper limbs, it is flexion of the wrist and fingers, pronation of

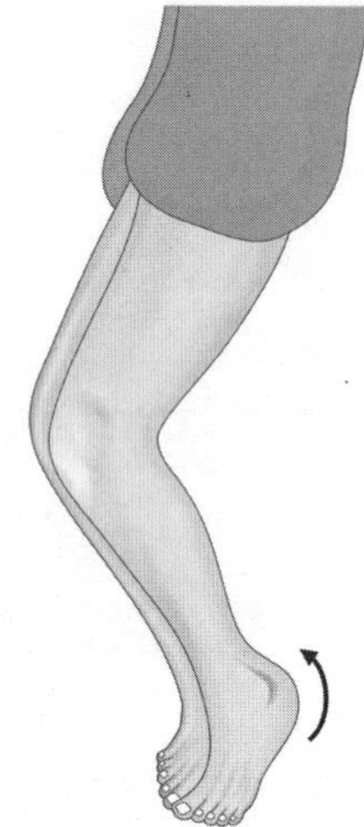

Fig. 27.1: Spastic contracture of the hip, knee and foot in cerebral palsy.

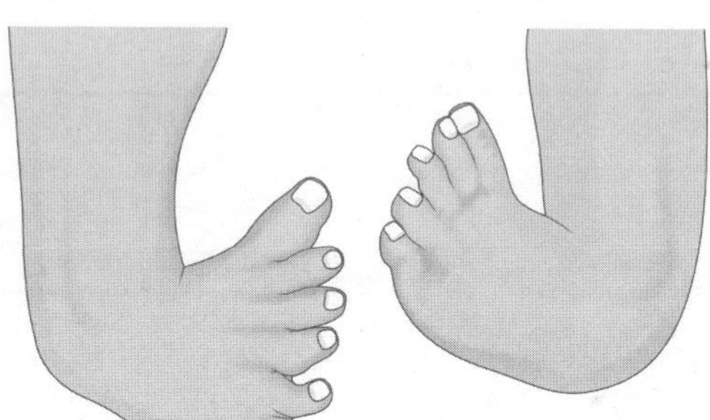

Fig. 27.2: Spastic equinovarus.

the forearm and thumb abduction. Variable muscle weakness leads to muscle imbalance and deformities. Sustained pressure helps overcome the spasticity at the joints only to return in toto with vengeance once the pressure is released. Involvement of extrapyramidal tract causes ataxia, athetosis, dystonia, etc., there could be one or more associated findings.

Treatment

Unfortunately, there is no cure for cerebral palsy. Hence, the *aim of treatment is to increase patient's assets as much as possible and minimize his or her defects.*

Order of preference to improve the quality of life in cerebral palsy is as follows:
❖ Education and communication is the first priority
❖ Training and assistance in the activities of daily life
❖ Mobility
❖ Ambulation

The role of orthopedic surgeon starts when the child is 12 months of age and seldom before.

Methods

❖ Motor age test.
❖ Physiotherapy, occupational therapy, speech therapy, etc., are the most important adjunctive treatment measures.
❖ Use of braces to:
  ◆ Improve function
  ◆ Control unnecessary movements
  ◆ Prevent and correct deformities
❖ **Drug therapy:** The role of drug therapy is disappointing. Muscle relaxants, antiepileptic may have a role.

❖ Surgery
  ◆ Not done till 5 years of age.
  ◆ Indicated to correct deformity in an ambulatory patient and to make him or her socially more acceptable.
  ◆ Commonly indicated in spastic type of CP.

<table><tr><td>Aim of surgery in cerebral palsy is</td></tr><tr><td>1. To correct the deformity.
2. To balance the muscle power.
3. To stabilize uncontrollable joints.</td></tr></table>

POLIOMYELITIS

Definition

This is a viral infection of the anterior horn cell of the spinal cord **(Fig. 27.3)** or nerve cells of brainstem, resulting in temporary or permanent paralysis. Common in children, often attacks young adults.

Viruses

The following Picorna group of viruses is known to cause poliomyelitis: Brunhilde (type I), Leon (type II), and ansing (type III).

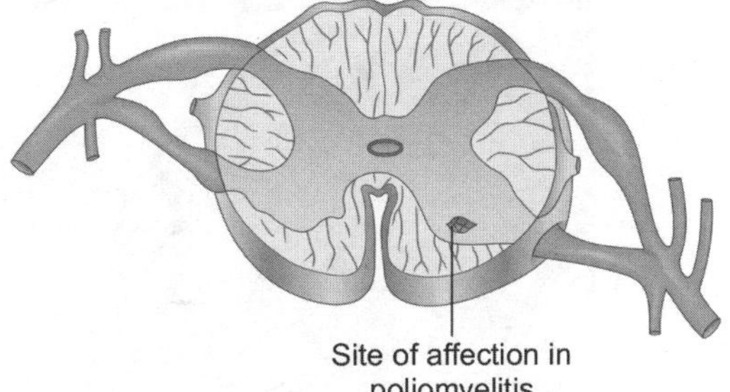

Fig. 27.3: Showing site of affection in polio.

<table><tr><td>Quick facts</td></tr><tr><td>In polio, the scene is set by the infection only something needs to pull the trigger to target the anterior horn cells. The trigger is let loose by one of the following events:
◄◄ Falls or any other trauma
◄◄ Intramuscular injections
◄◄ Any strenuous physical activity
◄◄ Surgeries like tonsillectomy, adenoidectomy, etc.
◄◄ Tooth extraction</td></tr></table>

Clinical Features

Polio usually affects children less than 12 months. There is a mild episode of fever, headache and diarrhea. On examination, there could be mild neck stiffness and the child may find it difficult to move the affected limb (pre-paralytic). The lower limbs are more commonly affected and the paralysis could be partial or total (paralytic stage).

The paralysis of the muscles whether spinal (75%) or bulbar (25%) usually lasts until 2 months. Then there may or may be not be recovery for a period of two years. Any residual paralysis after two years of affection is permanent with no chance of recovery. Bulbar poliomyelitis is rare and affects the respiratory muscles. It may be fatal.

Orthopedic Deformities

Orthopedic deformities encountered in poliomyelitis are shown in **Figures 27.4A to D.**

Treatment

Supportive treatment during the early stages of the disease.

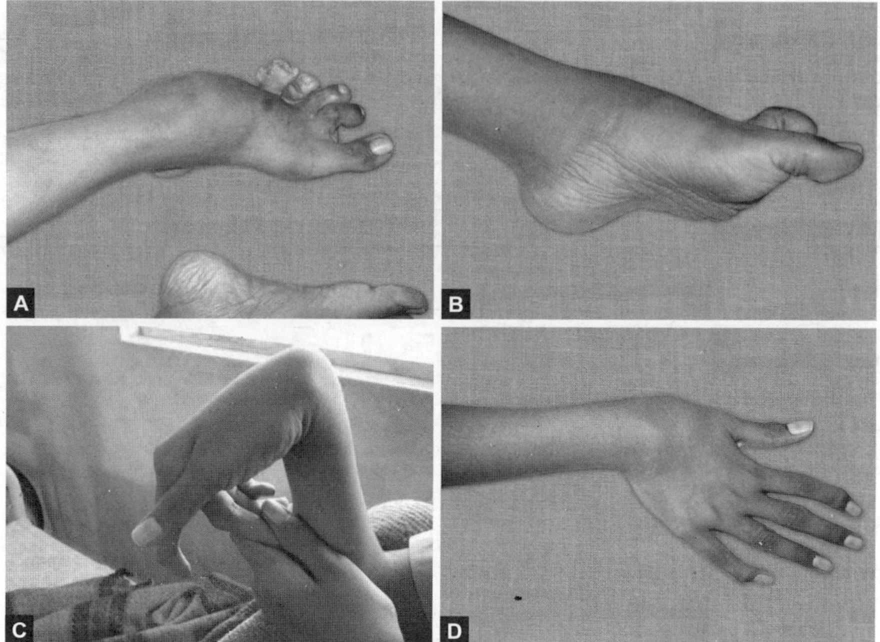

Figs. 27.4A to D: Showing various foot deformities (A and B) and hand deformities (C and D) in poliomyelitis.

1. To prevent deformities from developing.
2. To assist returning of muscle power by graduated exercises.
3. To reduce disability by appropriate appliance or by operations on joints and muscles.

Treatment Methods

Early stages: During the stages of onset, maximum paralysis and the stages of recovery, the child is admitted into the hospital and supportive treatment is given. The child is put on a ventilator support if there is respiratory paralysis due to bulbar polio. Warm and moist packs are given to the joints and all intramuscular injections are avoided during this phase. Plaster splints in functional positions immobilize the affected joints.

Recovery stages: In this stage, the joints are properly splinted through various appliances to prevent or correct the deformities.

Role of Appliances

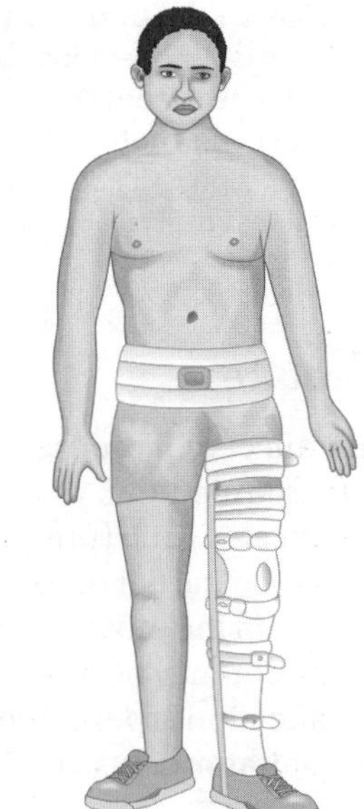

Fig. 27.5: Showing an above knee caliper (KAFO) in a polio patient.

The purpose of external appliances is to support joints that have lost their normal control. They are more often required for lower limbs rather than upper limbs **(Fig. 27.5).**

Stage of Post-polio Residual Paralysis

During this stage, the role of orthopedic surgeon is predominant and surgery is the treatment of choice.

Goals of Surgery

1. To obtain muscle balance.
2. To prevent or correct soft tissue contractures.
3. To prevent or correct bony deformities.

Surgical methods: These include soft tissue release for soft tissue contractures, tendon and bone surgeries like osteotomy, arthrodesis and ilizarov techniques for deformity corrections.

28
CHAPTER

Bone Neoplasias

Like other systems in the body, musculoskeletal system may also develop tumors, either as a **primary** from this system itself or as a **secondary** from a distant primary location. The *latter appears to be more common*. Some of the tumors are benign and others are malignant. The accurate diagnosis of a neoplasm is a must before planning the treatment strategy. Diagnosis is best established by history, a proper physical examination and investigations like histopathological examination, biochemical assays, X-ray, CT scan, MRI, bone scans, arteriography, ultrasound, biopsy (both frozen section and permanent paraffin section), etc.

Primary bone tumors may be benign or malignant. Tumors spreading secondarily to the bone are generally primary carcinomas of breast, kidney, thyroid and lung. These tumors are called *metastatic carcinomas* because the tissue of origin is ectoderm. Secondaries of the bone are always malignant. Let us explore only important tumor conditions in orthopedics.

OSTEOCHONDROMA

This is the most common benign bone tumor. It is an offshoot from the spongy bone tissue covered with a cartilaginous cap (size of the cap may vary from 1 to 40 cm).

Age

It is common during the growth period and ceases to grow once the growth plate fuses. Hence, it is not a true tumor.

Sex

It has a male preponderance.

Area

Location favors the sites of *tendinous attachments, which* are usually around the metaphysis of long bones in the region of knee, ankle, hip, shoulder and elbow.

Clinical Features

Symptoms

Usually, it is symptom less but patient may complain of pain, swelling, etc., once complications like bursitis, malignant change, fracture, etc., have developed **(Fig. 28.1)**.

Signs

A firm nontender swelling fixed to the bone around the joints is the most common clinical finding. A bursa if inflamed will give rise to tenderness and local warmth. Joint movements may be decreased because of the tumor causing a mechanical block rather than the extension of the tumor into the joint.

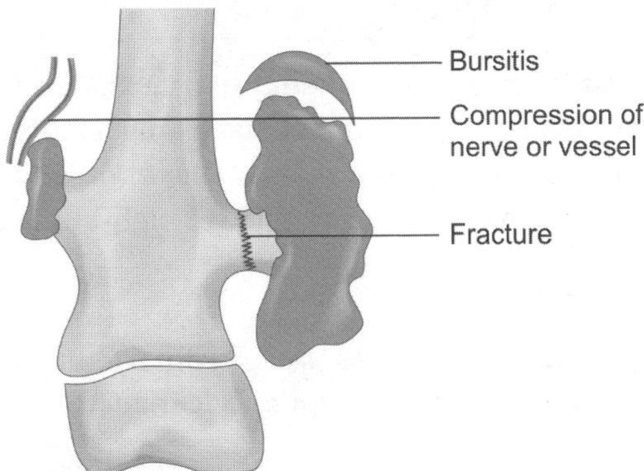

Fig. 28.1: Osteochondroma and some of its complications.

Radiographic Features

This consists of an outgrowth of bone at the metaphysis. This attachment is sessile or pedunculated. The tumor is composed of cortical and medullary portions, which *are continuous with the main bone.* The cartilage and capsules are not seen *unless it calcifies* **(Fig. 28.2)**.

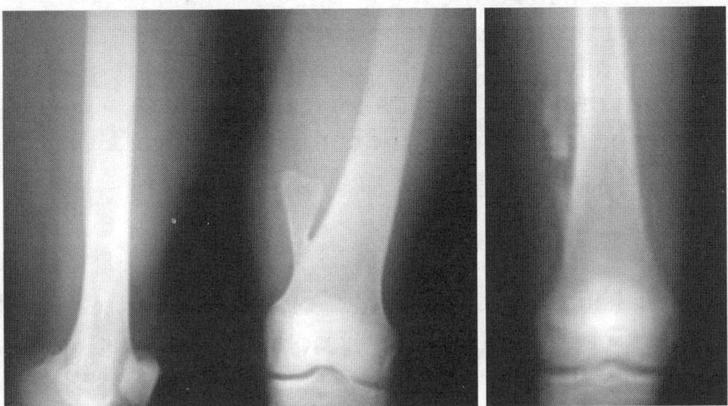

Fig. 28.2: X-ray showing osteochondroma.

Treatment

Usually, it requires no treatment but complete surgical excision is indicated in the following situations:

- ❖ **Joint interference** if the tumor is large and obstructing the joint movements, it needs excision of the tumor along with its periosteal cover to prevent recurrence of the tumor.
- ❖ **Painful bursitis** a bursa usually develops because of the constant friction between the tumor and the surrounding soft tissues. If inflammation develops within this bursa, it gives rise to pain necessitating its excision.
- ❖ **Fracture** of the bony stalk may occur due to trauma.
- ❖ **Malignant change** (1–2%) local irradiation may convert this benign tumor into malignant. It grows rapidly and has to be excised.
- ❖ **Pressure on the neighboring vessels** and nerves may give rise to neurovascular complications.

CHONDROSARCOMA

This is *second* in frequency to osteosarcoma. It arises from the cartilage cells. It is a malignant but *slow* growing tumor. It has a long history and a better prognosis. Unlike osteogenic sarcoma, there is *no neoplastic osteoid formation and alkaline phosphatase is usually not raised*. It ranges from being locally aggressive to high-grade malignancy.

Location

It is common at the sites of proximal femur, humerus, ribs, and scapula, in nominate bones, rare in hands and feet except in calcaneus, and occur in pelvis or upper femora.

Sex

Males are more commonly affected than females.

Age

Twenty to sixty years, rare below 20 years, peak in the sixth decade.

Symptoms

The duration of symptoms are usually less than 2 years in 75% of the cases and less than 5 years in the remaining 25%. Pain is usually not a prominent feature unlike osteogenic sarcoma. The central tumor remains entirely asymptomatic until it has eroded and penetrated the cortex or caused a pathological fracture. A palpable firm mass attached to the bone is the common physical sign. The tumor may assume large proportion **(Fig. 28.3)**.

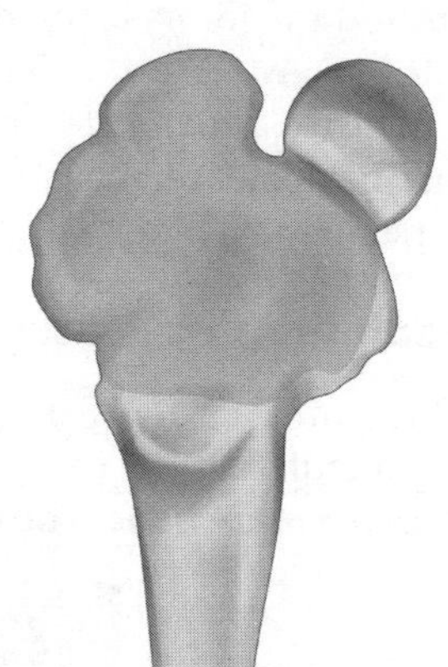

Fig. 28.3: Chondrosarcoma affecting the upper end of the femur.

Radiology

Central lytic lesion with calcification gives a fluffy, cotton wool, popcorn or breadcrumb appearance **(Fig. 28.4)**. Metaphysis or diaphysis of the long tubular bone is usually affected. Greater degree of calcification is observed in slow growing tumors.

Treatment

Surgery is the treatment of choice.
Low and medium grade lesions require wide excision, e.g., forequarter amputation (Thikor-Linberg) for the shoulder girdle; hindquarter amputation for the pelvic girdle.

High grade lesions require radical marginal excision. The role of systemic chemotherapy in chondrosarcoma is controversial.

Palliative radiotherapy is indicated when the tumor cannot be resected because of its enormous size or if the tumor is present in inaccessible region.

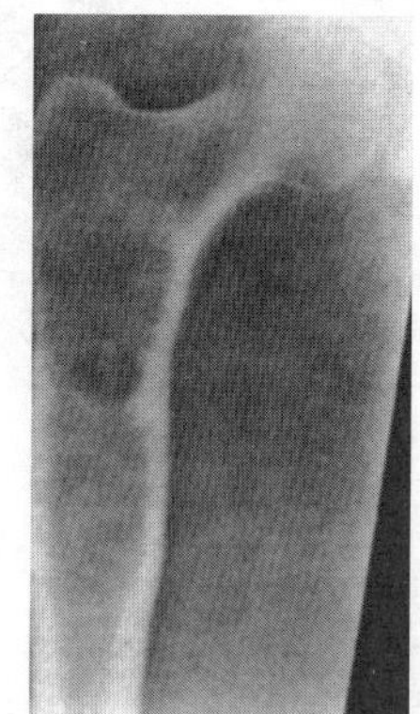

Fig. 28.4: Radiograph showing chondrosarcoma.

OSTEOID OSTEOMA

This is a benign osteoblastic tumor with a well-demarcated nidus of less than 1 cm surrounded by a distinct reactive bone **(Fig. 28.5)**. This tumor presents very interesting clinical features. It is a tumor of young adults, benign in nature and occurs in endochondral bones.

Age

It is common in young adults between 10 to 25 years of age

Sex

Male preponderance (M: F = 2:1)

Sites

The diaphysis of long bones usually tibia, femur are more commonly affected. The posterior vertebral elements are the other favorable sites.

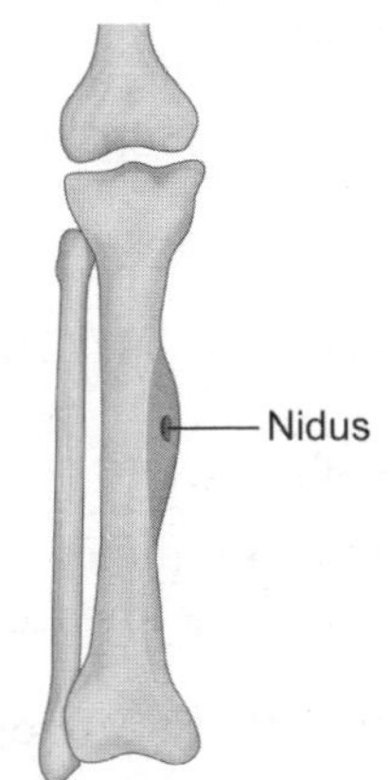

Fig. 28.5: Showing osteoid osteoma in tibia.

Clinical Features

Patient complains of vague and intermittent pain, which is more at night. The pain dramatically decreases after giving aspirin so much so that this is called the *therapeutic test*. Patient also complains of limp due to pain. There is a mild swelling, the local area may be tender, temperature is not raised, and the skin is not stretched, shiny or warm. When the lesion occurs in the spine, patient presents with acute low backache.

Radiology

It usually shows small-rarefied lesion < 2 cm in diameter found in either the cortex, subcortical or subperiosteal regions. It is surrounded by a thick sclerotic bone. A small dense center of ossification seen in the center as the *nidus* (**Fig. 28.6**). 5% of the cases of sciatica are due to osteoid osteoma. CT scan and MRI also help in diagnosing this tumor.

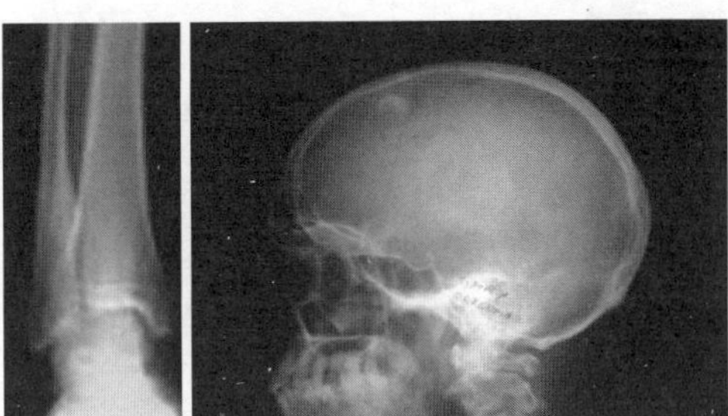

Fig. 28.6: Radiograph showing osteoid osteoma.

Treatment

Conservative line of treatment consists of rest to the part and analgesics. If the tumor is too troublesome, complete excision of the cortex, containing the nidus is sufficient.

Note: Osteoid osteoma is the commonest 'true' bone tumor.

OSTEOGENIC SARCOMA

Osteogenic sarcoma is a highly malignant primary bone tumor. Here tumor cells invariably form a neoplastic osteoid, bone, or both. It arises from a common multifactorial mesenchymal tissue and hence the tumor could be either *fibroblastic, osteoblastic* or *chondroblastic*. This is the most frequent primary bone tumor next only to multiple myeloma.

Age

It is common in the second decade, rare below 10 years of age, 75% of the cases are seen below the age of 25 years.

Sex

Male preponderance, when found in females it starts at an early age.

Incidence

Incidence is 1/75,000 population.

Site

90% of the tumor occurs in the metaphysial region of the ends of long bones. It has a predilection around the knee and upper humerus. It may affect the jaws in the aged.

Clinical Features

The patient usually presents with pain as the first symptom. It precedes the tumor, is seen first at night and is intermittent in nature. History of trauma is a common feature. Patient complains of tired feeling and limp. General condition is good till the late stages. Pyrexia is seen with increased WBCs. Patient is usually anemic than cachectic. Swelling develops later and the skin over the tumor is stretched, shiny and mobile **(Fig. 28.7)**. Local temperature is increased, consistency of the tumor is variable, dilated veins are present (and is evident at an early stage). Pathological fracture is not typical of osteogenic sarcoma since the swelling and pain keeps the patient off his or her feet. The nearest joint may show pain and effusion. Joint movements may be unimpaired but there could be a mechanical block caused by the tumor bulk. Neurovascular structures could be compressed.

Spread

1. It is mainly by blood spread, lungs are involved in 80% of the cases.
2. Lymphatic spread to regional lymph nodes is seen in 30% of the cases.

Investigations

Laboratory tests reveal Hb percentage decreased, alkaline phosphate (Alk PO_4) increased, ESR increased, WBCs increased, etc.

Special Radiographic Features

Sunray appearance seen in the subperiosteal space and it is due to deposition of tumor osteoid along the vessels.

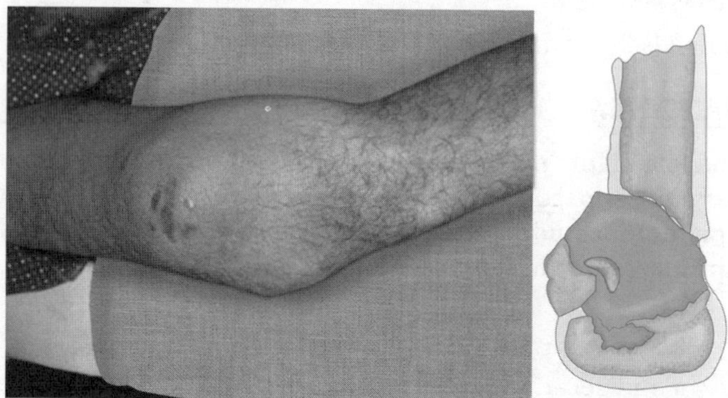

Fig. 28.7: Showing clinical photograph of osteogenic sarcoma lower end of femur.

Codman's triangle: This is a reactive bone formation parallel to the bone and is triangular, it is not specific to osteosarcoma as it is also seen in Ewing's sarcoma and chronic osteomyelitis (**Fig. 28.8**).

Pathological fracture: If the bone tumor grows fast, new bone formation is weak and pathological fracture may occur. It is commonly not seen.

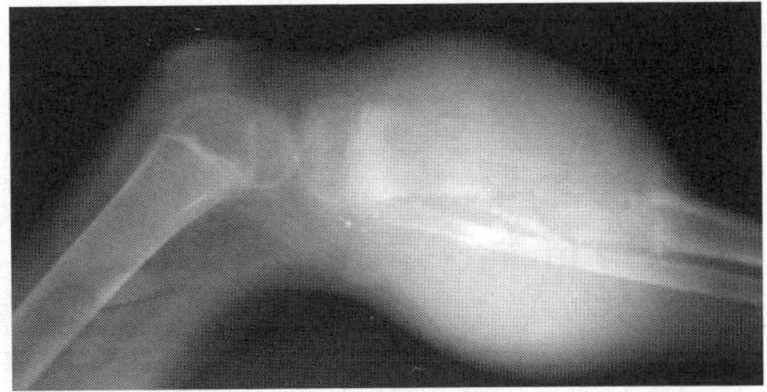

Fig. 28.8: Osteosarcoma upper end of tibia.

Other Investigations

a. **Tomograms** of the entire bone are done to define the extent of the tumor.
b. **Complete skeletal survey** is done using radioactive isotopes to determine the metastatic lesions elsewhere.
c. **Chest X-ray** helps to determine the lung metastasis.
d. *CT scan* helps to study the cross-section of the tumor and enables to detect the chest metastasis as small as 2 mm.
e. **MRI** helps to define the medullary spread and soft tissue involvement.
f. **Biopsy** of the tumor is very useful in arriving at a definitive diagnosis.

Principles

❖ Fine-needle aspiration cytology (FNAC) is preferred as incision may further provoke the spread.
❖ Hence, frozen section biopsy and ablative surgery carried out at the same time is logical.
❖ Biopsy material is obtained from the softer *peripheral* portion, as this is the most recently formed tumor whose malignant characteristics are not yet concealed by the formation of osteoid and new bone.

Treatment

General Principles

1. Early radical amputation is done to remove the primary tumor.
2. An attempt is made to prevent metastasis or control it if it has already formed by preoperative irradiation, chemotherapy or both.
3. Resection of large pulmonary metastasis is carried out.

Surgery

Early and radical ablation is the surgical procedure of choice. Having first established the diagnosis by biopsy, the level of amputation is determined after carrying out the various investigations mentioned above. Surgery is done at the *earliest* possible time.

Megavoltage Radiotherapy

Megavoltage irradiation is given pre-operatively before amputation to decrease the *viability* of the cells that may be disseminated into bloodstream by surgical trauma. It is a useful adjunct in the treatment of resectable tumors. Its efficacy is doubtful in the non-resectable tumors, e.g., vertebra. Irradiation destroys tumor cells with minimal effect on the uninvolved parts.

Chemotherapy (CT)

Earlier osteogenic sarcoma was refractory to chemotherapy. Nevertheless, it has now been found that high doses of methotrexate, citrovorum factor rescue (CFR) and Adriamycin are effective. By using the above drugs in short cyclical courses, toxic effects can be held to a minimum. Addition of an alkylating agent like cyclophosphamide has increased the interval between the administrations of individual drugs. This has markedly reduced the toxicity of the drugs. The treatment triads in order of sequence are shown in **Figure 28.9**.

In summary, after having established the diagnosis of osteogenic sarcoma with certainty, patient is initially put on chemotherapy. Local irradiation of the tumor is done next. Early radical surgical ablation is then carried out at the appropriate time.

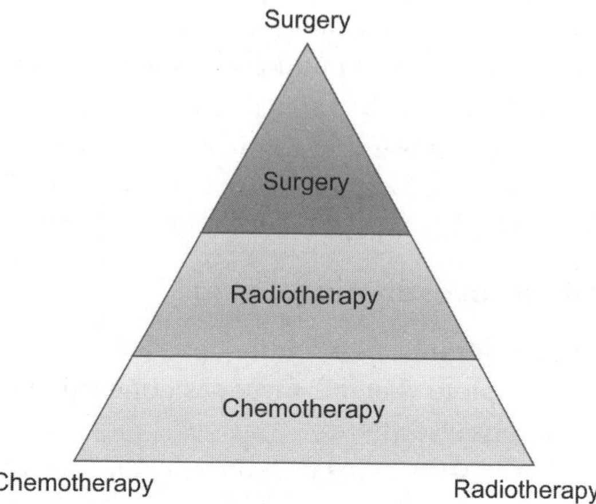

Fig. 28.9: Triad of treatment in osteogenic sarcoma.

Prognosis

Prognosis of osteogenic sarcoma has dramatically improved by the combined approach of ablation, megavoltage irradiation and chemotherapy. In untreated cases, survival time after pulmonary metastasis has developed is around 2.9%. With the combined approach of chemotherapy, radiotherapy and pulmonary resection, the five-year survival rate has increased by 60%.

BENIGN GIANT CELL TUMOUR (GCT) (SYN: OSTEOCLASTOMA)

Benign giant cell tumor is an osteolytic tumor arising from the *epiphysis* and is common in young adults. Though it is benign, it is *locally* malignant. The presence of *tumor giant cells* is the hallmark of this tumor.

Sex

The male: female ratio is 1.5:1.

Age

It is common between 15 and 35 years 80% occur in more than 20 years of age and the average age group is 35 years.

Areas affected are asymmetric portions of the epiphysis of long bones. About 75% of GCT occurs in lower end of femur, upper end of tibia, fibula and the distal end of radius.

Pathology

Gross

The tumor consists of ragged, friable, bleeding tissue filled with old or fresh blood clots with various sized cysts and cavities. Color varies from red to brown. Epiphyseal end of the bone is distorted. Tumor extension into the joint cavity is usually not seen and there is no evidence of periosteal reaction.

Microscopy

The tumor is encompassed by a fibrous capsule at the periphery. Presence of abundant tumor giant cells is quite characteristic. These cells are characterized by their larger size, multiple nuclei more than 150 in number, which are distributed through out the cell. Appearance of spindle cells indicates *malignant* potential.

Clinical Features

The course of the tumor is chronic. Unlike osteogenic sarcoma, pain is not the presenting feature but trauma is, the patient complains of swelling which is situated on one side of the bone. Skin over the tumor is stretched but there are no dilated veins. Tenderness is moderate or absent, *egg shell crackling* sensation may be present or absent. Limitation of joint movements is not seen till the late stages. There is no increase in joint fluid and the joint is rarely invaded. Pathological fracture is a late feature.

Radiology

- ❖ An eccentrically situated swelling.
- ❖ An osteolytic area is seen near the epiphysis **(Fig. 28.10)**.
- ❖ The cortex is expanded and thin.
- ❖ There is no periosteal new bone formation.
- ❖ Thin septa of bone traverse the interior and produce a *soap-bubble appearance* **(Figs. 28.11A and B)**
- ❖ The cortex may be disrupted in late stages
- ❖ Joint extension is rare.
- ❖ There is no calcification within the tumor.

Malignant GCT

Primary

This develops as a frank sarcomatous lesion.

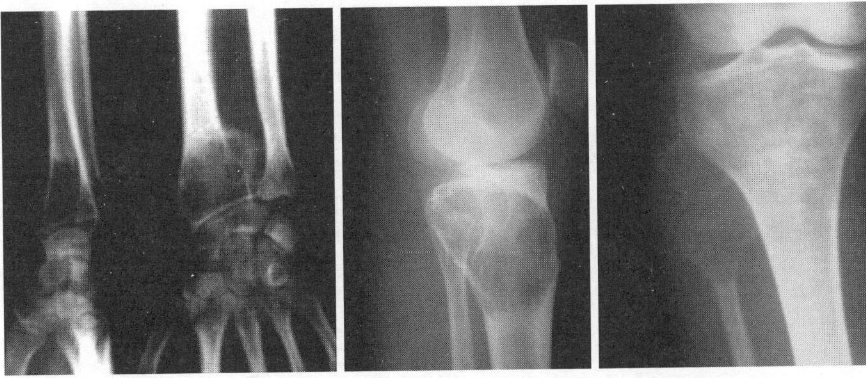

Fig. 28.10: Giant cell tumor of the lower end of radius and upper end of tibia and fibula.

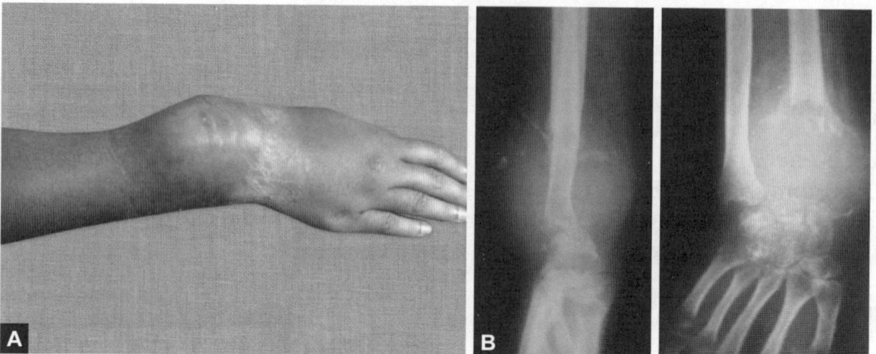

Figs. 28.11A and B: Showing clinical photograph of GCT lower end of radius and radiograph showing malignant GCT.

Secondary

This develops at the site of previously treated GCT.

Treatment

Surgical Methods

Approach that is more aggressive is adopted for lesions that are more aggressive and the surgical methods described are curettage and bone grafting, enbloc excision, curettage and acrylic bone cementation, curettage and cryosurgery, excision and curettage, excision and reconstruction, etc., depending on the extent of the lesion.

Irradiation Therapy

Irradiation therapy induces malignant change if it is given to the benign lesion. Megavoltage therapy is permissible only for inaccessible lesions located in the spine, sacrum, pelvis, etc. The recommended dosage is 1,500–5,000 rads for 5–6 weeks.

Metabolic Bone Disorders

RICKETS

Definition

It is a metabolic bone disease of childhood in which the osteoid, the organic matrix of bone, fails to mineralize due to interference with calcification mechanism. It is usually common between 6 months and 2 years.

Types of Rickets

1. **Fetal rickets:** It is commonly seen in osteomalacic mothers.
2. **Infantile rickets (nutritional rickets):** This is rare before 6 months and is the most common form of rickets, seen in 6 months to 3 years of life.
3. **Late rickets or rachitis tarda:** This is late onset rickets, familial, and it is vitamin D resistant rickets.

Quick facts
Varieties of rickets
Type I This is due to dietary deficiency or defects in metabolism of vitamin D.
Type II This is due to low serum phosphorus due to dietary phosphate deficiency or defective tubular resorption.
Type I *Dietary deficiency of vitamin D is the most common variety of rickets.*

Clinical Features

Symptoms

Patient complains of bone pain during rest, and excessive perspiration in upper half of the body **(Fig. 29.1)**. He or she loathes using the limb and the weakness of proximal muscles of the lower limbs produces waddling gait. There is evidence of catarrh of mucus membranes (recurrent diarrhea, constipation, bronchitis). Irritability of CNS produces convulsions, laryngismus, spasmophilia, Chvostek's sign, opisthotonos, etc.

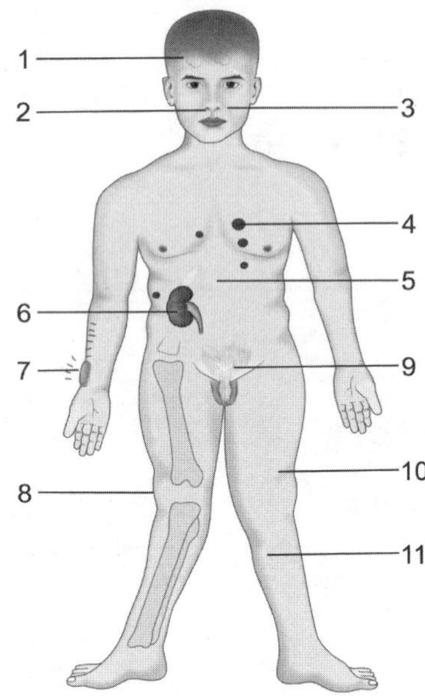

Fig. 29.1: Showing features as seen in nutritional rickets: (1) Frontal bossing, (2) Dentition changes, (3) Chvostek's sign, (4) Chest changes, (5) Malabsorption, (6) Aminoaciduria, (7) Expanded wrist, (8) Genu valgum, (9) Pelvic obliquity, (10) Myopathy, (11) Skin changes.

Deformities of Rickets (from Head to Toe) (Fig. 29.2)

Skull

❖ Broadened forehead
❖ Skull squared (caput quadratum)

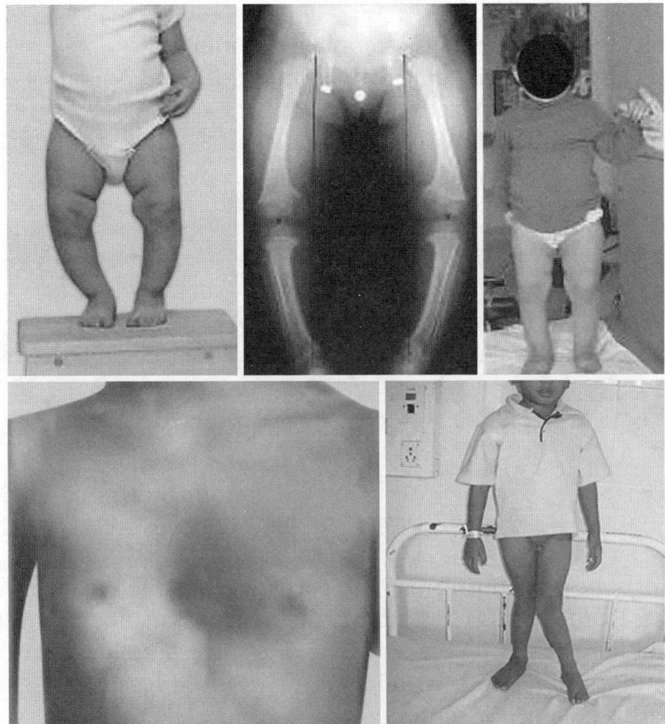

Fig. 29.2: Deformities of rickets.

❖ Frontal and parietal bossing—seen after the age of 6 months.
❖ Craniotabes is a ping-pong sensation on compressing the membranous bones of the skull.

Chest

❖ Pigeon chest due to prominent sternum.
❖ Narrow chest.
❖ Rickety rosary (enlargement of costochondral junction).
❖ Harrison's sulci due to diaphragmatic pull on the soft ribs.

Bones

❖ *Enlargement of the metaphysical segments* of long bones like radius, tibia, costochondral junction, etc., seen in children between 6 and 9 months of age.
❖ *Vertebral columns* show exaggerated curvature.
❖ *Pelvis* is trefoil shaped.
❖ *Coxa vara*
❖ *Femur* is bent anteriorly and laterally.
❖ *Knock knee (genu valgum)*
❖ *Bowed tibia.*

Other Features

Other features encountered in rickets are wizened look, delayed dentition, prominent abdomen, separation of recti, pale and flabby skin, and incomplete fractures, etc.

Investigation

X-rays of the distal, of the forearm, and around the knees show characteristic changes typical of rickets. These changes help in the early detection of ricket (*see* **Box**).

> **Remember**
>
> **Characteristic X-ray findings (Figs. 29.3 and 29.4)**
> ◄◄ Delayed appearance of epiphysis and widening of the epiphyseal plates.
> ◄◄ Champagne glass appearance (widening and cupping of the distal ends of long bones) also called 'trumpeting'.
> ◄◄ Space between diaphysis and epiphysis is increased.
> ◄◄ Deformity and bowing of the ends of long bones.
> ◄◄ Thickened epiphysis.
> ◄◄ Decreased density of cortex (rarefaction).
> ◄◄ Trabecular pattern is course.

Biochemistry

❖ Calcium is normal or decreased (due to compensatory hyperparathyroidism).
❖ Serum phosphorus is low.
❖ Alkaline phosphatase is normal.
❖ Urinary calcium is low (excretion <5 mg/kg/24 hour).
Importance of biochemical values in this condition is their return to normal upon correct therapy.

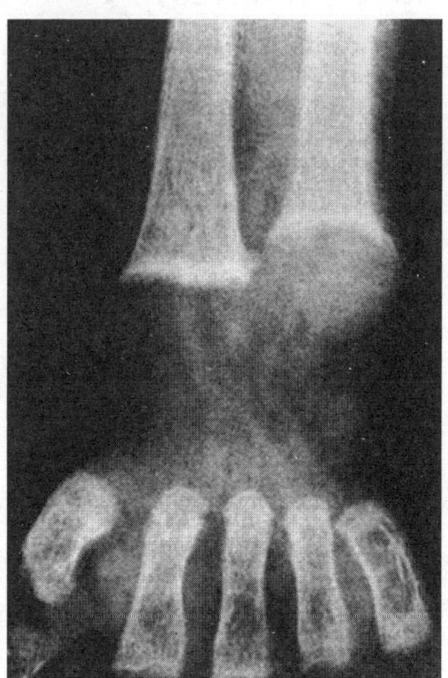

Fig. 29.3: Typical X-ray of the wrist metaphyseal cupping and irregularity of epiphyseal plates seen in rickets.

❖ Levels of 25-hydroxyvitamin D if low will indicate effectiveness of treatment.

Treatment

Medical treatment in the initial stages aims to bring about quick healing. A single oral dose of 6 lakh IU of vitamin D is given. A second same dose may be required after 3–4 weeks of treatment if no sclerotic (healing sign) change is seen on the radiograph at the metaphyseal side of the growth plate. A maintenance dose of 4,000 IU of vitamin D may be required if the child responds to the above treatment regimen.

Absolute and strict bed rest, rickets splints, etc., can do prevention of deformity.

Treatment of Established Deformity

Correction by splints (Mermaid splint): This is mainly useful when the disease is active and the deformity is slight. It is very effective in children and in preventing deformities concerning the lower limbs. However, it is slow and requires continual supervision.

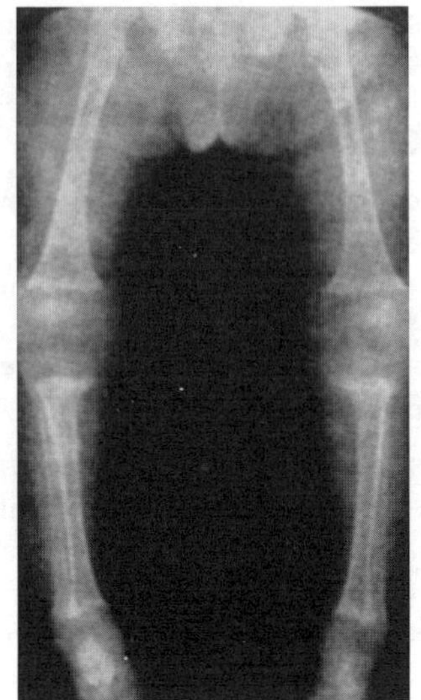

Fig. 29.4: Radiographic features of the knee in rickets.

Correction by osteotomy: It is indicated when deformity is near the joint and when the growth stops. It is done during III stage (Lovett's) (nonunion follows if done before).

Note: *At least 6 months of medical treatment should have elapsed before contemplating surgical correction.*

Differential diagnosis: Acute poliomyelitis, congenital syphilis, septic arthritis, infantile scurvy, etc.

OSTEOMALACIA

It is the adult counterpart of rickets and is characterized by failure of mineralization and an excess of osteoid due to an interference with calcification mechanism. *The osteoid is increased at the cost of mineralized bone. It is primarily a Vitamin D deficiency disease* (**Figs. 29.5A and B**).

Etiology

1. Decreased vitamin D intake or defective absorption from the intestine.
2. Derangement of vitamin D and phosphorus metabolism (hereditary or acquired).
3. Lack of explain to sunlight: This is common in Muslim women who practice purdah system and this remain unexposed to sun for greater part of their lives.

Clinical Features

Patient complains of generalized skeletal pain and muscle weakness. There may be acute pain due to fracture. Other symptoms related to causative factors like dietary, renal and GIT may be seen. The following deformities are encountered, scoliosis, kyphosis, coxa vara, protrusio acetabuli, thighs and legs are bent, pelvis is trefoil, etc.

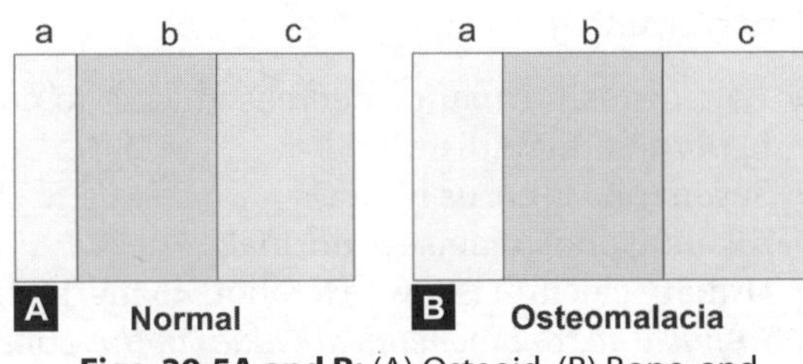

Figs. 29.5A and B: (A) Osteoid, (B) Bone, and (C) Marrow.

Radiographic Features (Fig. 29.6)

Reveal generalized demineralization, loss of transverse trabeculae, no subperiosteal resorption of bone, etc. Presence of Looser's zones is quite characteristic of osteomalacia.

❖ **Spine:** The bodies of spine are biconcave and are called "codfish spine".

❖ **Hip:** Show protrusio acetabuli and triradiate pelvis.

Laboratory Investigation

The following changes are seen in the blood: Serum calcium is normal or decreased, serum phosphatase is normal or decreased, alkaline phosphatase is slightly increased (rarely exceeds 200 IU), and serum PTH is increased.

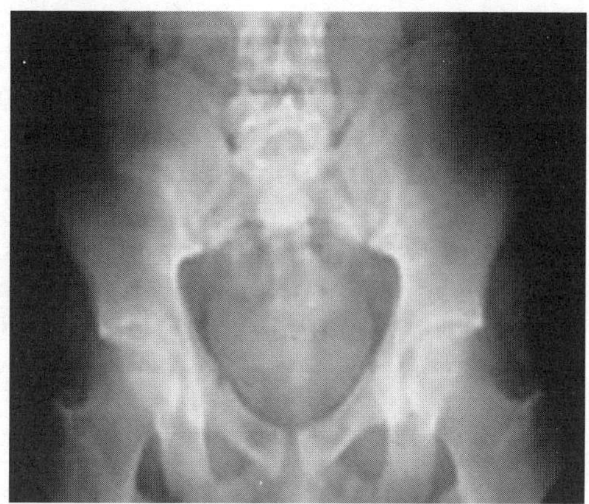

Fig. 29.6: Showing looser zones in the pelvis in osteomalacia.

Conservative Treatment

Calium is given at 0.5 to 3 g/day, vitamin D 10,000 IU/day, and high protein diet. In vitamin D deficiency, 10,000 IU of vitamin D followed by a daily maintenance dose of 400 IU is recommended. In renal diseases, alfacalcidol is the drug of choice. Calcium needs to be supplemented in daily divided doses of 0.5–3 g. The gastrointestinal tract errors are also corrected simultaneously.

OSTEOPOROSIS

Definition

It is a generic term referring to a state of decreased mass per unit volume of a normally mineralized bone due to loss of bone proteins.

Remember

About osteoporosis
It is the most common skeletal disorder in the world, next only to arthritis. In osteoporosis, there is a long latent period before clinical symptoms develop. Most prevalent complications are fractures of vertebral bodies, ribs, proximal femur, humerus, distal radius with minimal trauma. Most common cause is involutional bone loss in perimenopausal age group.

Causes

❖ Senility
❖ Postmenopausal women
❖ *Disuse*
  ◆ Prolonged bed rest or inactivity
  ◆ Prolonged casting or splinting
  ◆ Paralysis, space travel, etc.
❖ *Diet*
  ◆ Calcium, protein, vitamin C low in the diet

- ◆ Chronic alcoholism
- ◆ Anorexia nervosa.
- ❖ *Drugs* whose prolonged use causes osteoporosis are heparin, methotrexate, ethanol, glucocorticoids, etc.
- ❖ *Idiopathic* variety is seen in adolescent and middle-aged male population.
- ❖ *Genetic* role is seen in osteogenesis imperfecta.
- ❖ *Chronic illness* like rheumatoid arthritis, cirrhosis, sarcoidosis, renal tubular acidosis, etc.
- ❖ *Neoplasm* like bone marrow tumors (myeloma, lymphoma, leukemia).
- ❖ *Endocrine abnormalities* Hyperparathyroidism, increased levels of glucocorticoids, estrogens, etc.

> **Remember**
>
> **In osteoporosis**
> - ◀ Decreased density is due to deficiency of protein matrix in which calcium is laid down
> - ◀ Here rate of bone resorption is greater than bone formation
> - ◀ Most commonly it is due to ageing process
> - ◀ But the most common cause is involutional bone loss in perimenopausal women

Clinical Features (Fig. 29.7)

Osteoporosis most of the times does not produce any symptoms and hence is called a "silent disease". However, in the event of complications, patient presents with the following complaints:

Early Symptoms

Patient complains of acute pain in middle or low thoracic or high lumbar region. Sudden movement, sitting, sneezing, cough, etc. increases pain. Rest **(Fig. 29.7)** relieves it. *Most common symptom of osteoporosis is back pain secondary to vertebral compression* **(Fig. 29.8)**. However, in some cases, fractures of axial skeleton may be seen with trivial trauma. Round type of gibbus due to compression of thoracic vertebrae is commonly seen. Patients with osteoporosis exhibit progressive loss of height.

Investigation

- ❖ *Radiology* Changes seen in the spine are:
  - ◆ Loss of vertebral height due to symmetric transverse compression **(Fig. 29.9)**.
  - ◆ Biconcave central compression (codfish spine) due to the pressure of the bulging disc into the bodies.
  - ◆ Anterior wedge compression.

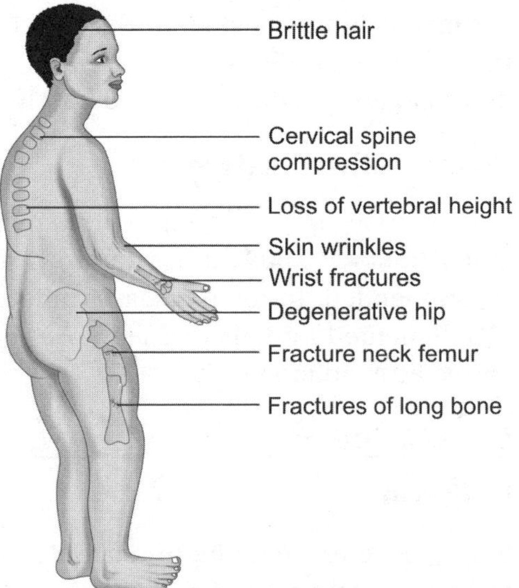

Fig. 29.7: Clinical features of osteoporosis.

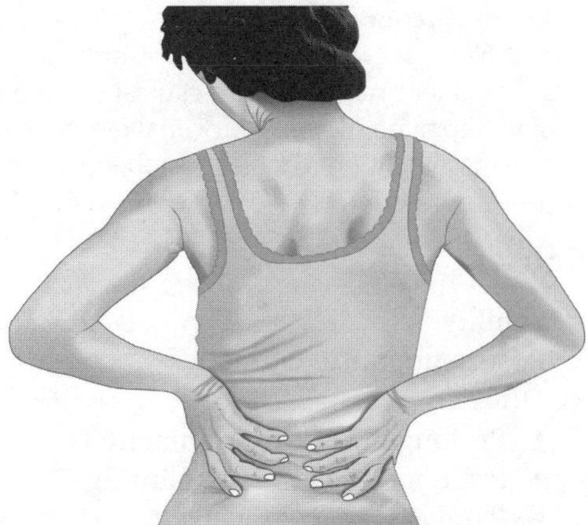

Fig. 29.8: Backache is the most common presentation in osteoporosis.

Other bones
- Ground glass appearance due to generalized rarefaction.
- *Singh's index:* This is the grading of trabecular pattern **(Fig. 29.11)** of the neck of femur from 1 to 6.
- Metacarpal index, etc.
- Pathological fractures.

❖ Techniques for bone mass measurement is by densitometry **(Fig. 29.10)**.
- Single photon absorptiometry is used to assess the amount of cortical bone mineral in appendicular skeleton **(Fig. 29.12)**.
- Dual photon absorptiometry and quantitative CT scan helps to assess the mineral status of axial skeleton. *Note: Dual photon absorptiometry is the gold standard.*

❖ Total body neutron activation analysis to determine calcium content of the entire body.

❖ **Transiliac bone biopsy:** It is an important diagnostic tool in patients of >50 years in postmenopausal diseases.

❖ **Blood chemistry:** Serum calcium, phosphorus and alkaline phosphatase levels are normal.

Management of Osteoporosis

The following treatment regimen is recommended:

❖ **High protein diet** will help increase the organic matrix of the bone.

❖ **Diet:** Calcium rich foods like Ragi, dairy products like Milk, curds, butter, cheese etc.

❖ **Calcium supplementation** in those who do not take calcium rich foods. Calcium carbonate is the most commonly used calcium supplement.

❖ **Rest and drugs** like analgesics and anti-inflammatory drugs. Muscle relaxants and supports like belt, collar, etc.

❖ **Spinal orthosis** when patient is erect and mobile to prevent and correct spine deformities.

❖ **Postural exercises** and back care **(Fig. 29.13)**.

❖ **Hormone replacement therapy (HRT):** Estrogen supplementation is the single most effective measure to prevent postmenopausal osteoporosis. It preserves positive calcium balance by bone remodeling.

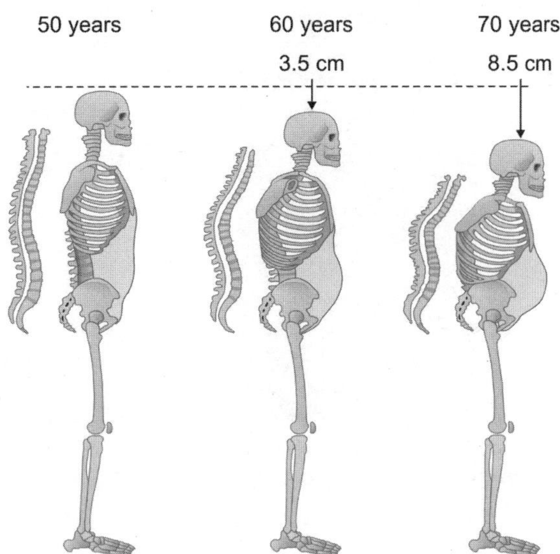

Fig. 29.9: Showing progressive loss of height due to osteoporosis.

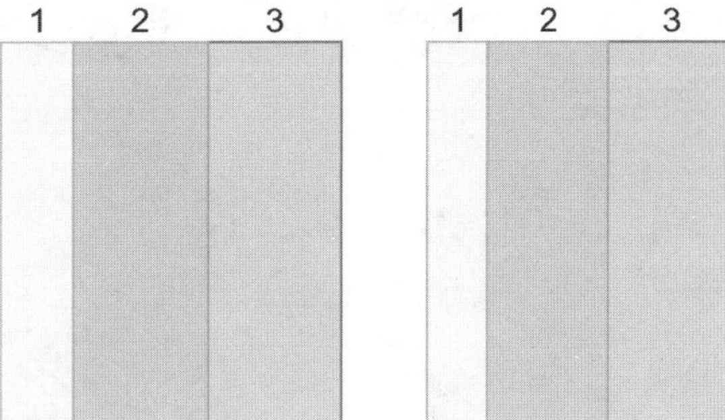

Fig. 29.10: (1) Osteoid, (2) Bone, and (3) Marrow.

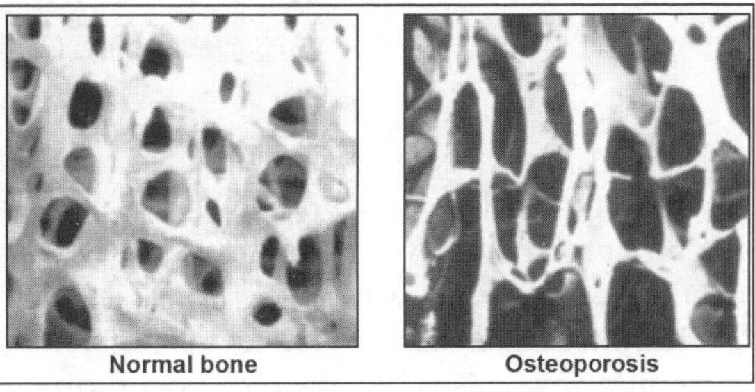

Fig. 29.11: Showing trabecular pattern in osteoporosis.

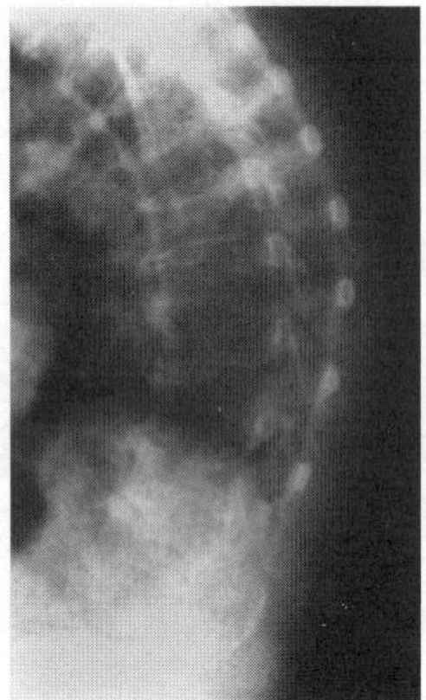

Fig. 29.12: Radiograph showing kyphotic deformity in osteoporosis.

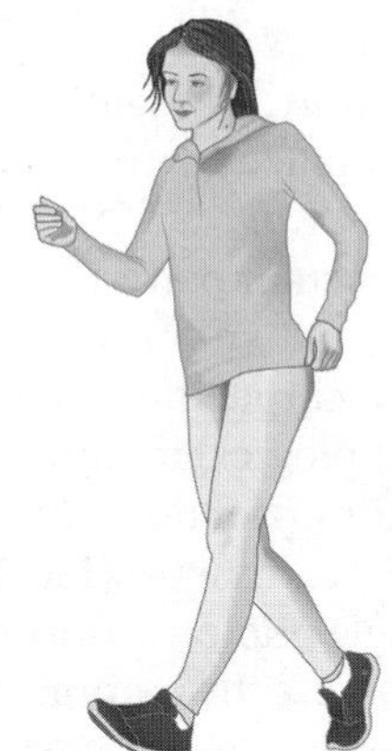

Fig. 29.13: Regular exercises as walking is of great help in elderly patients suffering from osteoporosis.

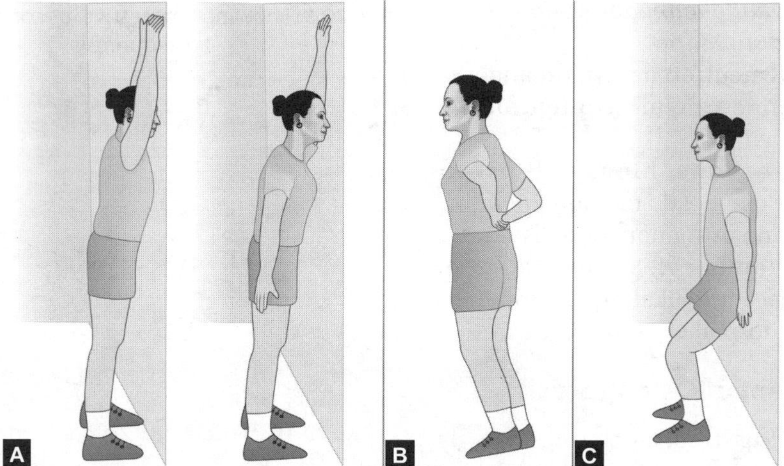

Figs. 29.14A to C: Showing various posture correction exercises in osteoporosis patient. (A) Wall arching; (B) Back bending; (C) Wall sliding exercises.

- ❖ **Alendronate:** It is a bisphosphonate drug and is useful in male patients and in those women who refuse HRT or in whom HRT is contraindicated.
- ❖ **Calcitonin** has been recently used for prevention of postmenopausal osteoporosis. It inhibits bone loss by bone resorption.
- ❖ **Vitamin D and calcium** intake in sufficient quantities.
- ❖ **Regular exercises** like walking, swimming help **(Figs. 29.14A to C)** to improve the bone strength.

Regional Orthopedic Conditions

UPPER LIMB

LATERAL TENNIS ELBOW

It is a lesion affecting the tendinous origin of common wrist extensors **(Fig. 30.1)** from the lateral epicondyle arising of the humerus.

Causes: A number of pathological conditions in and around the elbow joint can lead to these conditions. However, the most common incriminating cause is single or multiple tears in the extensor carpi radialis brevis tendon.

Seen in
- All levels of tennis players.
- In world class players "SERVE" appears to be the cause.
- In less than world class players "backhand stroke".
- Seen in other sports also.
- May be occupational, carpenters, miners, etc.

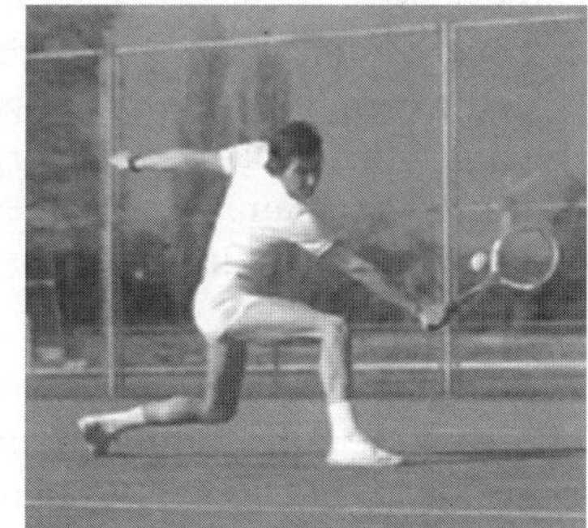

Fig. 30.1: Repetitive stress at common extensor origin in tennis players.

ETIOLOGY

Problems in tennis players: More than one-third tennis players all over the world are affected with this problem over 35 years of age are obviously due to faulty playing techniques.

Nontennis players: Ironically tennis elbow is more common is nontennis players. This unfortunate group is comprised of homemakers, carpenters, miners, drill workers, etc. India's Cricketing Legend Sachin Tendulkar has made Tennis Elbow very popular across the country and the world.

Indian housewives: This is the third largest group suffering from this condition. The household chores like washing, booming, cooking, etc., require repeated extension of the elbow leading to the development of this condition **(Fig. 30.2)**.

Fig. 30.2: Tennis elbow is common in Indian housewives.

Computer related injuries: This is emerging as a recent epidemic among computer professionals across the globe due to repetitive stress while using laptops, mouse, etc.

Clinical features: Patient complains of pain on the outer aspect of the elbow and has difficulty in gripping objects and lifting them. Sportspersons will have difficulty in extending the elbow. The following are some of the useful clinical tests:

❖ Local tenderness on the outside of the elbow at the common extensor origin with aching pain in the back of the forearm **(Fig. 30.3)**.

❖ *Cozens test:* Painful resisted extension of the wrist with elbow in full extension elicits pain at the lateral elbow **(Fig. 30.4)**.

Investigations: Routine AP and lateral view of the elbow radiographs are usually normal. However, in few cases status may be seen in the victory of the lateral epicondyle.

Treatment

Conservative management: It consists of rest and physiotherapy. In tennis players exercises, light racket, smaller grip, elbow strap, etc., are helpful **(Fig. 30.5)**. Injection of local anesthetic and steroid are useful in 40% of cases.

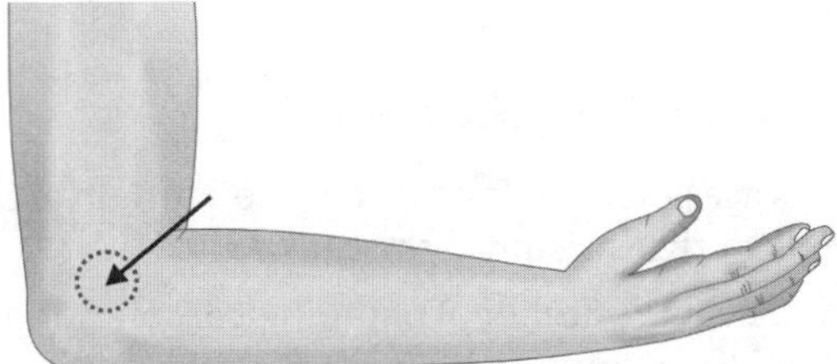

Fig. 30.3: Arrow showing site of tenderness in tennis elbow.

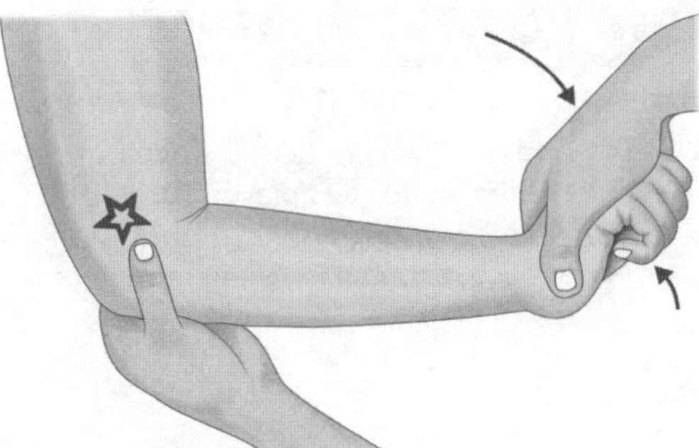

Fig. 30.4: Showing Cozen's test.

Surgical management: This is reserved for intractable cases that are unresponsive for the routine conservative regimen.

Surgical Methods

❖ Percutaneous release of epicondyle muscles.
❖ Bosworth technique of excision of the proximal portion of the annular ligament, release of the origin of the extensor muscles, excision of the bursa and excision of synovial fringes.

GOLFER'S ELBOW (SYN: EPITROCHLEITIS, MEDIAL TENNIS ELBOW)

It is a tendinopathy of the insertion of the epitrochlear muscles (flexors of the fingers of the hand and pronators). Epitrochleitis is very similar to lateral epicondylitis (tennis elbow) but occurs on the medial side of the elbow, where the pronator trees and the flexors of the wrist and fingers originate. Tensing of these muscles by resisted wrist and finger flexion in pronation will provoke the pain. *Tenderness is often less well localized than in tennis elbow* (**Fig. 30.6**).

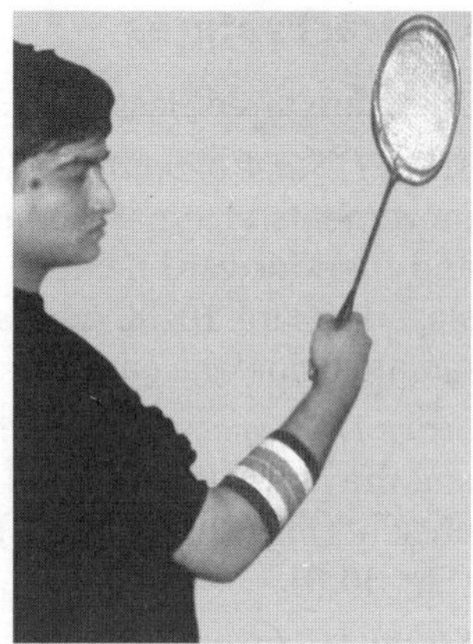

Fig. 30.5: Showing the elbow supports to be used in tennis elbow.

> **Did you know?**
>
> Tennis elbow is nine times more common than Golfer's elbow.

Treatment: It is the same as for tennis elbow but the treatment is even less satisfactory.

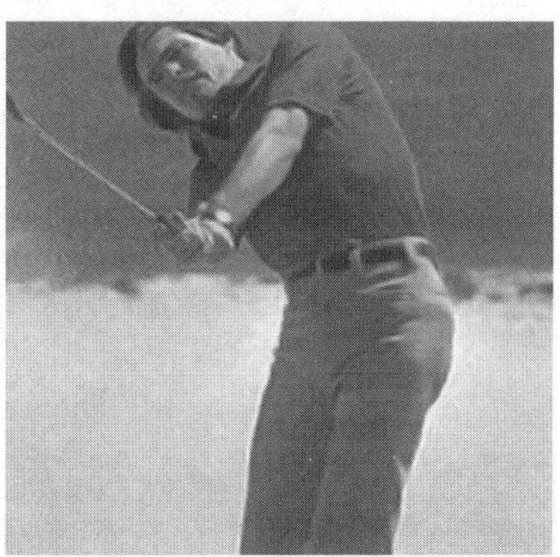

Fig. 30.6: Golfer's elbow is common in Golf players.

FROZEN SHOULDER (SYN: PERIARTHRITIS, ADHESIVE CAPSULITIS)

It is defined as a clinical syndrome characterized by *painful restriction of both active and passive shoulder movements* due to causes within the shoulder joint or remote (other parts of the body).

Causes

Shoulder causes problems directly related to shoulder joint which can give rise to frozen shoulder are tendinitis of rotator cuff, bicipital tendinitis, fractures and dislocations around the shoulder, etc.

Nonshoulder causes problems not related to shoulder joint like:
❖ Diabetes (more common and severe in diabetics)
❖ Cardiovascular diseases with referred pain to the shoulder which keeps the joint immobile.
❖ Reflex sympathetic dystrophy, frozen hand shoulder syndrome, a complication of Colles' fracture can all lead to frozen shoulder.

The reason in all the cases mentioned above could be prolonged immobilization of the shoulder joint due to voluntary immobilization of the shoulder, referred pain, etc.

Pathology: During abduction, and repeated overhead activities of the shoulder, long head of biceps, and rotator cuff undergo repeated strain. This results in inflammation, fibrosis and consequent thickening of the shoulder capsule which results in loss of movements.

Clinical Features

There are three classical stages in frozen shoulder:

Stage I (Stage of pain): Patient complains of acute pain, decreased movements, external rotation greatest followed by loss of abduction and then forward flexion. *Internal rotation is least affected.* This stage lasts for 10–36 weeks. Pain due to frozen shoulder will not radiate below the elbow unlike is cervical spondylitis **(Fig. 30.7)**.

Stage II (Stage of stiffness): In this stage pain gradually decreases and the patient complains of stiff shoulder. Slight movements are present **(Figs. 30.8A and B)**. Certain routine activities are affected. **(Fig. 30.9)**.

Stage III (Stage of recovery): Patient will have no pain and movements will have recovered but will never be regained to normal. It lasts for 6 months to 2 years.

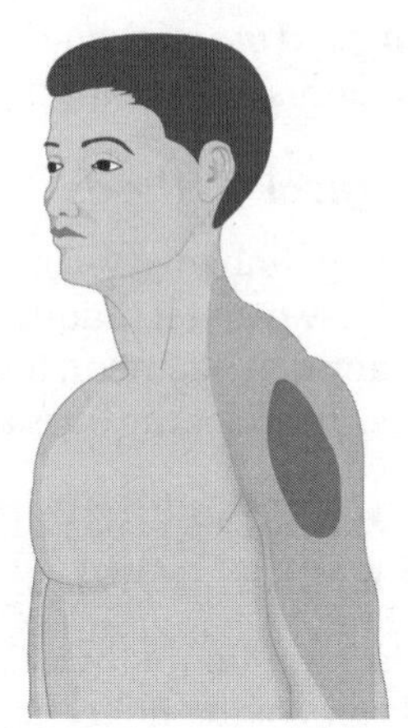

Fig. 30.7: Showing region of distribution of pain in frozen shoulder.

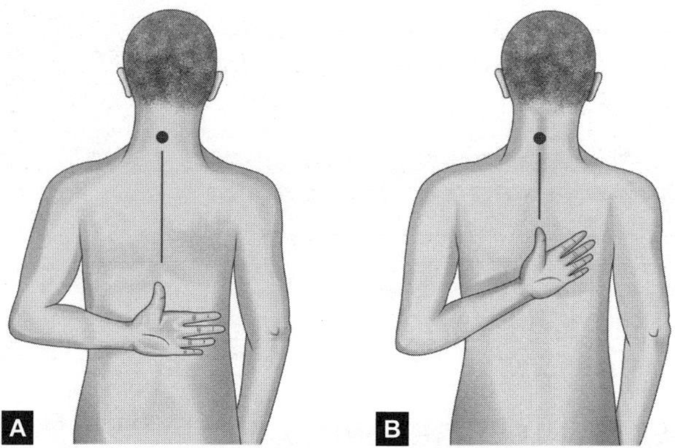

Figs. 30.8A and B: Showing degrees of internal rotations: (A) Normal, (B) Frozen.

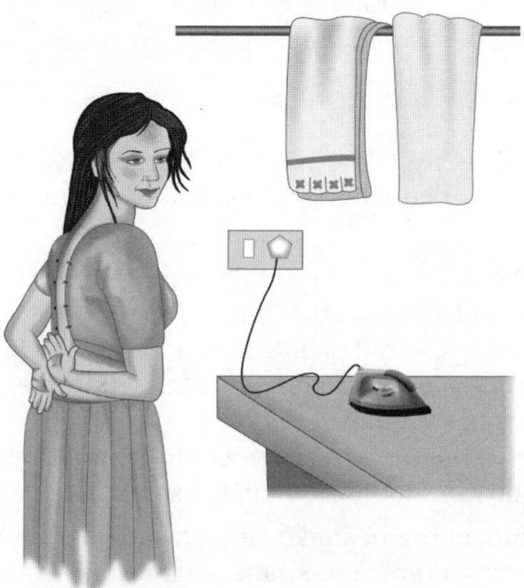

Fig. 30.9: Activities like these are not possible in frozen shoulder.

Treatment

Stage I: In this stage long-acting once a day NSAIDs are usually preferred as this condition usually runs a long course (10–36 weeks). Intra-articular steroids may help.

Stage II: In this stage since the pain will have reduced considerably, exercises both active and passive are gradually begun followed by physiotherapy, ultrasound, heat and shoulder wheel exercises. The role of manipulation of the shoulder is controversial but can be attempted under general anesthesia in this stage.

Stage III: In this stage active and passive exercises, physiotherapy consisting of short wave diathermy, ultrasound, etc., are continued.

Mercifully frozen shoulder is a self-limiting disease and abates after 6–9 months of agonizing experience to the patient. Some stiffness may remain as a sequel.

REGIONAL ORTHOPEDIC CONDITIONS OF THE KNEE

Deformities around the knee joint could be in two planes. In the coronal plane we may encounter genu valgum and genu varum deformities and in the sagittal plane antevertum and recurvatum deformities.

GENU VALGUM (KNOCK KNEE)

Definition: It is an outward deviation of the longitudinal axes of both tibia an ' femur. Apex of tl.e curve or angulation of the knee is medial **(Fig. 30.10)**.

Incidence: 75% children have genu valgum up to 4 years of age. This is called physiological genu valgum, which usually disappears by 7 years.

Types: It is broadly classified into physiological and pathological, the latter could be unilateral or bilateral.

Clinical features: The primary deformity in a genu valgum is *a medial angulation of the knee.* In response to this, secondary deformities develop in the femur, tibia and foot.

Assessment of genu valgum deformity: *Clinical assessment* the severity of the deformity is measured by noting the intermalleolar distance, and studying the plums line. The methods are classified in the section on clinical examination of the knee.

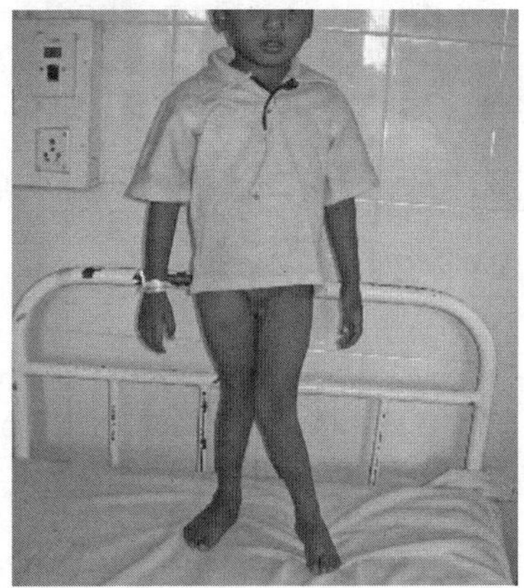

Fig. 30.10: Genu valgum or knock-knee deformity.

Treatment of Genu Valgum

- ❖ **Mild cases:** Child is seen at intervals of 3 months and the progress is recorded. These cases usually require no treatment, and raising the inner side of the heels by 4–5 mm may possibly relieve strain on ankles. The knock-knee braces may be useful.
- ❖ **Severe cases:** If by the age of 4 years, intermalleolar distance is 10 cm or more, operation may become necessary.

Surgical Methods

- ❖ Epiphyseal stapling is done on the medical side and before skeletal maturity
- ❖ *Osteology*: After skeletal maturity a lateral closed wedge osteotomy is done.

GENU VARUM (BOW LEGS)

Definition

It is defined as *a lateral angulation of the knee. The longitudinal axis of femur and tibia deviates medially.* The deformity involves tibia alone or the femur or tibia and fibula **(Fig. 30.11)** both.

Measurements of the Deformity

Child: The deformity is clinically assessed by noting the intercondylar distance and drawing the plumb line (methods described in clinical examination of the knee).

Adults: The angle of genu varum is calculated on a standing radiograph of the whole limb.

Clinical features: The primary deformity in genu varum is *lateral angulations of the knee.* In response to this, secondary deformities develop in the tibia and the foot.

Treatment: Treatment should be conservative until 4 years of age. Knee-ankle-foot orthosis with the medial bar and the lateral strap is used.

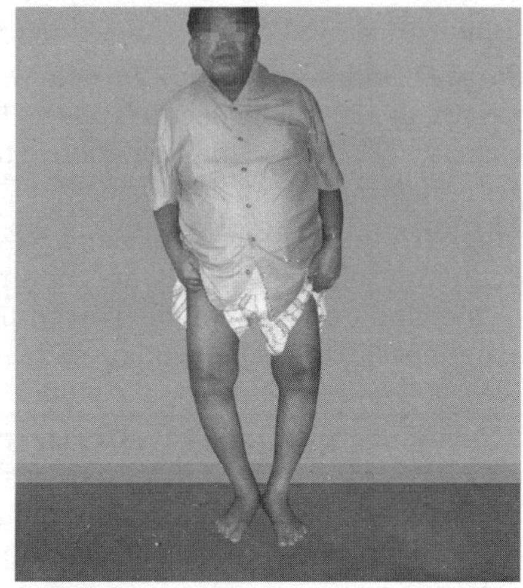

Fig. 30.11: Showing genu varum with increased intercondylar distance. Genu varum is said to exist if there is approximately 3 cm gap between the medial femoral condyles when the malleoli are together.

BURSAE AROUND THE KNEE

Anterior

- ❖ *Suprapatellar* always communicates with the knee joint
- ❖ *Prepatellar bursitis* (housemaid's knee) is seen in the lower half of patella and upper half of ligamentum patella. The mechanism is shown in **Figure 30.12**. Clinical presentation is shown in **Figure 30.13**.
- ❖ *Infrapatellar* seen in the lower half of ligamentum patella. It is seen commonly in Clergyman's, Parson's, or carpet layer's knee **(Fig. 30.14)**. Clinical presentation is seen in **Figure 30.15**.

Lateral: Cyst of lateral meniscus.

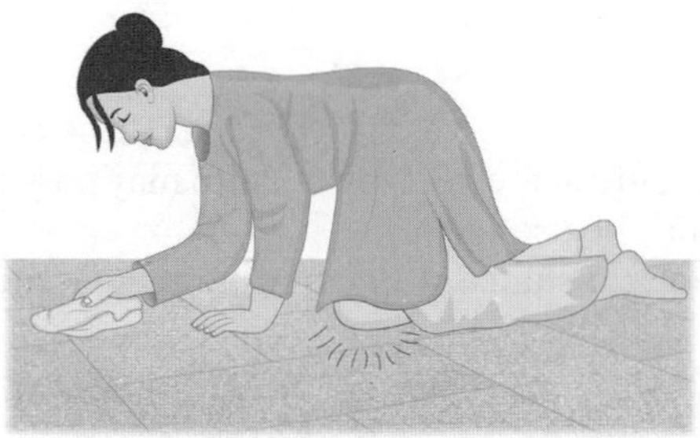

Fig. 30.12: Showing mechanism of housemaid's knee.

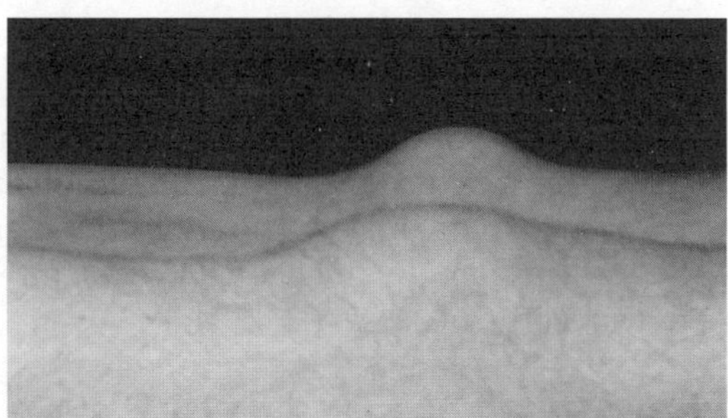

Fig. 30.13: Clinical photograph of housemaid's knee.

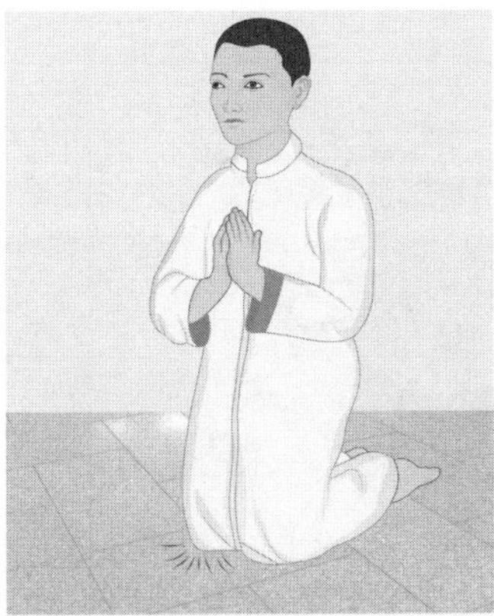

Fig. 30.14: Showing mechanism of formation of clergyman's knee.

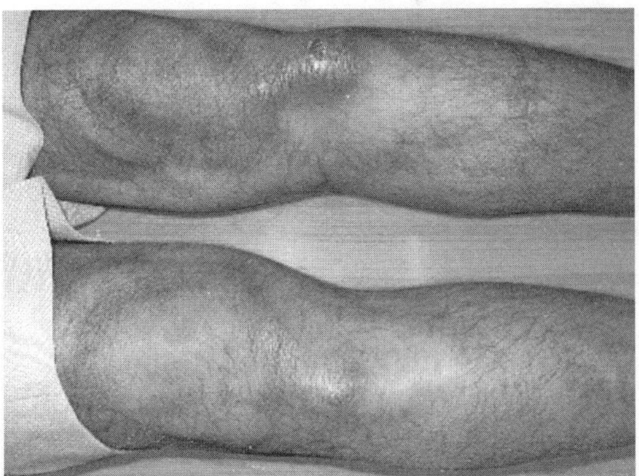

Fig. 30.15: Showing clergyman's knee.

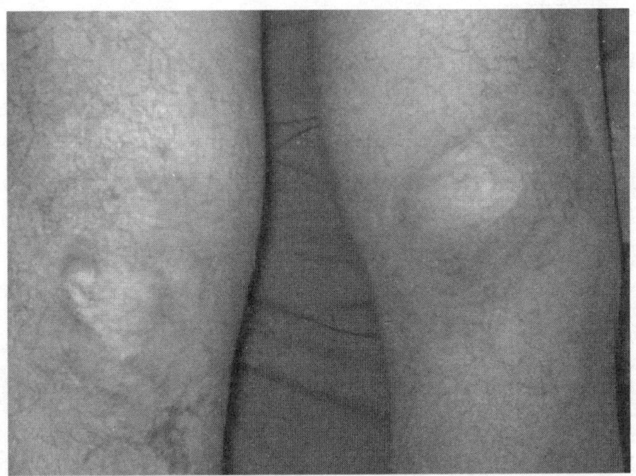

Fig. 30.16: Baker's cyst arises from the herniation of the synovial membrane through the capsule.

Popliteal cyst (Baker's cyst): This was first described by Adam in the year 1840 and later by Baker in 1877. Commonly symptoms are seen in bursa of the medial head of gastrocnemius and semimembranosus bursa.

Causes: Though the exact cause is unknown are children in adults it could be secondary due to rheumatoid arthritis or osteoarthritis.

Clinical features: These are similar to internal derangement of the knee, like pain, stiffness, swelling, giving way, etc. **(Figs. 30.16).** The swelling is seen in the middle of the popliteal fossa. It disappears or flexion and appears or extension. The fluctuation and transillumination tests are positive.

Treatment: The treatment of choice is excision of the bursa and closer of the capsular orifice by:
❖ Scarification of the edges and suture.
❖ To close the gap by a graft from tendinous part of the gastrocnemius, etc.
　One-third to one-half of patients with Baker's cyst is children. It is rare after seventh year of life. Hence, delay in excision is followed by gradual disappearance of the cyst.

CHONDROMALACIA PATELLA

It is defined as a blistering, cystic change of the patellar cartilage and it usually affects the medial facet of the patella.

Clinical features: Patient complains of generalized deep pain in the knee. The knee may be swollen with a chronic effusion of synovial fluid and there will be a positive patellofemoral grinding test when the condition is severe **(Fig. 30.17)**. The patella will appear out of alignment and there may well be a high 'Q'-angle. The vastus medialis

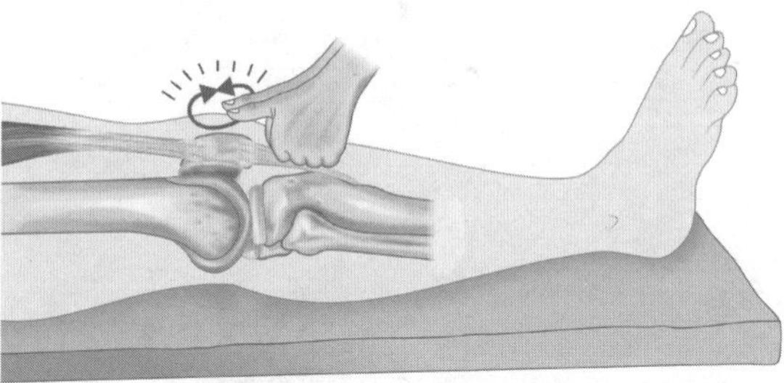

Fig. 30.17: Showing method of performing a grinding test in chondromalacia patella.

will be weak, radiographs will occasionally show spurring and the patient will be unable to do squats.

Movie sign or theater sign: This is quite characteristic of chondromalaciace. Prolonged sitting as in watching a movie herald is the onset of knee pain **(Fig. 30.18)**.

Investigations: Radiographs of the knee shows irregular retro patellar surface. Arthroscopy is an extremely useful diagnostic technique **(Fig. 30.19)**.

Differential diagnosis: Chronic synovitis of the knee, sprain of the retinacula, etc.

Treatment: Treatment consists of ice and ultrasound massage of the painful area, realignment of the maltracking of the patella by orthotic therapy and arthroscopic shaving of the retropatellar surface gives excellent results.

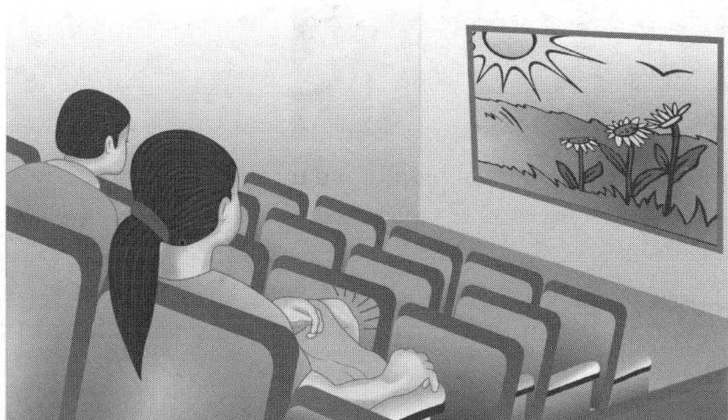

Fig. 30.18: Showing the typical "movie or theater sign" in chondromalacia patella.

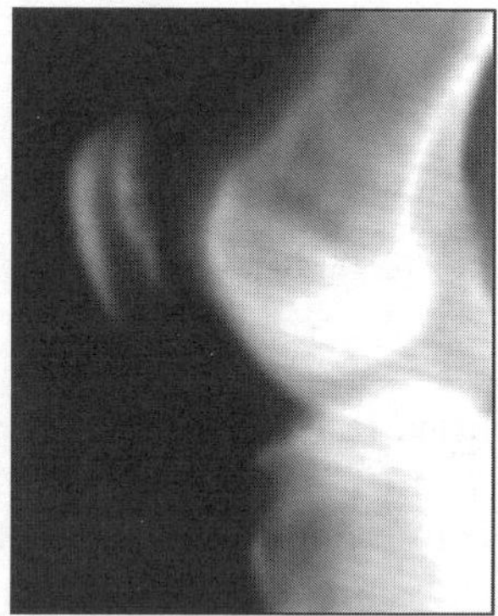

Fig. 30.19: X-ray of the knee showing chondromalacia of the patella.

REGIONAL ORTHOPEDIC CONDITIONS OF THE NECK

TORTICOLLIS (WRY NECK)

Torticollis is defined as the rotational deformity of cervical spine that causes turning and tilting deformity of the head and neck **(Fig. 30.20)**.

Causes

- *Congenital*
- *Infective*: Tuberculosis of cervical spine, acute respiratory tract infection, etc.
- *Traumatic*: Sprain, dislocation and fracture of the cervical spine.
- *Myositis or fibromyositis* of sterno-cleidomastoid, exposure to cold causes myositis.
- *Spasmodic* painful, persistent or intermittent sternomastoid muscle contraction.
- *Unilateral muscle paralysis,* e.g., polio
- *Neuritis* of spinal accessory nerve.
- *Ocular disturbances* child turns head to one side to compensate for defective vision.

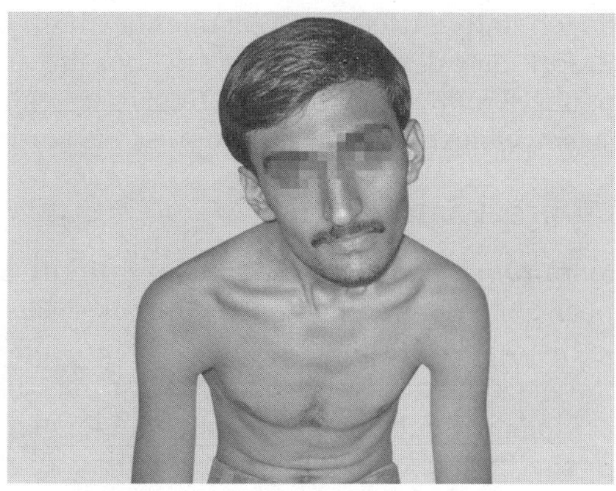

Fig. 30.20: Clinical presentation of wry neck.

Clinical features: Head of the patient is tilted toward the affected side while the chin points to the other side. Sternocleidomastoid muscle is prominently seen. In the later stages, the patient may develop facial asymmetry and macular disturbances in the eye. *Among the acquired causes of torticollis, spasmodic muscle contraction of the sternocleidomastoid is the most common cause.*

Management: Conservative management is the first line of treatment. This consists of nonsteroidal anti-inflammatory drugs (NSAIDs), muscle relaxants drugs, etc. Physiotherapy like ultrasound, heat, massage is advocated. In acute pain, patient is encouraged to wear a collar. Gradual neck strengthening exercises are advised once the acute symptoms subside.

Surgical management is advised after the failure of conservative treatment. It consists of release of sternomastoid muscle from its clavicular attachment as in congenital torticollis and intradural section of both spinal accessory and three cervical roots in cases of torticollis due to spasmodic or neural causes.

CERVICAL DISC SYNDROMES

The cervical region consists of seven cervical vertebrae with their intervening discs. The disc is made up of central nucleus pulposus and annulus fibrosus at the periphery. The disc functions as an effective shock absorber and also gives the cervical spine more mobility. If the disc material herniates **(Fig. 30.21)** because of trauma or old age it gives rise to the cervical disc syndrome.

More than 90% of the disc lesions in the cervical spine occur at the C_5 and C_6 levels as these are the most mobile segments.

Pathogenesis: Advancing age, improper neck postures; neck misadventures we indulge day is and day out (e.g., our habit of using thick pillows, etc.) takes its toll or the neck structures particulars the intervertebral discs. Over the years disc degenerates disc space narrow, fact joints

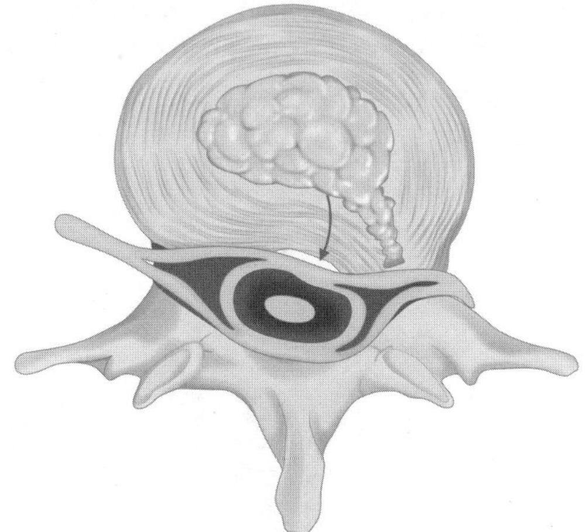

Fig. 30.21: Cervical disc herniation compressing the nerve root.

degenerate muscles and ligaments stiffen causing pain in the neck. Consequent to all this unfortunate developments, extra bone growths called osteophytes develop heralding the onset of nerve root compression. A tragic saga called cervical spondylitis thus unfolds. Catastrophe sets in when osteophytes compress the cord and the nerves.

Clinical Features

Symptoms: Patient complains of *pain* in the neck which is gradual or acute in onset. There is history of morning stiffness. Extension of the neck increases the pain. Patient may also complain of radiating pain to the shoulder, elbow or the fingers. *Tingling and numbness in the fingers* develops if the nerve root is compressed but it does not follow the dermatomal pattern.

Signs: Movements of the neck are decreased due to pain. Pain **(Fig. 30.22)** increases on hyperextension. There is localized tenderness over the spinous process. Trigger point tenderness at the scapular region is present. Pressure against the top of the head increases pain. If the nerve root is compressed by the disc herniation sensory, motor and reflex changes occur and follow the dermatomal pattern **(Fig. 30.23)**. *Cord compression could lead to features of UMN lesion.*

Investigations

X-ray **(Fig. 30.24):** Normal in soft lesions but in hard lesions it shows, narrowing of disc space, anterior and posterior osteophyte formation, and narrowing of IV foramen.

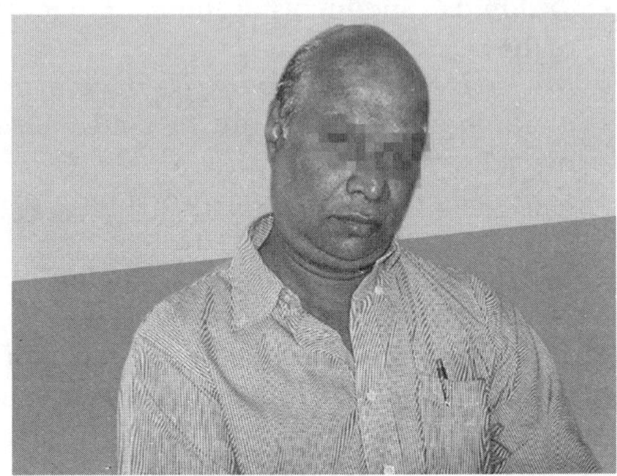

Fig. 30.22: Showing a clinical photograph of the cervical spondylitis.

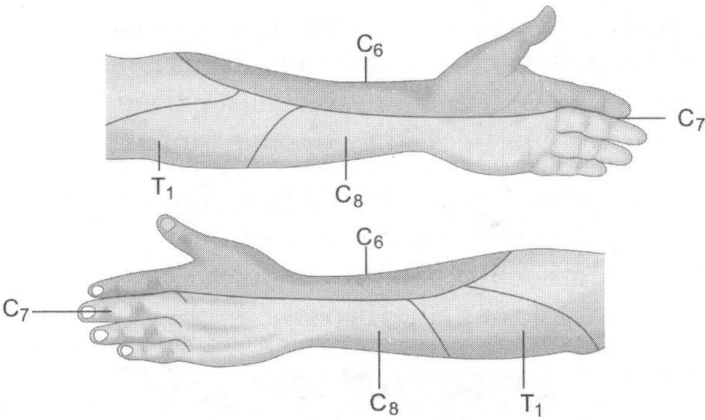

Fig. 30.23: Dermatome pattern of upper limb.

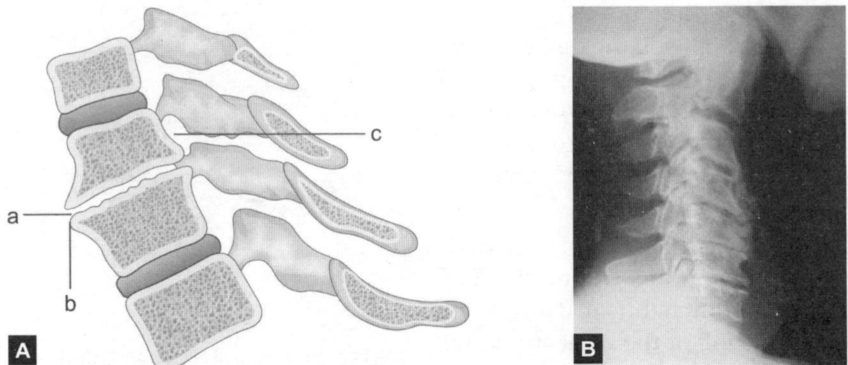

Figs. 30.24A and B: Diagrammatic representation of radiograph in findings in cervical disc syndrome: (a) disc space narrowing, (b) osteophyte formation, and (c) narrowing of intervertebral foramina.

Myelography: It helps in localizing the lesion but is invasive.

MRI: This is useful, as it is noninvasive, and helps localize the lesion, but its high cost is prohibitive **(Fig. 30.25)**.

CT scan: It is more useful in evaluating traumatic conditions of the neck than degenerative conditions.

EMG discography, thermography are occasionally used.

Treatment conservative *treatment* is the more accepted form of treatment in cervical disc syndrome. It consists of rest which is the cornerstone of the treatment as it allows soft parts to heal by reducing the inflammation. Cervical traction could be continuous or intermittent depending on the severity of the symptoms. Traction helps by reducing the muscle spasm, increasing the disc space and reducing the tension on the nerve roots. Wearing cervical collar helps to relieve pain and muscle spasm during acute exacerbation of chronic spondylitis **(Fig. 30.26)**. Physiotherapy like short wave diathermy, ultrasound, and infrared rays are useful. NSAIDs once a day are usually preferred. After the pain decreases, patient is encouraged to perform gradual graded isometric neck exercises **(Figs. 30.27A to E)**.

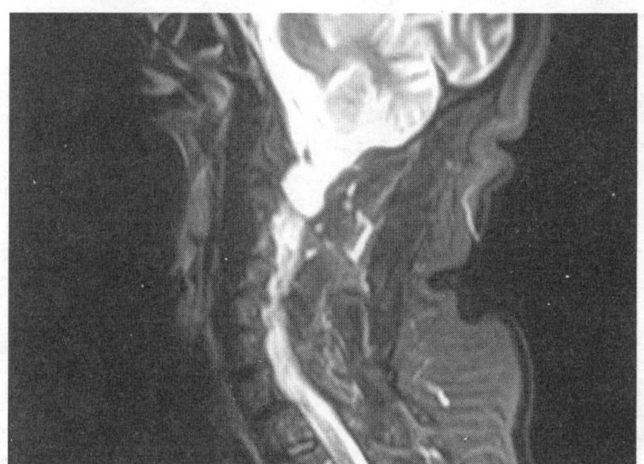

Fig. 30.25: Showing MRI features of cervical spondylitis.

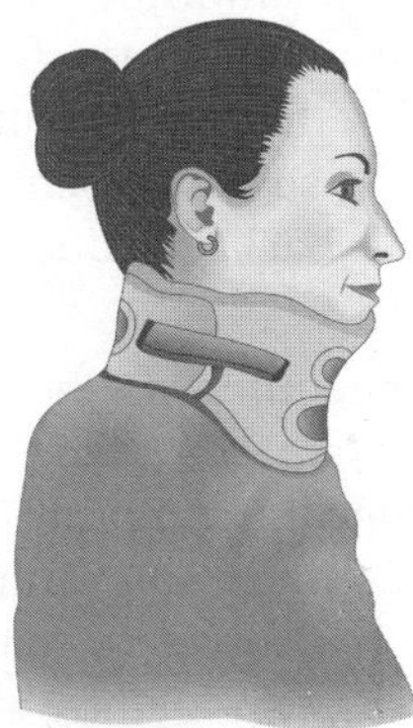

Fig. 30.26: Wearing a cervical collar is a popular method of treatment of cervical spondylitis.

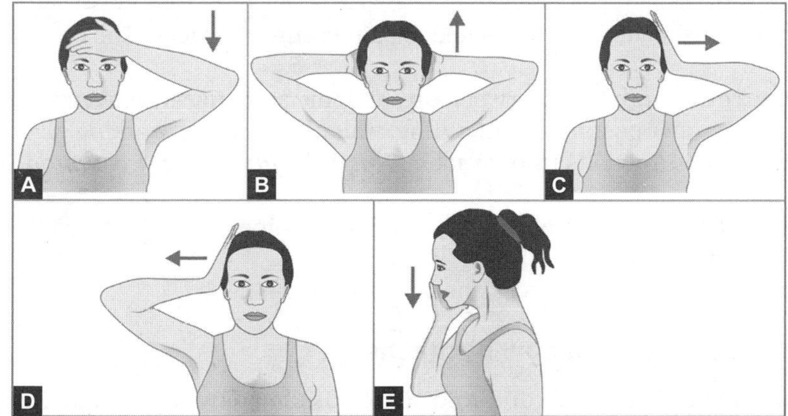

Figs. 30.27A to E: Different self-resistive isometric neck exercises. (A) Neck flexion; (B) Neck extension; (C) Lateral flexion; (D) Neck rotation; (E) For neck flexion.

Important Preventive Measures

❖ Practicing proper neck fractures
❖ Avoiding thick pillows and using proper sized pillows (2")

Surgical treatment: Less than 5% of the cases of cervical spondylitis require surgery and is usually indicated in cases of chronic pain, failed conservative treatment and neurological deficits due to root or cord compressions. The surgical procedure usually consists of removal of the cervical disc through an anterior approach and cervical interbody fusion by placing an autologous iliac bone graft. Excision of large osteophytes can also be done through this route. Excision of one or two cervical bodies (corpectomy) may be justified in multiple level disc pathology. Laminectomy usually does not produce the desired results.

LOW BACKACHE

Backache, which was known as an ancient curse, is now known as a modern international epidemic. It is an extremely common malady afflicting the human race across the globe cutting the geographical boundaries, race, culture, etc. 80–90% of the human population will suffer from some form of backache, mild or severe in their lifetime. Among the galaxy of causative factors, both spinal and extraspinal, the most common cause of low backache seems to be mechanical or common low backache due to postural problems.

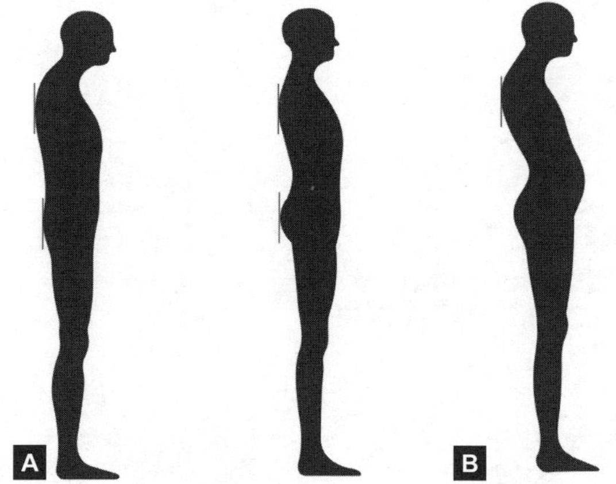
Figs. 30.28A and B: Posture: (A) normal posture, and (B) bad posture due to protruding belly.

Posture: *It is defined as the positional relationship of the different regions of the body to each other.* Proper posture is about maintaining an erect and balanced spine. Thus, it can be concluded that postural defects, overloading and abrupt unbalanced movements are frequently responsible for backache **(Fig. 30.28)**.

Causes of Backache

A variety of conditions related and unrelated to spine cause backache. The common causes of backache are:

❖ *Unaccustomed activities* a sedentary person suddenly adopting an active form of life, etc.
❖ *Poor posture* improper posture during sitting, walking, standing, working places enormous load on the back and results in backache. *This is by far the most common cause of low backache.*
❖ *Occupational backache* certain occupation places enormous stress on the back, e.g., garbage collectors, porters, etc.
❖ *Obesity:* Protruding abdomen places enormous strain on the back.

Other Important Causes for Low Backache

❖ *Uncommon causes:* These are due to diseases of the spine like congenital anomalies, inflammatory conditions, infections, tumors, etc.

- *The facet joint osteoarthritis* due to old age, repeated bending and twisting activities lead to arthritis of facet joints.
- *Spinal stenosis:* Spinal stenosis due to degenerative process is another common cause.

Common Low Backache (Accounts for 80%)

This includes back muscle strain, ligament sprain, and prolapsed disc:
- *Muscle strain* after backache is due to strain of the back muscles during, sudden unaccustomed activity, sports, trauma, etc.
- *Ligament sprain:* Back ligaments are strained during sudden lifting or twisting activities.
- Prolapsed *lumbar intervertebral disc:* This is the second most common cause for low back pain after muscle strain. Discussed at great length earlier.

Clinical Features

Age: Backache is more common in middle-aged and elderly people (usually degenerative). In young adults, it is due to trauma and in children; it is usually due to organic lesions such as TB, etc.

Sex: Osteoporosis, rheumatoid arthritis, etc., are more common in females. Ankylosing spondylitis, trauma, secondaries, etc., are more common in males.

Occupation: People with sedentary jobs and heavy manual laborers are frequently prone for backache.

Presenting Complaints

Pain: Over 90% of the patients complain of pain in the back. The following points should be enquired.

- *Nature of pain* is it sudden (trauma) or gradual (spondylosis)? Did weight lifting, sudden bending, etc., precede it? Is there remissions and exacerbations (disc disease) or is it continuous (tumors)? Is there history of night cries (e.g., TB spine)? Does rest relieve it? Does it radiate to the lower limbs, etc. **Figure 30.29** shows various day to day activities that can lead to lower back pain.
- *Remember*: In ankylosing spondylitis and other SSA, pain becomes worse after rest! In common low backache rest relieves pain and muscle spasm.
- *Site*: Is the pain in the middle of the spine or paravertebral muscles. Is it in the dorsolumbar spine (trauma or tumor) or in the lumbar spine (disc disease)?

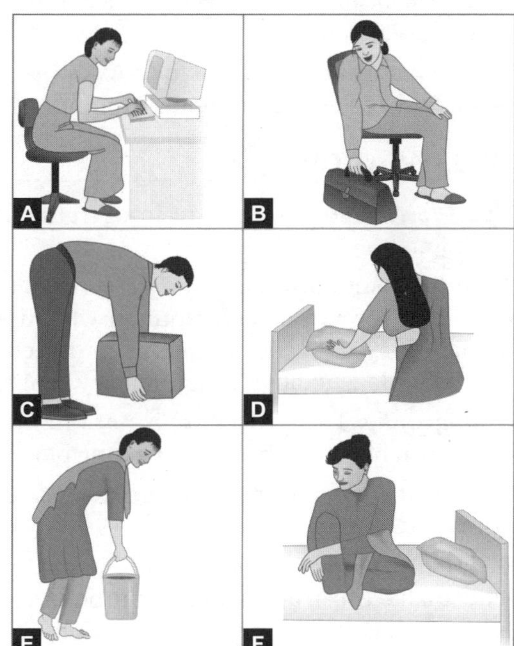

Figs. 30.29A TO F: Showing various activities than can lead to lower back pain.

- *Sciatica and its causes*: Sciatica is defined as a radiating pain along the course of the sciatic nerve and is felt in the back, buttocks, posterior of the thigh, legs and the foot. It is commonly due to disc prolapse.
- *Neurological symptoms*: These consist of paresthesia, muscle weakness, disturbance of sphincters, cauda equina syndrome, etc.

❖ *Facet syndromes*: Here patient complains of chronic backache, early morning stiffness, difficulty in getting out of bed, standing, sitting or climbing.
❖ *Other complaints*: There may be history of stiffness, pain in other joints (e.g., rheumatoid arthritis), constitutional symptoms (e.g., tuberculosis, malignancy, etc.), genitourinary complaints, etc.

Physical Signs

Stance and gait: Does the patient stand with a normal stance or has deformities like scoliosis, kyphosis, lordosis or pelvic tilt. Is the gait normal or altered?

Spasm: This is seen in acute painful conditions of the spine. The patient complains of pain in the paravertebral muscles and painful restriction of all the spine movements.

Movements: There may be restriction of the spine movements due to the organic lesions affecting the back or due to muscle spasm, disc lesions, etc.

Swelling: It may be due to cold abscesses following TB spine.

Tenderness: It may be present over the spinous process, in between the spinous processes, over muscles, ligaments, facet joints, etc., for method of eliciting tenderness.

Neurological examination: This consists of examinations of the various dermatomes for sensations, myotomes for muscle power and reflexes.

SLRT and tension signs: This is to know the effects of disc prolapse on the sciatic nerve and is already discussed.

Other examinations: It include examinations of the adjacent joints, peripheral pulses, abdominal, rectal or paravaginal examinations.

INVESTIGATIONS

Blood tests: These are useful in detecting metabolic, hormonal, infective and malignant conditions.

Radiology: Routine plain radiographs of the lumbar spine are advised. Both anteroposterior and lateral views are usually required. Oblique views are helpful in detecting the fracture of pars. Though X-rays are not very helpful in detecting the disc prolapse, it is of value in diagnosing metabolic, degenerative, inflammatory, malignant conditions affecting the spine.

Myelography: This procedure is not routinely used anymore because of its complications. However, it has a role in demonstrating blocks due to disc prolapse.

CT scan: It is a noninvasive procedure and helps to identify the bone and soft tissue problems with greater accuracy.

MRI scan: This is the gold standard in the investigations of the spine. It is noninvasive and is better than CT scan in diagnosing the bone and soft tissue problems around the spine. However, its high cost is prohibitive and is available only in major cities and centers.

Treatment: The underlying cause has to be detected and managed accordingly. The general treatment for backache consists of drugs like NSAIDS, muscle relaxants, physiotherapy, traction, use of belts and corsets **(Fig. 30.30)**. proper postural habits, back exercises and back education go a long way in preventing the backache. Surgery is done for specific indications and specific surgical techniques have been dealt in relevant sections.

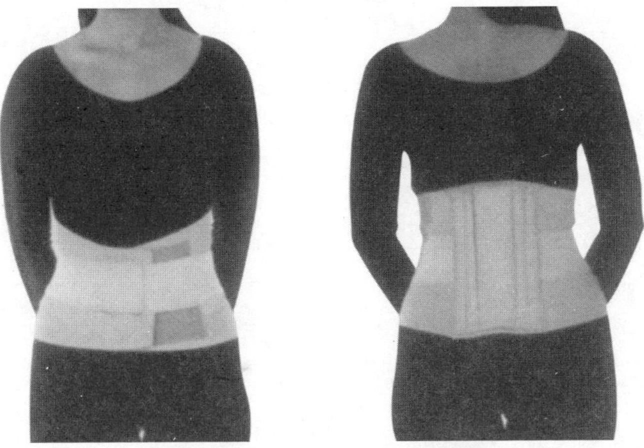

Fig. 30.30: Showing lumbar belts.

Ways to prevent recurrence: This is the most important aspect of the management of backache. Like in all other diseases, so in backache prevention is better than cure. Backache can be prevented largely by observing the following measures:

- Adopting proper posture and creating awareness that it is in the erect position that the back can withstand strain the best.
- *Back exercises:* These aim to strengthen the abdominal, pelvic, back and thigh muscles. Strong healthy muscles reduces load on the discs and other structures.
- *To avoid:* All sports including the aerobic ones. Swimming and walking are encouraged.
- *Back education:* Stress on the back is less when it is properly used during sitting, walking, etc. These proper habits have to be cultivated with practice.

Arthroplasty

ARTHROPLASTY

This essentially means replacement of joints and this could be partial or total. When only one part of the joint is removed, it is called partial and is known as Hemi replacement arthroplasty. When complete joint is replaced it is called Total Joint replacement and when one half of the joint is replaced it is called Unicondylar replacement of the joint. When only diseased surface is resected and resurfaced it is called Resurfacing procedure.

Types of Prosthesis

❖ Metallic prosthesis on one or both sides of the joints
❖ High density polyethylene
❖ Ceramic

Choice of Prosthesis

❖ Both metals
❖ Both Ceramics
❖ One metallic (Femoral) and one poly (Acetabular)

Fixation: It could be cemented or uncemented. The former is used in older people and the latter in younger individuals.

Total knee and hip arthroplasty has become the definitive treatment for end stage osteoarthritis. They have proved to be reliable and successful allowing patients to resume normal activities.

TOTAL HIP REPLACEMENT

Total hip replacement has stood the test of time and today commands its own place as an effective option for end stage arthritis of the hip joint. Hip arthroplasty can be performed without cement as in young patients, using cement or biologic fixation in elderly and osteoporotic patients. In cement fixation there is mechanical interlock of methyl methacrylate to the interstices of bone. Biological fixation can be either a porous-coated metallic surface that provides bone ingrowths fixation or by a grit-blasted metallic surface that provides bone ongrowth fixation.

Indications

* Severe osteoarthritis **(Fig. 31.1)**
* Rheumatoid arthritis
* Secondary osteoarthritis
* Avascular necrosis of the head of femur
* Failed Hemi replacement arthroplasty
* Ankylosed hip
* Tuberculosis hip

Contraindications

* Infection is an absolute contraindication
* Poor medical risk
* Poor anesthetic risk
* Obesity
* Neuropathic joints

Complications

* DVT
* Fat embolism
* Infection
* Breakages of implants
* Loosening of implants
* Osteolysis
* Periprosthetic fractures
* Dislocation
* Heterotrophic ossification
* Vascular and nerve injuries

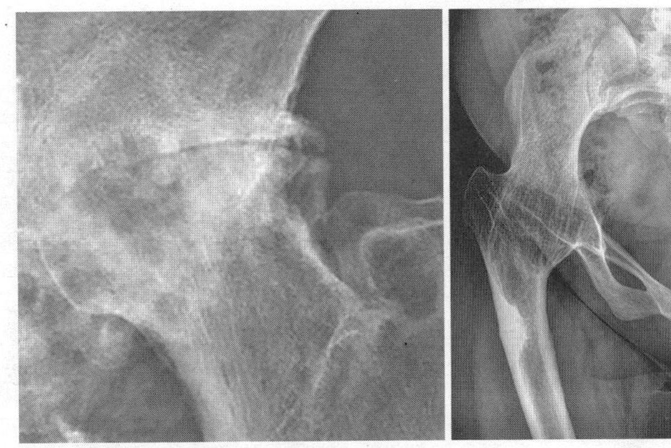

Fig. 31.1: Showing severe OA hip and ankylosed hip which require total hip replacement.

The Choice of Cup and Stem

The choice of method of fixation remains controversial. In hip arthroplasty the tendency is towards the use of uncemented prosthesis in younger active patients because cemented prosthesis have reported a higher loosening rate in long term follow up. In total knee arthroplasty the cemented prosthesis have reported good results in long term follow up and is more widely used than the cement less ones.

Articular bearing in hip arthroplasty is mainly on "hard on soft couple" which include metallic heads coupled with polyethylene cup. The other hard on soft couple is ceramic head with polyethylene cup. Titanium alloy heads should be avoided because it is liable to scratching which will cause rapid wear of the polyethylene surface. In knee arthroplasty the majority of articular bearing components are metallic femoral surface (cobalt, chromium) coupled with polyethylene tibial surface.

Types of THR

The hip replacement surgeries can be hemiarthroplasty which is now used as a salvage procedure in very old and inactive patient, bipolar hip replacement, total hip replacement or Birmingham hip resurfacing surgeries **(Fig. 31.2)**.

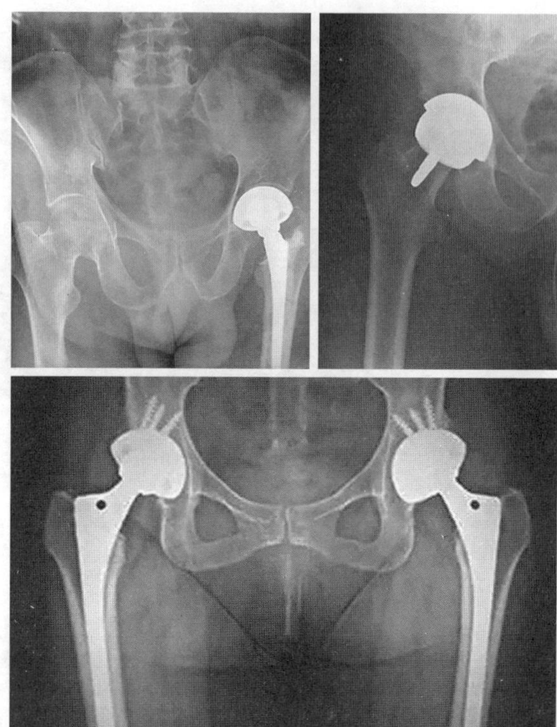

Fig. 31.2: Showing different types of hip surgeries: Bipolar hip replacement, total hip replacement and Birmingham hip resurfacing surgery.

TOTAL KNEE REPLACEMENT

This is increasingly gaining popularity thanks to the high incidences of osteoarthritis of the knee joints worldwide. Though not as popular or as successful as total hip replacement, TKR nevertheless is catching the attention of both orthopedic surgeons and patients alike and is being commonly performed across the country.

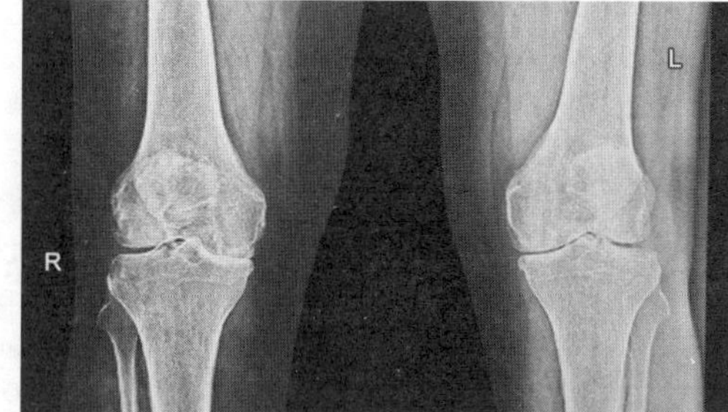

Fig. 31.3: Showing advanced OA knees, an indication for TKR.

Indications

- ❖ Advanced osteoarthritis of the knee (**Fig. 31.3**)
- ❖ Rheumatoid arthritis
- ❖ Advanced post-traumatic secondary osteoarthritis
- ❖ Failed Hemi replacement arthroplasty
- ❖ Ankylosed knee

Types

- ❖ **Unicondylar replacement:** Here only one compartment of the knee joint, usually the medial tibiofemoral compartment is replaced in unilateral OA knee and in young patients (**Fig. 31.4**).

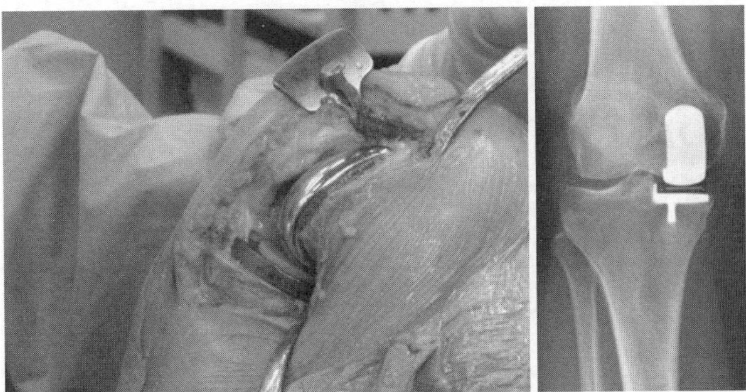

Fig. 31.4: Showing unicondylar knee replacement indicated in isolated medical compartment OA knees.

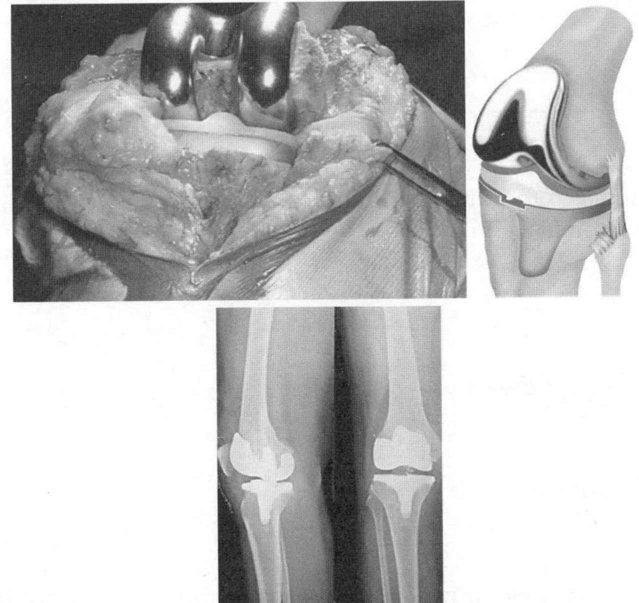

Fig. 31.5: Showing total knee replacement in advanced OA knees.

❖ **Total knee replacement:** This could be cemented or uncemented, PCL sacrificing or sparing or rotating platform **(Fig. 31.5)**.

Components

❖ A metallic femoral component
❖ Tibial base plate
❖ A plastic component
❖ A patellar component
Indications, contraindications and complications more or less remain the same as for THR.

32
CHAPTER

Amputations

AMPUTATION

Definition

Amputation is defined as removal of the limb through a part of a bone. Disarticulation is the removal of the limb through a joint.

Incidences

Age

Common in 50–75 years age group.

Sex

About 75% men, 25% women.

Limbs

About 85% is through the lower limbs, 15% is through the upper limbs. Injuries leading to amputations are the ones which are severe and leave the limbs badly mutilated. High speed RTA's, major falls, and crushing injuries due to industrial or agricultural accidents spell unmitigated disaster to the limbs making amputation a logical solution. However, in children, congenital anomalies and in the elderly, peripheral vascular disease is the common causes of amputations.

Remember

The only real absolute indication for amputation is irreparable loss of blood supply of a diseased or injured limb.

Quick facts: Common indications for amputations versus age

- Children—Congenital anomalies
- Young adults—Injuries
- Elderly patients—Peripheral vascular disease

AMPUTATION LEVELS

Upper Limbs

Various levels of amputation at the upper limbs **(Fig. 32.1)**

- ❖ Shoulder disarticulation
- ❖ Short above elbow
- ❖ Standard above elbow
- ❖ Elbow disarticulation
- ❖ Very short below elbow
- ❖ Medium below elbow
- ❖ Long below elbow.

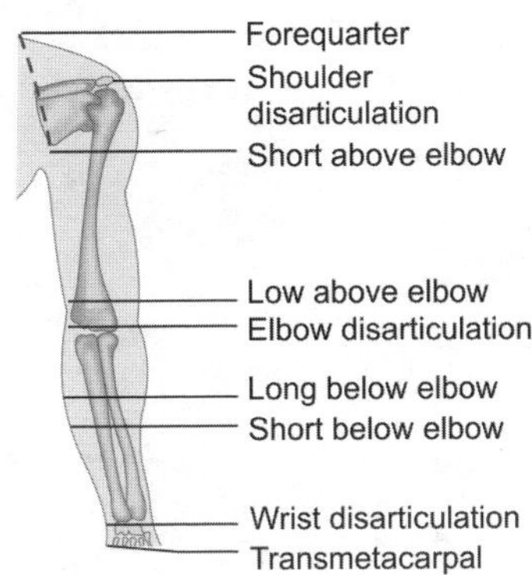

Fig. 32.1: Showing the levels of upper limb amputations.

Lower Limbs

Various levels of amputations at the lower limbs are **(Fig. 32.2)**:

- ❖ Hip disarticulation
- ❖ Very short above knee
- ❖ Short above knee
- ❖ Medium above knee
- ❖ Long above knee
- ❖ Very long above knee
- ❖ Knee disarticulation
- ❖ Very short below knee
- ❖ Short and below knee.

Ankle Amputation

- ❖ **Syme's amputation:** Here the level of bone section is 0.6 cm proximal to the ankle joint
- ❖ **Sarmiento's amputation:** Here the level is 1.3 cm proximal to the joint.
- ❖ **Wagner's:** It is two-stage Syme's amputation.
- ❖ **Boyd's:** This consists of talectomy and calcaneotibial arthrodesis.
- ❖ **Pirogoff's amputation:** In this only anterior part of the calcaneum is removed.

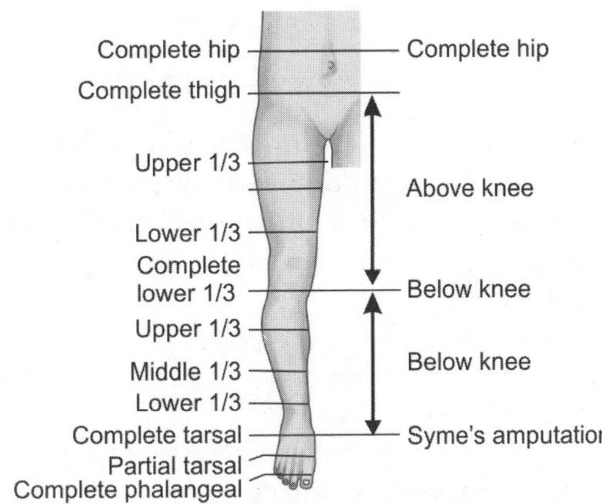

Fig. 32.2: Showing different levels of lower limb amputations.

Foot Amputation

- ❖ Amputation of great toes and other toes.
- ❖ Amputation through the metatarsal bones.
- ❖ **Lisfranc's operation:** Amputation is at the level of the tarsometatarsal joints.
- ❖ **Chopart's operation:** Amputation is through the midtarsal joints.

PRINCIPLES AND TYPES OF AMPUTATIONS

Closed Amputation

This is done most of the times as an elective procedure and may be above knee or below knee, above elbow and below elbow, etc. **(Fig. 32.3)**. In this, the skin is closed primarily after amputation.

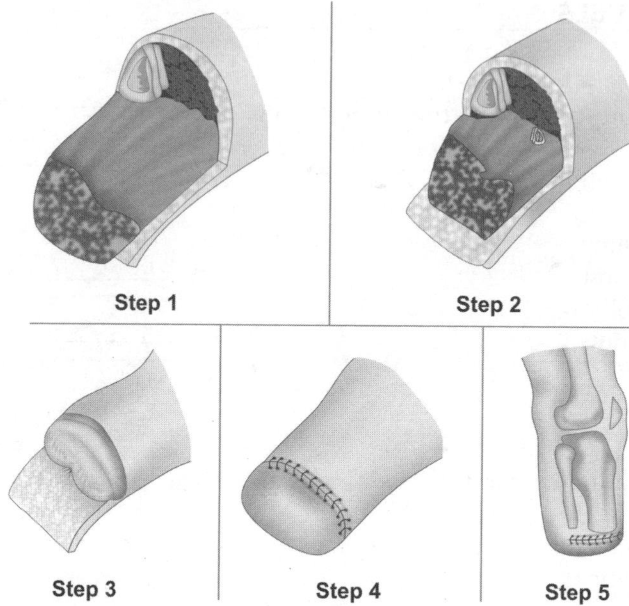

Fig. 32.3: Showing closed amputation.

1. **Tourniquets** these are desirable except in ischemic limbs.
2. **Level of amputation** as in the past the level of amputation is no longer important, thanks to the modern and sophisticated present day prosthesis.

> **Remember**
>
> **The cardinal rule**
> Amputate through the tissues that will heal satisfactorily and preserve all possible lengths consistent with good surgical judgment.

- ❖ **Skin flaps:** Good skin coverage for the amputation site is of vital importance. The skin should be mobile and sensitive. Location of the scar is not important.
- ❖ **Muscles:** The muscle is divided at least 5 cm distal to the level of intended bone section and sutured.

> **Remember**
>
> **Two methods of muscle suture**
> **Myodesis:** Here muscle is sutured to the ends of the bone stump.
> **Myoplasty:** Here muscles are sutured to the opposite muscle group under appropriate tension.

Note: *These are unpreferred methods in peripheral vascular disease.*

These two techniques of *myodesis and myoplasty* helps improve the function of the muscles and circulation in the stump and thereby helps to prevent phantom pain.

- ❖ **Nerves:** The nerves are pulled down and cut proximally and allowed to retract. Larger nerves like the Sciatic nerve needs to be ligated before cutting.
- ❖ **Blood vessels:** Blood vessels are doubly ligated with non-absorbable sutures and cut.
- ❖ **Bone:** The bone is sectioned above the level of muscle section. Ragged irregular bone edges need to be smoothened before closure.
- ❖ **Drains:** Drains are removed after 48–72 hours to prevent stump edema.

COMPLICATIONS OF AMPUTATIONS

Hematomas

These are due to slipping of ligatures, inadequate hemostasis etc. This delays the wound healing and acts as a culture media for the growth of the organisms. The treatment consists of aspiration and pressure bandaging.

Infections

This is more common in peripheral vascular disease and diabetics. Appropriate antibiotics needs to be given.

Necrosis

Necrosis of the skin flaps are usually due to insufficient circulation and require revision amputations or redesigning of the skin flaps.

Contractures

This is largely preventable by positioning the stump properly. Physiotherapy and severe ones by surgery can correct mild contractures.

Neuromas

Neuromas form always on the end of a cutaneous nerve and any pain from a neuroma is usually caused by traction on a nerve when it is embedded within the scar tissue.

Phantom Sensation

This is a pseudo feeling of the presence of the amputated limb. It could be of a painless or a painful variety. This is predominantly felt during the early stages of amputation. Treatment is challenging.

Causalgia

It is due to division of the peripheral nerves. Even local stimulus stimulates pain.

Remember

- 85% amputations are through the lower limbs.
- Severe injury forms the most common indication in adults PVD is elderly and congenital in children.
- Level of amputation is no longer important as in the past due to efficient prosthesis.
- The latest concept is to preserve as much stump length as possible.
- Guillotine amputations are salvage procedures for life-threatening infections.
- Stump care is very vital to prevent postamputation problems.

Prosthetics and Orthotics

PROSTHESIS

Definition

Prosthesis in Greek means "in addition". Thus, prosthesis is *defined as a replacement or substitution of a missing or a diseased part.* Prosthetics is the theory and practice of the prescription, fitting, design, assessment and production of prosthesis.

Classification

End Prostheses

These are implants internally used in orthopedic surgery to replace joints, e.g., Austin Moore prosthesis.

Exoprosthesis

These are for external replacement for the lost part of a limb. They are more extensively used in the lower limbs.

PARTS OF PROSTHESIS (LOWER LIMBS)

It has three components, the proximal, middle and the distal parts.

Proximal Part

This consists of two components namely, socket and suspension.

Socket

This is the lodging space for the stump and is usually double walled. The sockets are usually designed according to the shape of the stump, first by taking a plaster of Paris mould and finally the plastic mould. The final fit should be comfortable. If the weight bearing is through the end of the sump, it is called "End bearing stump" and if it is through the entire stump area, it is called the "Total Contact Socket". The other important component of the proximal part is the suspension which holds the socket to the stump.

Middle Part

This is the link between the proximal and distal parts and consists of joints and an extension, which is a link between the middle and distal parts.

Distal Part

This belongs to the prosthetic foot. Traditionally it is the SACH foot, with a wooden core and peripheral rubber components. SACH foot is designed to look like a normal foot and make walking on uneven surfaces easier. Indian modification to the SACH foot is the 'Jaipur Foot'. **(Fig. 33.1)**. Modifications are done keeping the Indian interest of 'barefoot walking' in mind. We all should be proud of our very own Dr PC Sethi of Jaipur whose pioneering work in devising Jaipur foot has come as a boon to our fellow citizens.

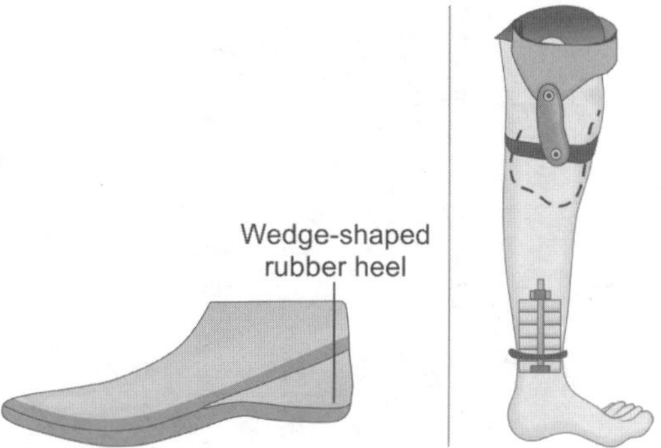

Fig. 33.1: Showing SACH foot and Jaipur foot.

Recent Trends

Use of computers in designing lightweight materials, battery and electronically operated devices etc., has revolution prosthetic designing and wear.

Types

1. **Temporary prosthesis (e.g., Pylon):** These are used following an amputation till the patient is fitted with permanent prosthesis **(Fig. 33.2)**.
2. **Permanent prosthesis:** PTB prosthesis Symes' prosthesis, SACH foot, Jaipur foot are some of the examples of permanent prosthesis.

Prosthesis for the lower limbs: Prosthesis for the lower limbs is required in the following situations:

❖ For disarticulation of hip and hemipelvectomy **(Fig. 33.3)**.

❖ Following transfemoral amputations: Two types of prostheses are recommended.

   a. *Suction-socketed limb* this is useful in young adults and is best suited for cylindrical stumps. It snuggly fits and has a two-way valve mechanism to maintain negative pressure.

   b. *Non-suction-socketed limb* Here no negative pressure is employed to hold the prosthesis, but pelvic bands or harness are made use of for holding.

❖ **Prosthesis for through knee amputation.**

❖ **Prosthesis for below knee amputations** two varieties are described:

   ◆ *Patellar tendon bearing (PTB) prosthesis:* In this, the socket is made in such a way that it fits exactly over the patellar tendon and the sides of the tibial condyles **(Fig. 33.4)**.

   ◆ *Conventional type prosthesis:* This consists of the thigh corset, the side steels, the knee joint, shin piece, ankle joint unit and the foot piece.

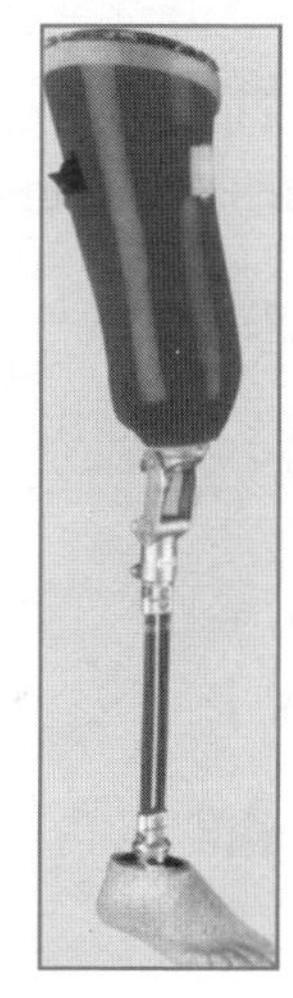

Fig. 33.2: Showing a temporary prosthesis.

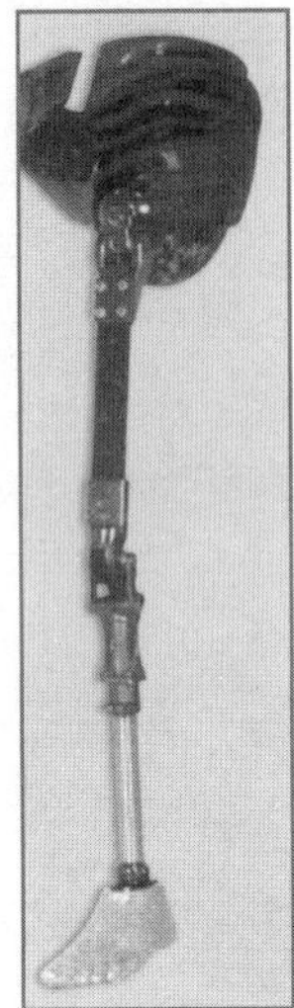

Fig. 33.3: Showing prosthesis for hemi-pelvectomy and hip disarticulation.

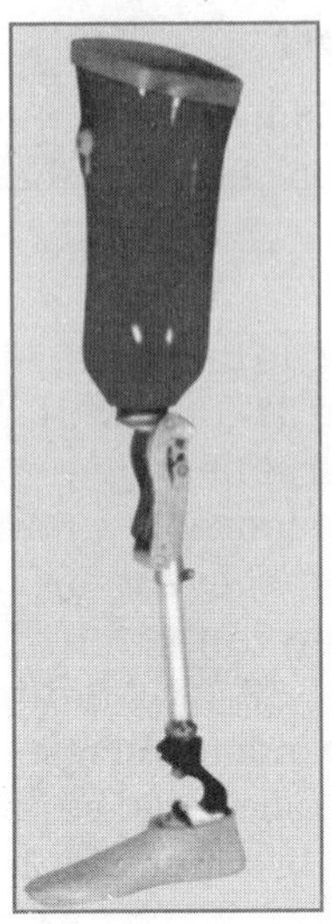

Fig. 33.4: Prosthesis for above-knee amputation.

❖ **Prosthesis for Syme's amputation:** This is a below knee prosthesis used after Syme's amputation **(Fig. 33.5)**. These prostheses may have closed sockets or open sockets and may be full weight bearing or modified end bearing.

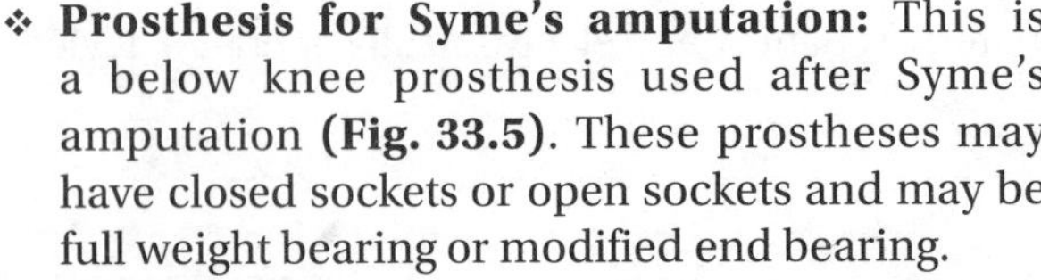

Remember

Aims of prosthetic fitting
- ◀◀ To substitute for a lost part.
- ◀◀ To restore a lost function.
- ◀◀ In lower limbs it must provide a comfortable ambulation with minimal expenditure of energy.

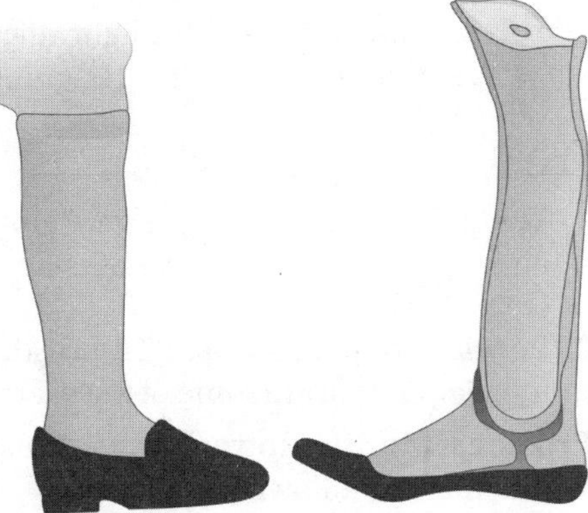

Fig. 33.5: Showing PTB prosthesis and syme's prosthesis.

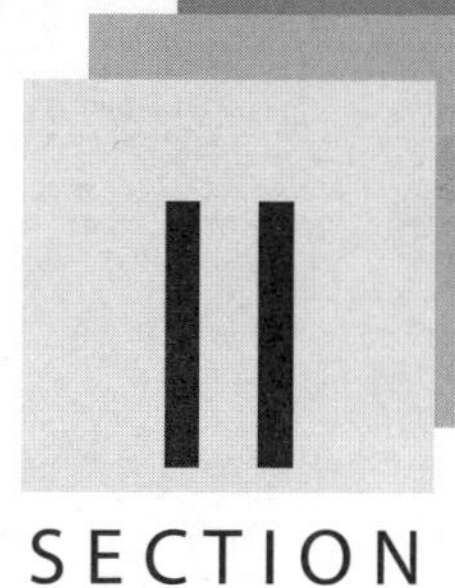

SECTION

PRACTICAL ORTHOPEDICS

SECTION OUTLINE

Upper Limbs

Lower Limbs

Upper Limbs

Upper Limb Fractures

This chapter deals with the step-by-step practical techniques of managing the common upper limb injuries.

1. Fracture Clavicle

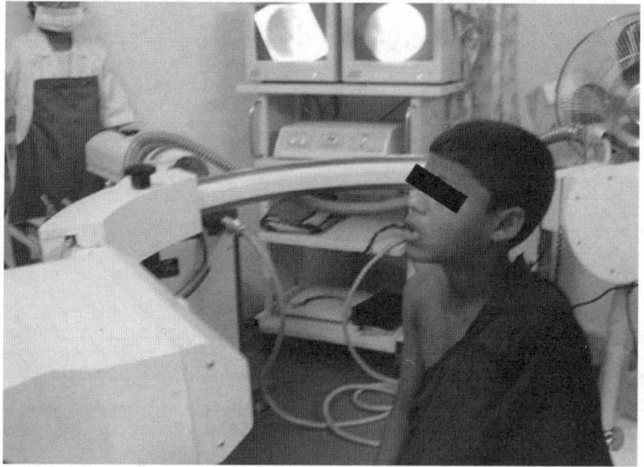

Fig. 34.1: Checking under C arm.

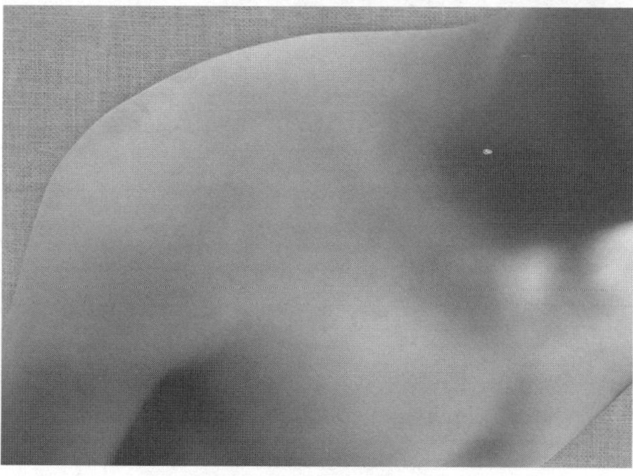

Fig. 34.2: Deformity.

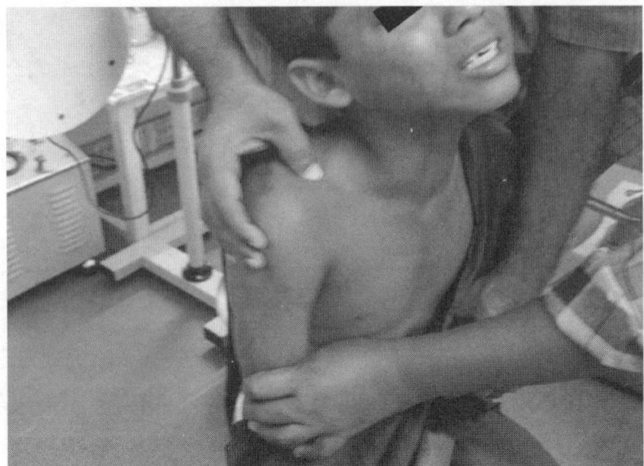

Fig. 34.3A: Elevation of the arm and bracing back of the shoulder.

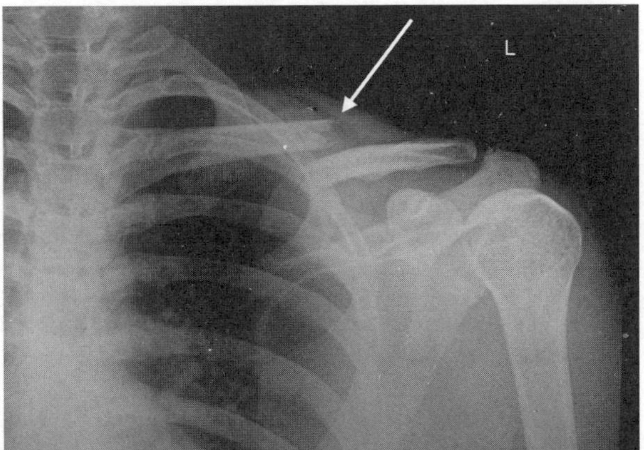

Fig. 34.3B: Plain X-ray of fracture clavicle.

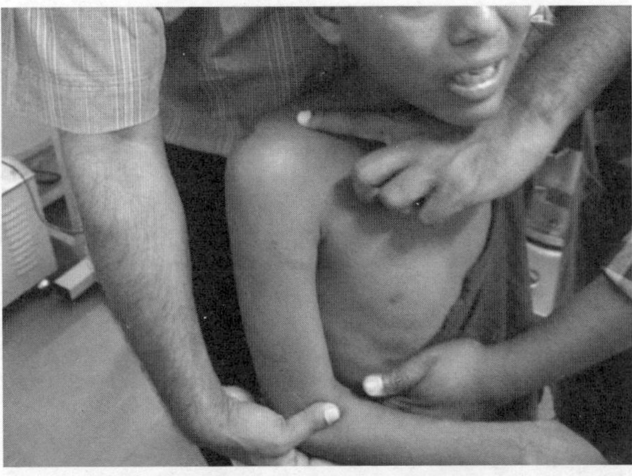

Fig. 34.4: Reduction technique.

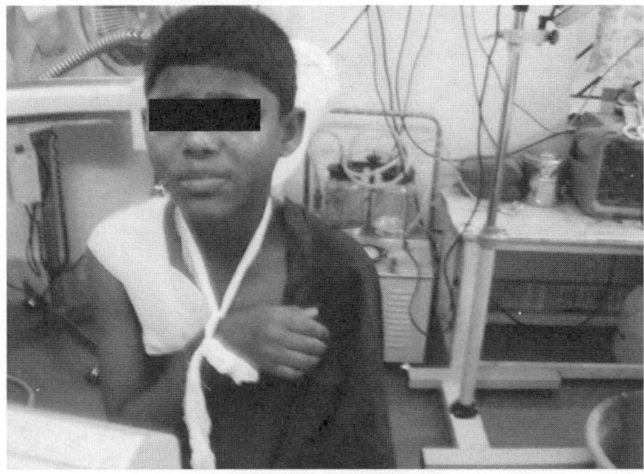

Fig. 34.5: Strapping and sling post-reduction.

2. Anterior Shoulder Dislocation—Reduction

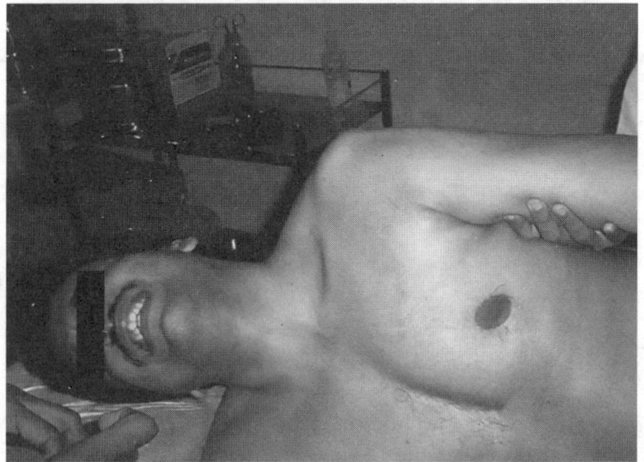

Fig. 34.6: Clinical photo.

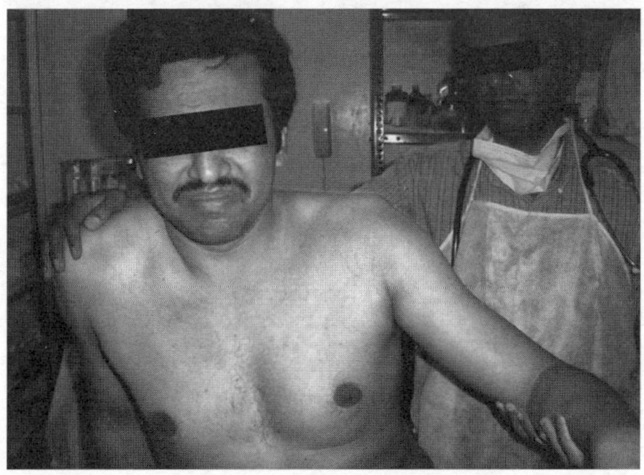

Fig. 34.7: Deformity.

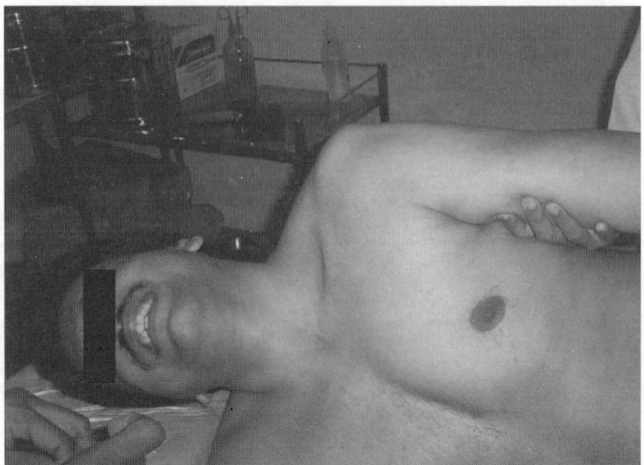

Fig. 34.8A: Loss of contour.

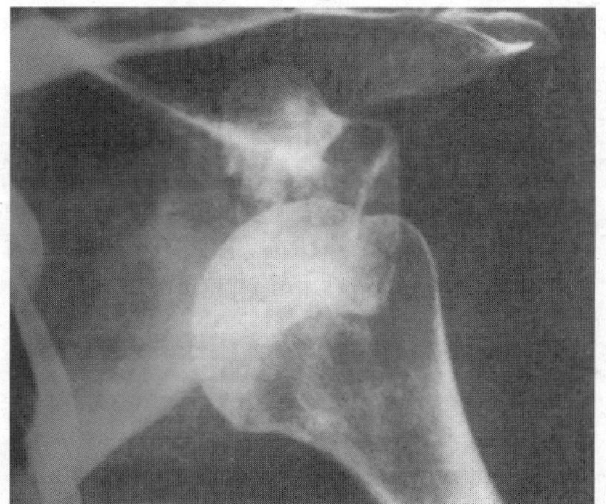

Fig. 34.8B: Plain X-ray showing anterior dislocation of shoulder.

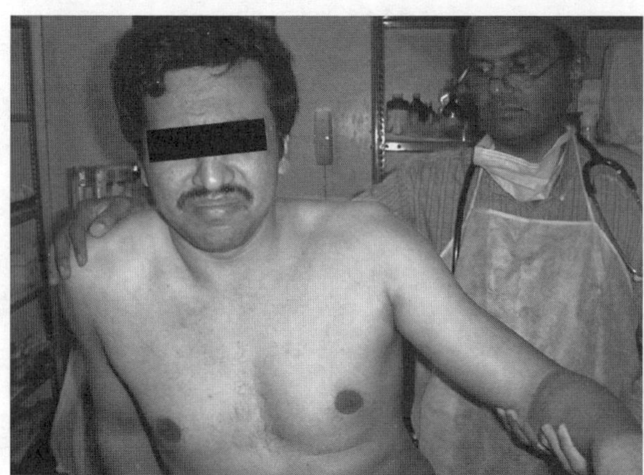

Fig. 34.9: Shoulder droop.

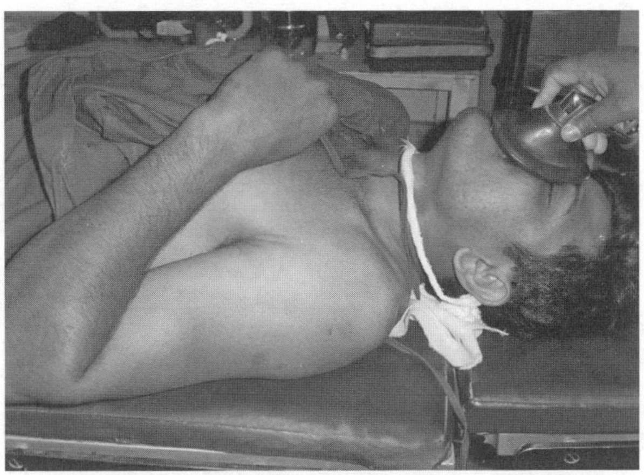

Fig. 34.10: Patient is under general anesthesia.

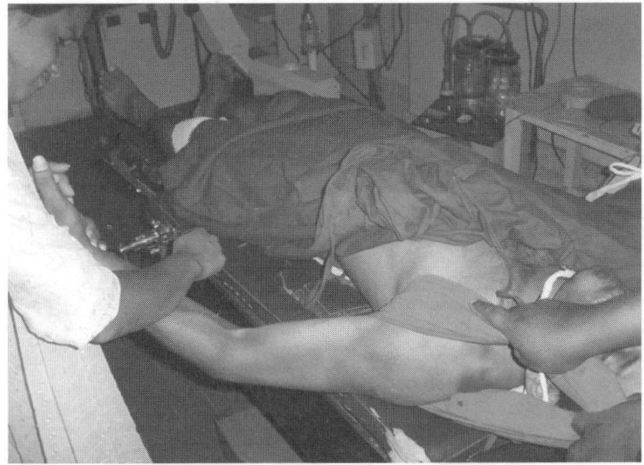

Fig. 34.11: Kocher's technique Step 1 longitudinal traction.

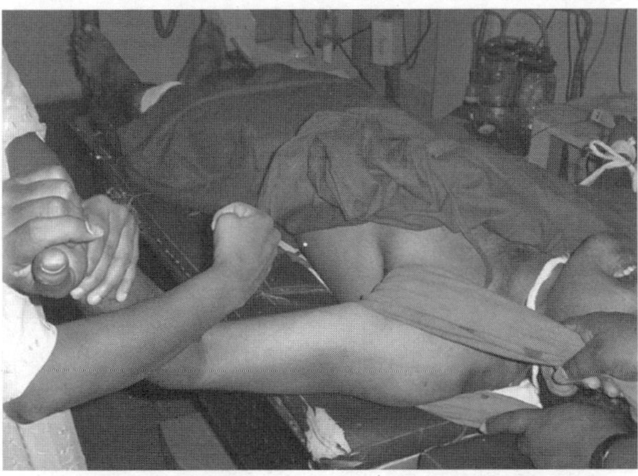

Fig. 34.12: Step 2 traction and counter traction.

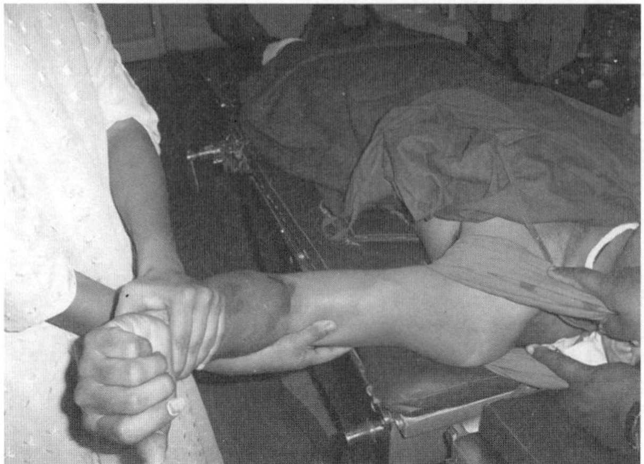

Fig. 34.13: Step 3 external rotation.

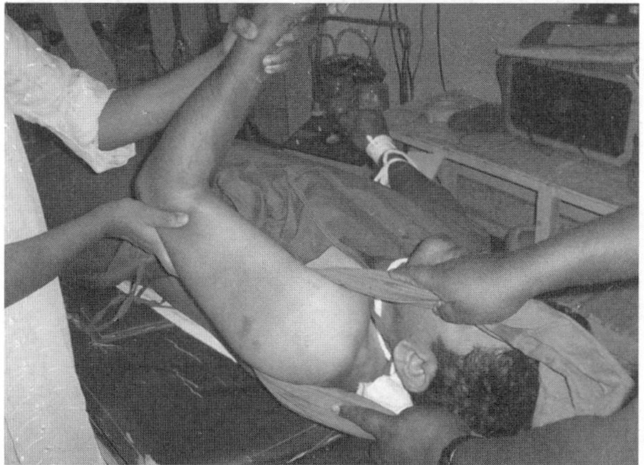

Fig. 34.14: Step 4 adduction.

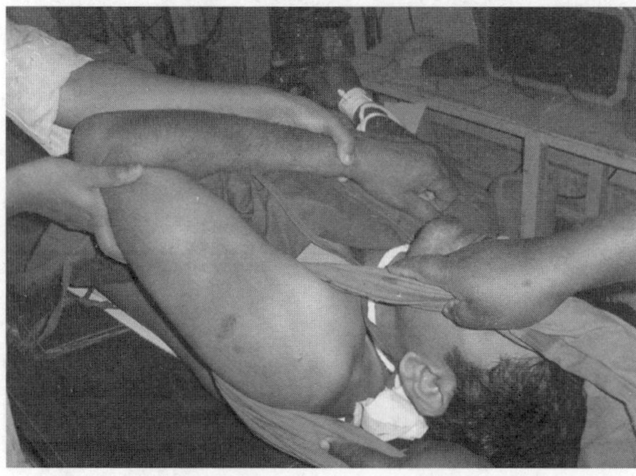

Fig. 34.15: Step 5 internal rotation.

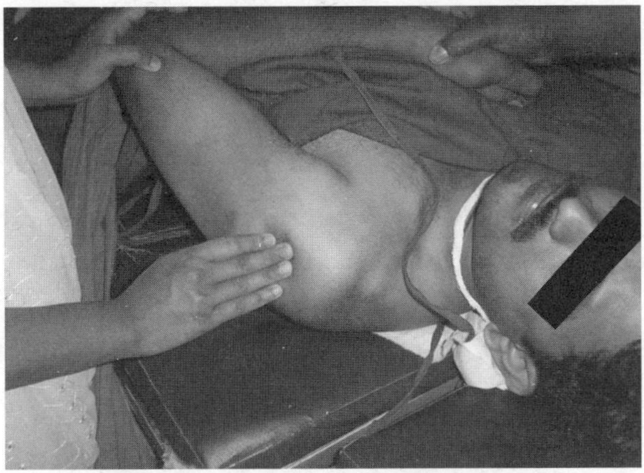

Fig. 34.16: Shoulder contour restored.

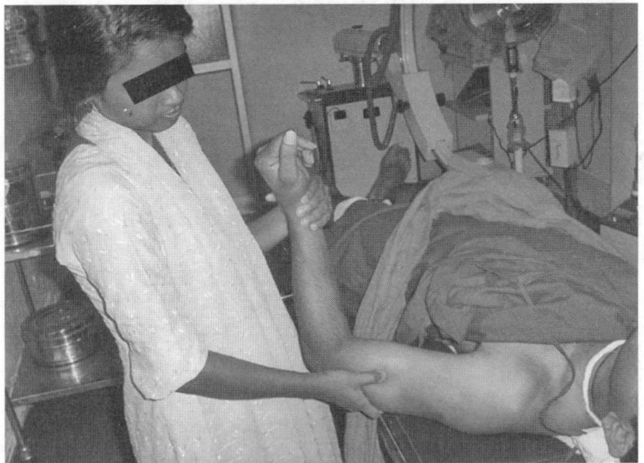

Fig. 34.17: Checking for the stability post-reduction.

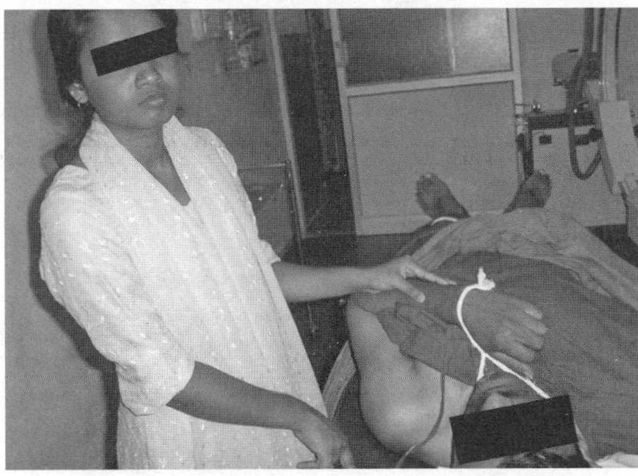

Fig. 34.18: Cuff and sling.

POSTERIOR FRACTURE DISLOCATION

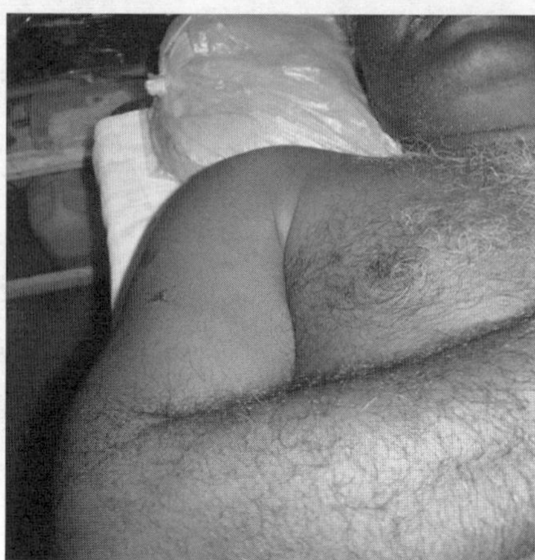

Fig. 34.19: Anterior contour lost.

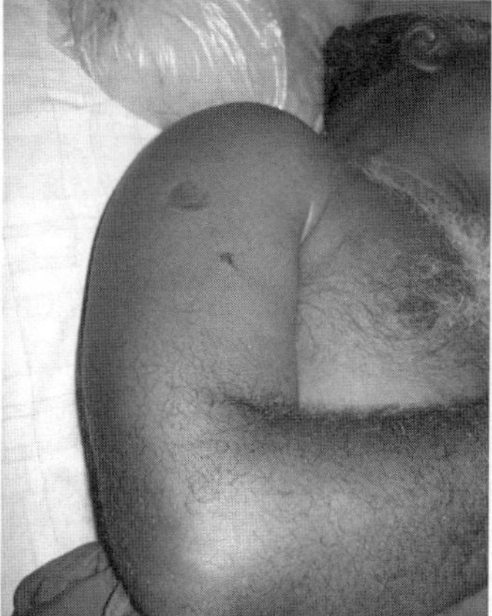

Fig. 34.20: Deformity.

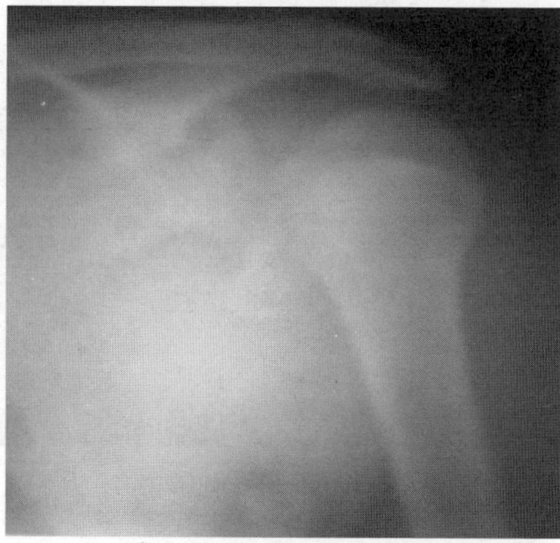

Fig. 34.21: Fracture seen.

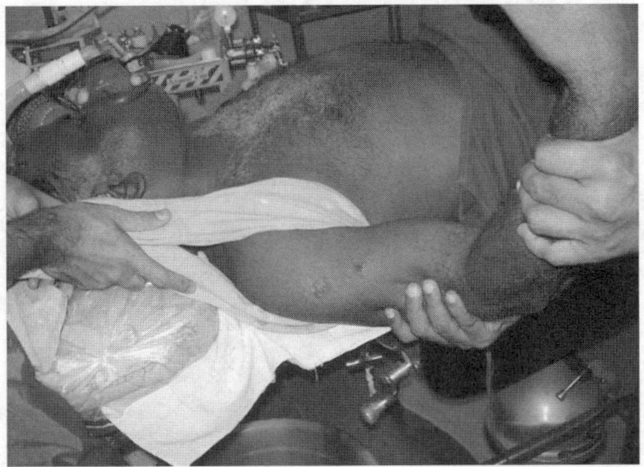

Fig. 34.22: Traction and countertraction provided.

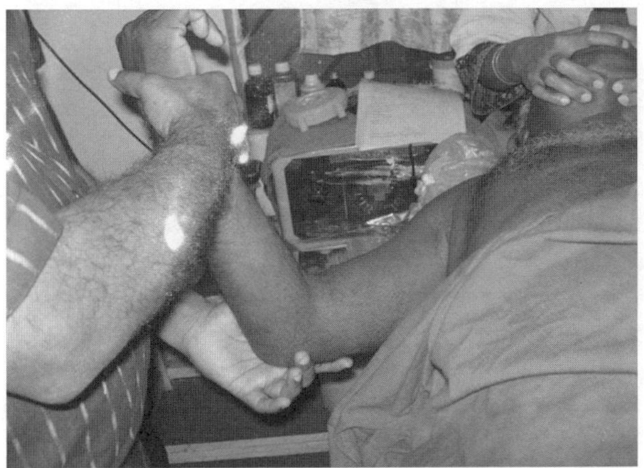

Fig. 34.23: Traction continued.

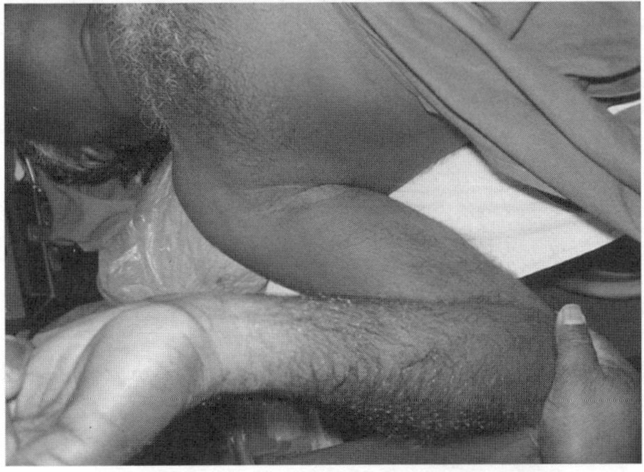

Fig. 34.24: Traction and external rotation.

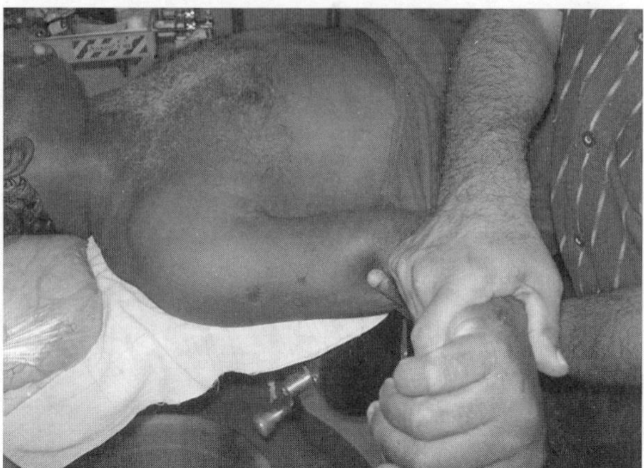

Fig. 34.25: Reduction achieved.

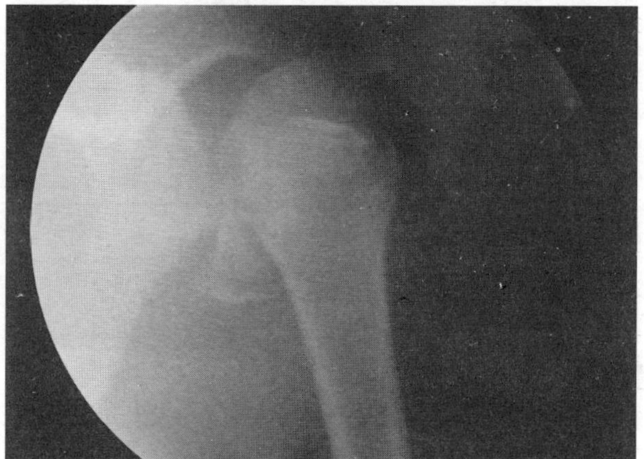

Fig. 34.26: But Image shows attempt unsuccessful.

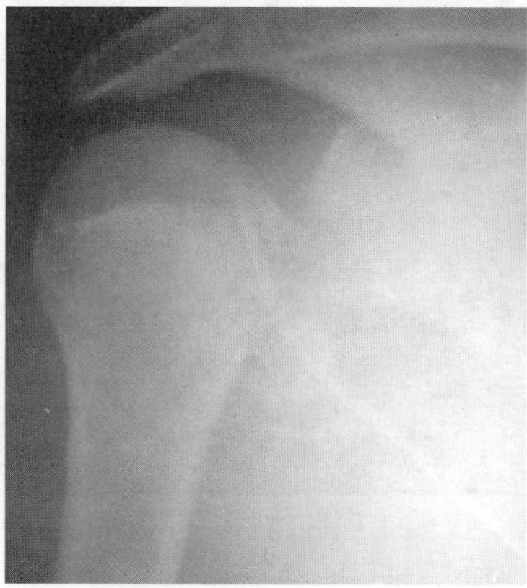

Fig. 34.27: X-ray vacant glenoid sign.

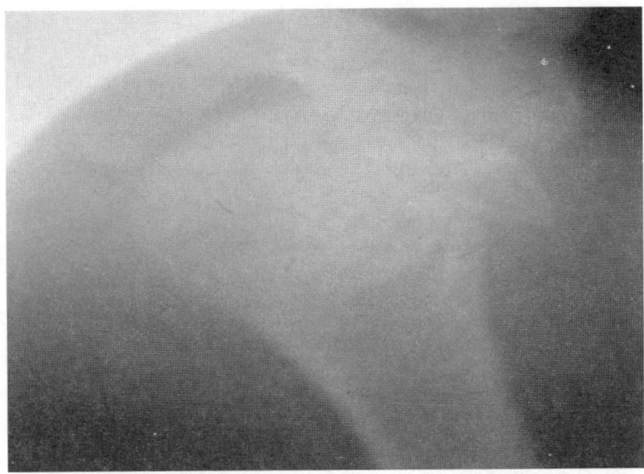

Fig. 34.28: Head in acetabular socket.

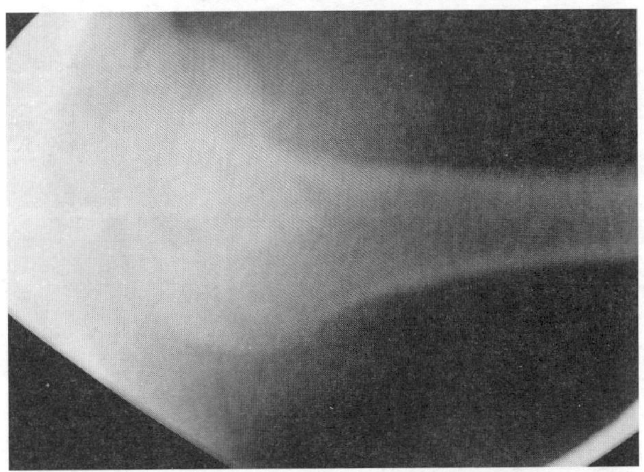

Fig. 34.29: Reduction attempted again.

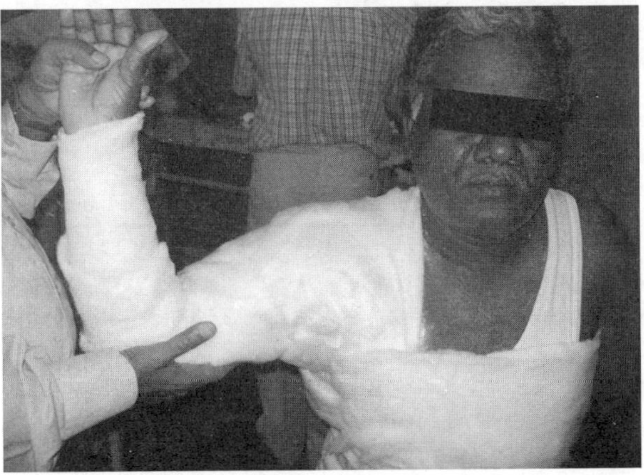

Fig. 34.30: Immobilization in external rotation.

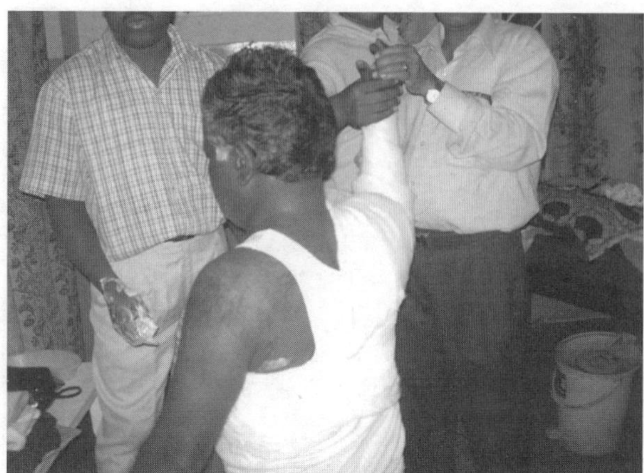

Fig. 34.31: Shoulder spica being applied.

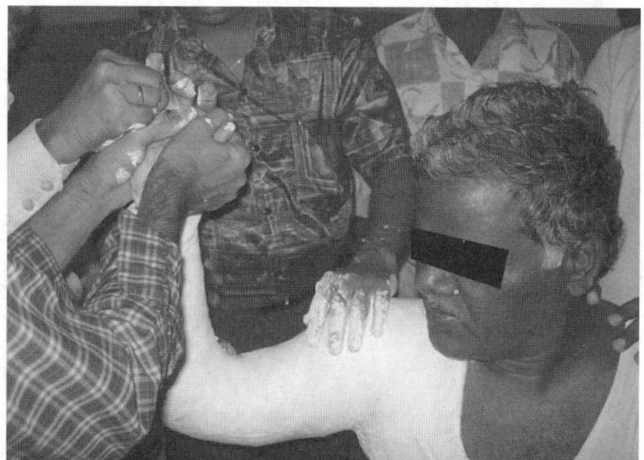

Fig. 34.32: Application continued.

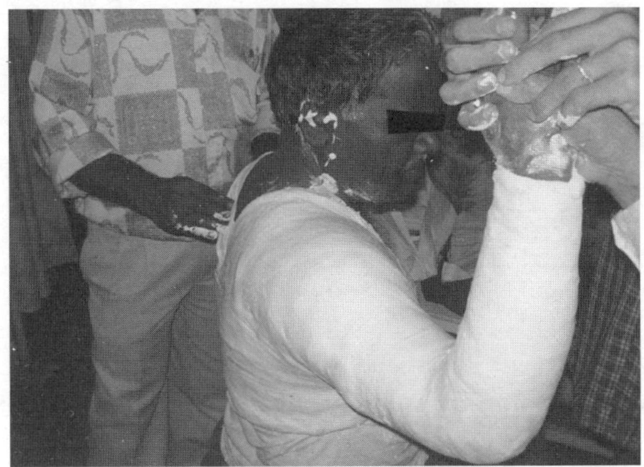

Fig. 34.33: Application completed.

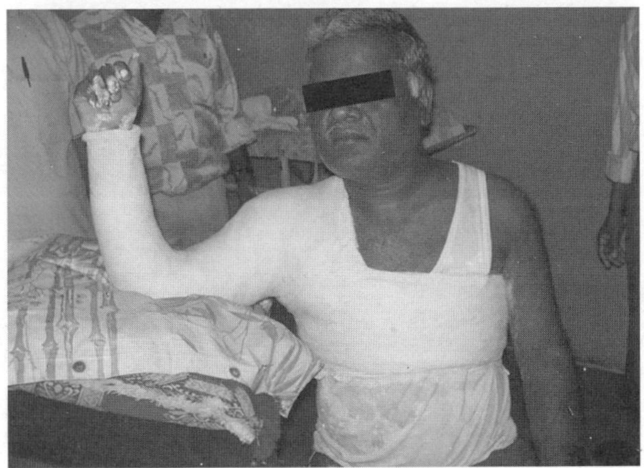

Fig. 34.34: Final position.

Forearm Fracture

This chapter deals with the step-by-step practical techniques of managing the common forearm injuries.

BOTH BONES FOREARM FRACTURE IN OLDER CHILD

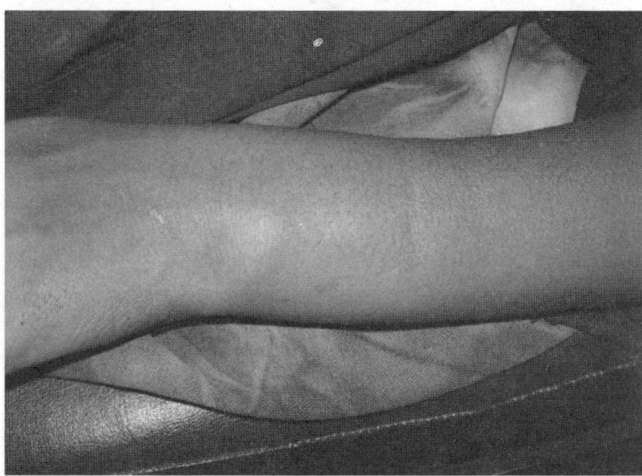

Fig. 35.1: Deformity.

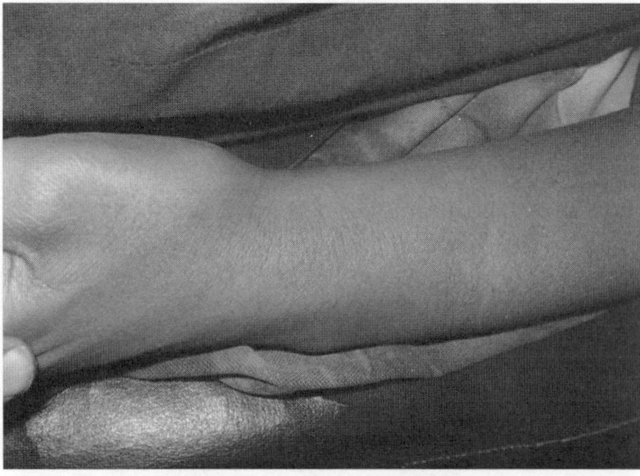

Fig. 35.2: Deformity side view.

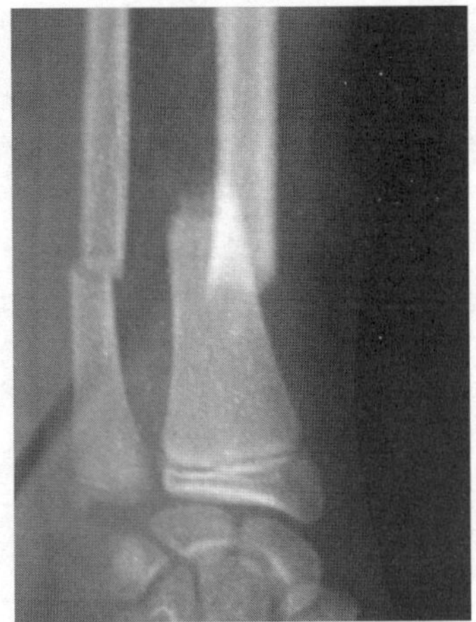

Fig. 35.3: X-ray—AP view.

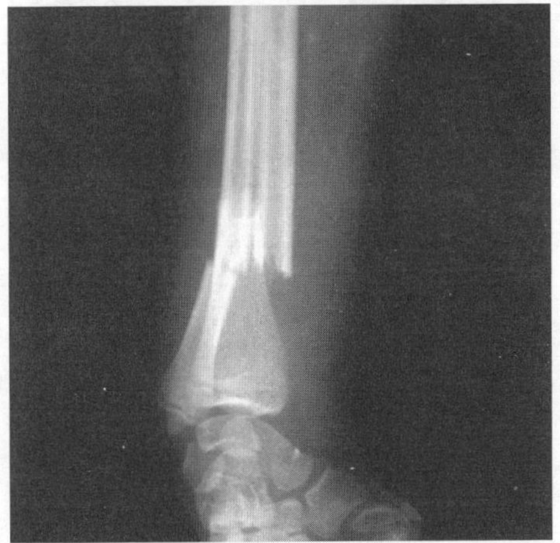

Fig. 35.4: X-ray—lateral view.

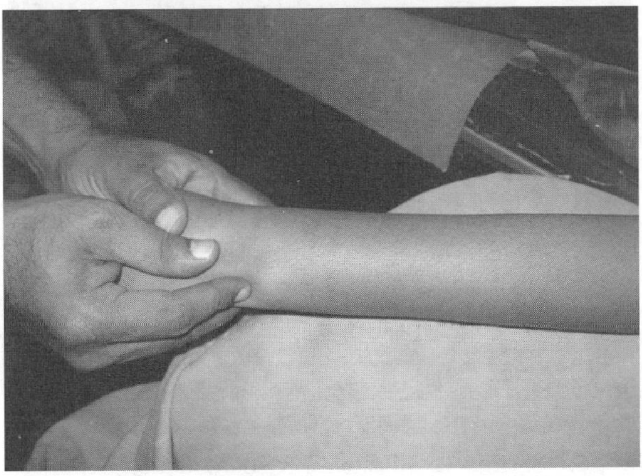

Fig. 35.5: Reduction Step 1—traction.

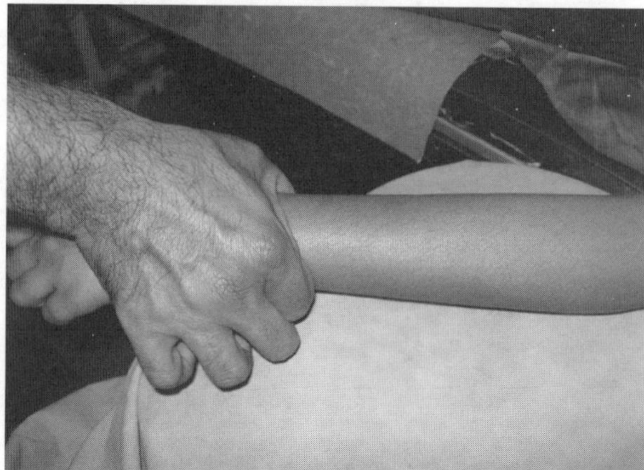

Fig. 35.6: Reduction Step 2—manipulation of the fracture.

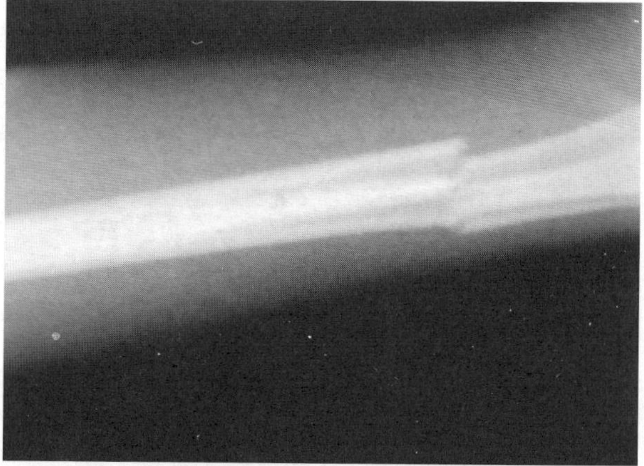

Fig. 35.7: C-arm—preplaster check of reduction—lateral view.

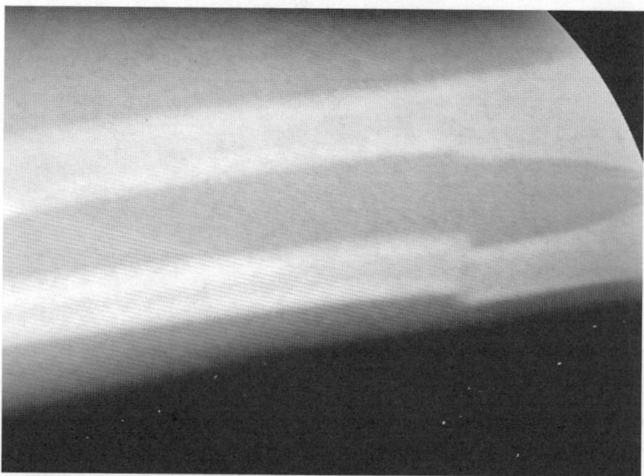

Fig. 35.8: C-arm—preplaster check of reduction—AP view.

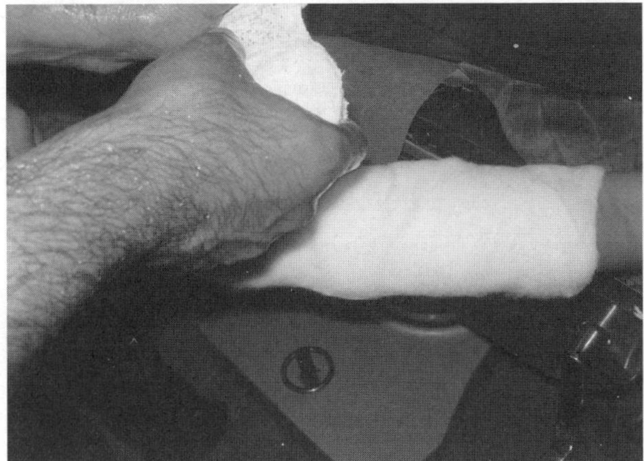

Fig. 35.9: Application of soft ban.

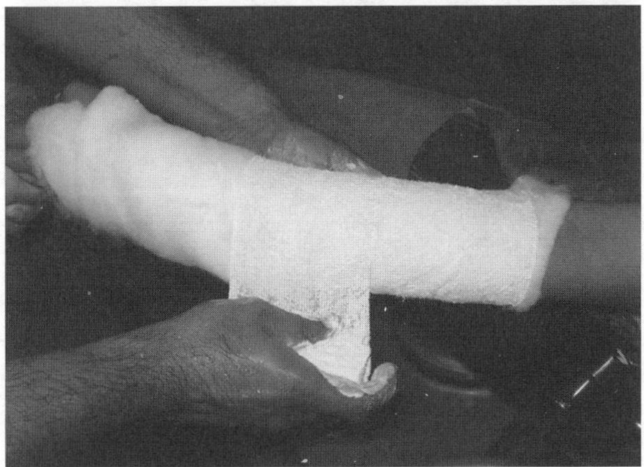

Fig. 35.10: Rolling of POP.

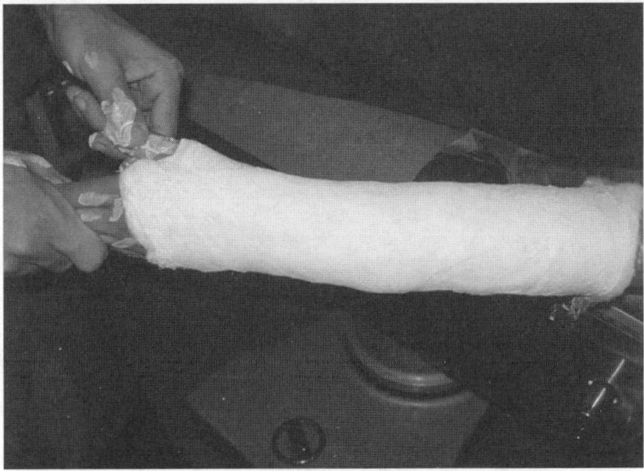

Fig. 35.11: Application of POP completed.

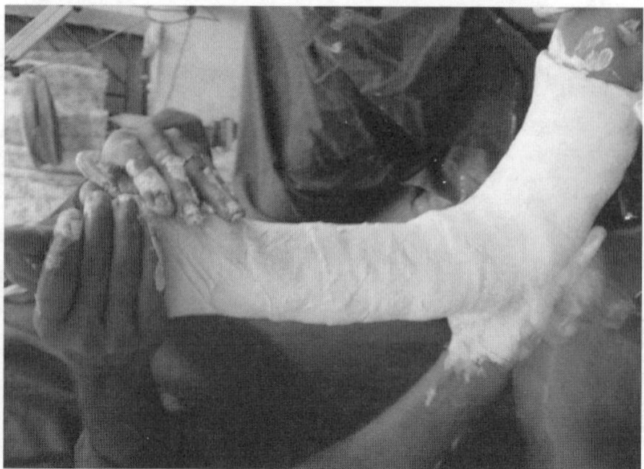

Fig. 35.12: Above elbow POP applied.

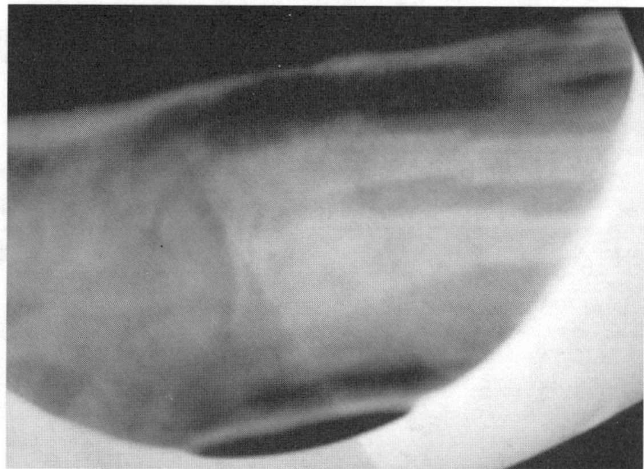

Fig. 35.13: Post-plaster C-arm picture.

DISTAL FOREARM BOTH BONES FRACTURE

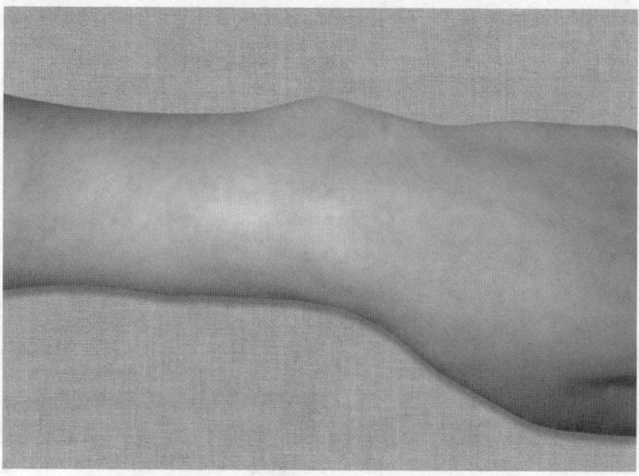

Fig. 35.14: Deformity of the forearm.

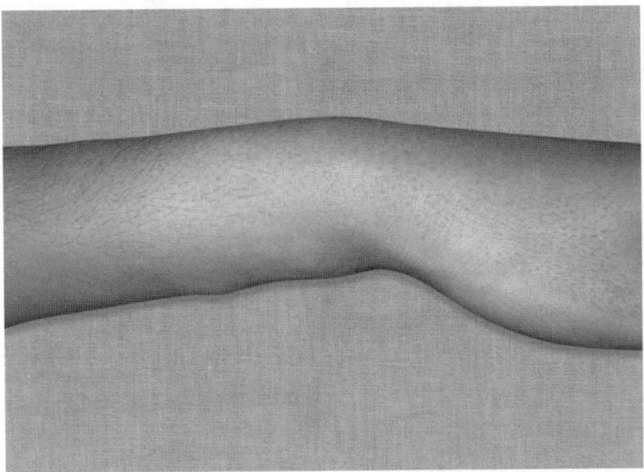

Fig. 35.15: Deformity from the sides.

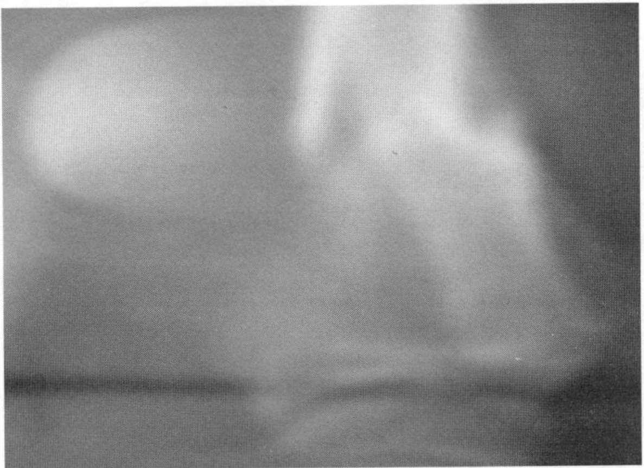

Fig. 35.16: X-ray showing displaced fracture.

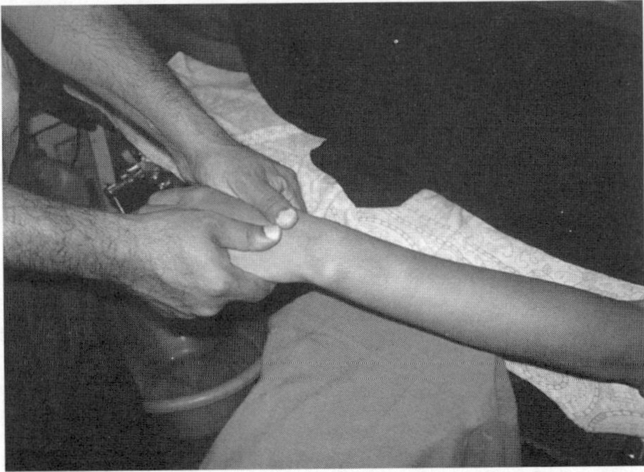

Fig. 35.17: Closed reduction Step 1—longitudinal traction.

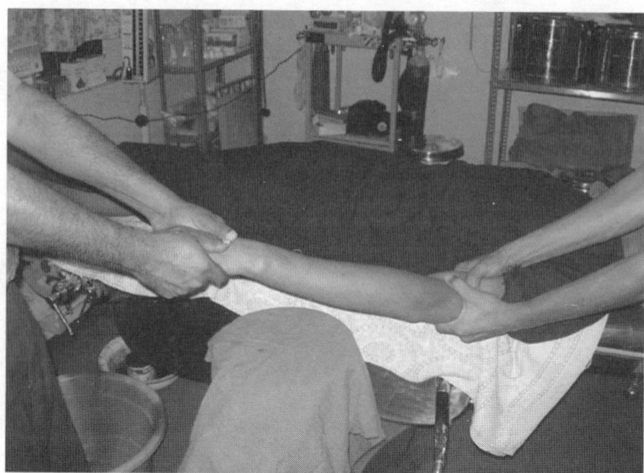

Fig. 35.18: Step 2—counter traction.

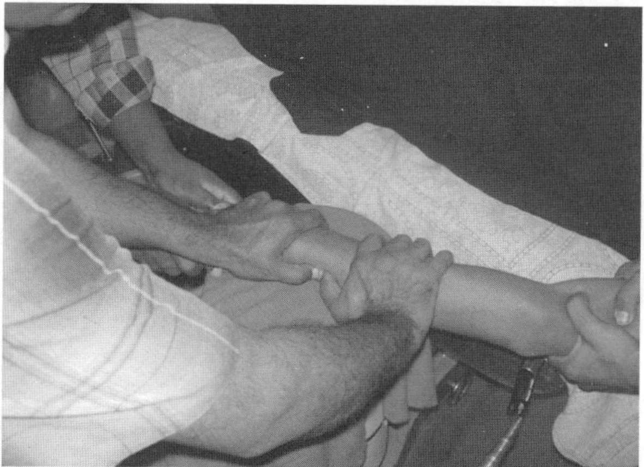

Fig. 35.19: Manipulation of the fractures.

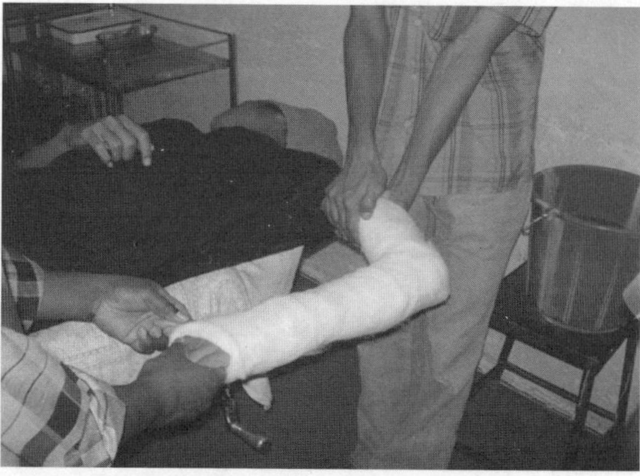

Fig. 35.20: Application of soft ban.

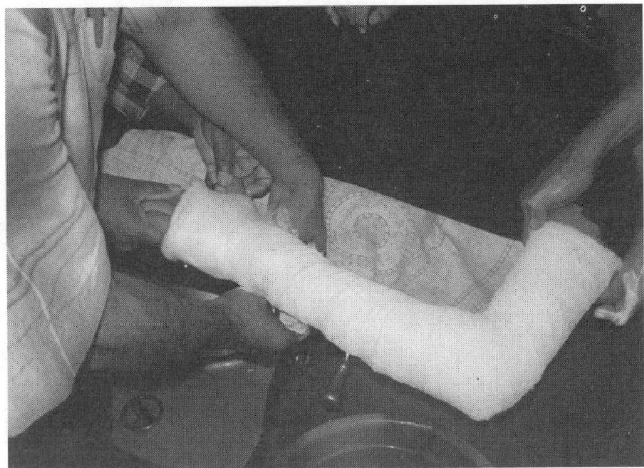

Fig. 35.21: Commencing plaster application.

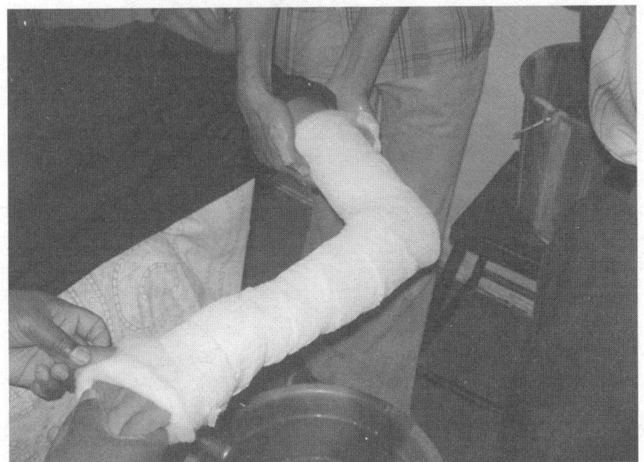

Fig. 35.22: Application continued.

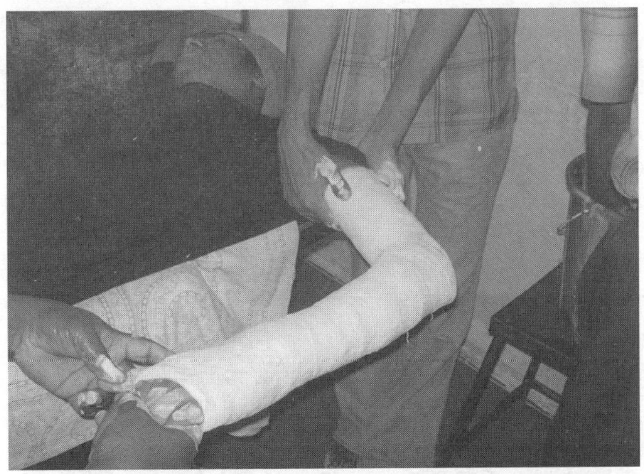

Fig. 35.23: Completion of the above elbow cast.

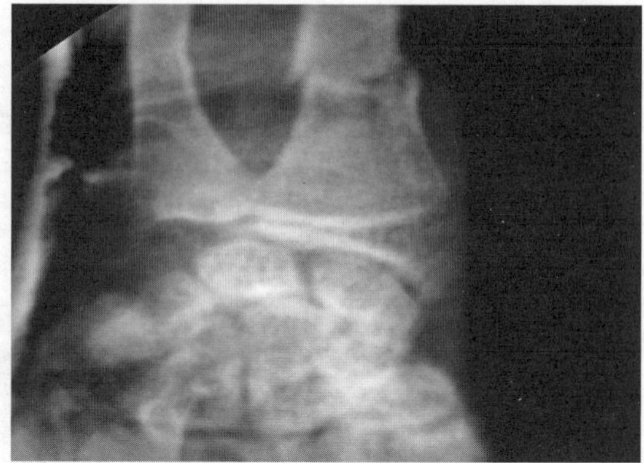

Fig. 35.24: Post-reduction X-ray satisfactory.

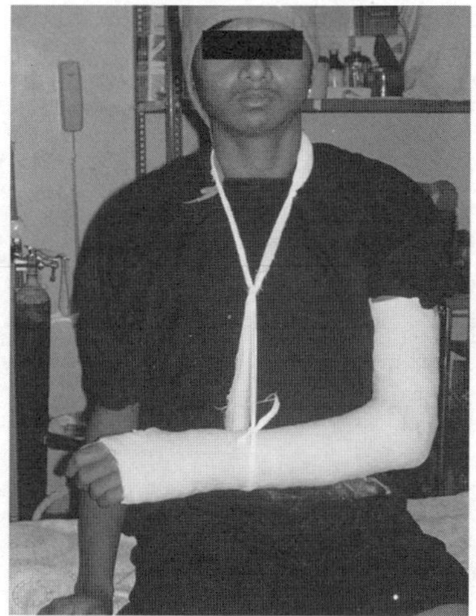

Fig. 35.25: Final presentation with sling.

GREENSTICK BOTH BONES FOREARM FRACTURE (PINPOINT COMPOUND)

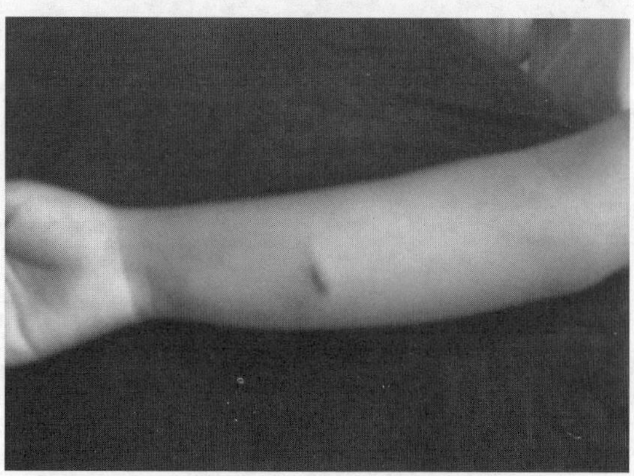

Fig. 35.26: Pinpoint compound fracture.

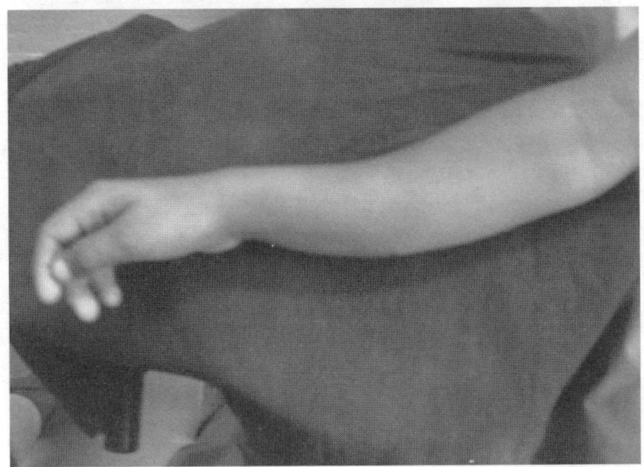

Fig. 35.27: Deformity.

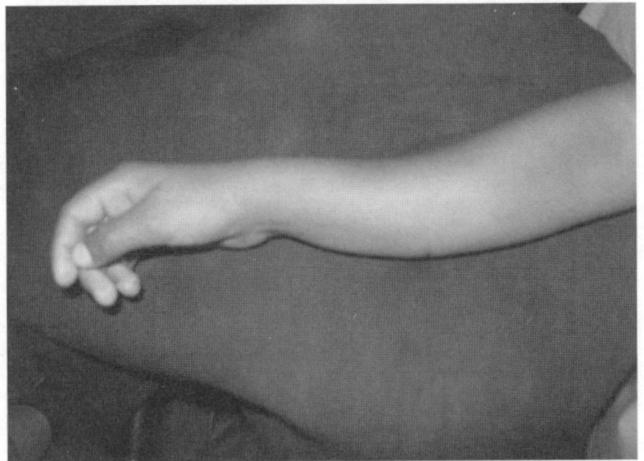

Fig. 35.28: S-shaped deformity due to Greenstick fracture.

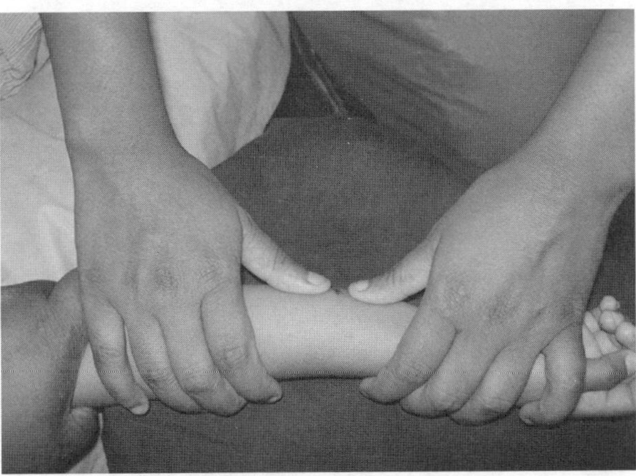

Fig. 35.29: Fracture manipulation.

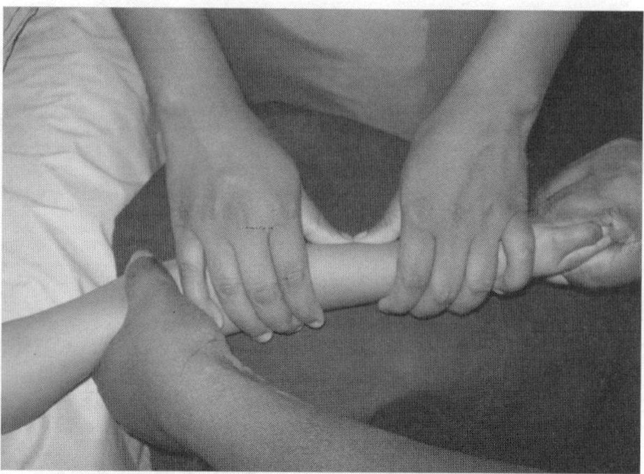

Fig. 35.30: Breaking the other cortex.

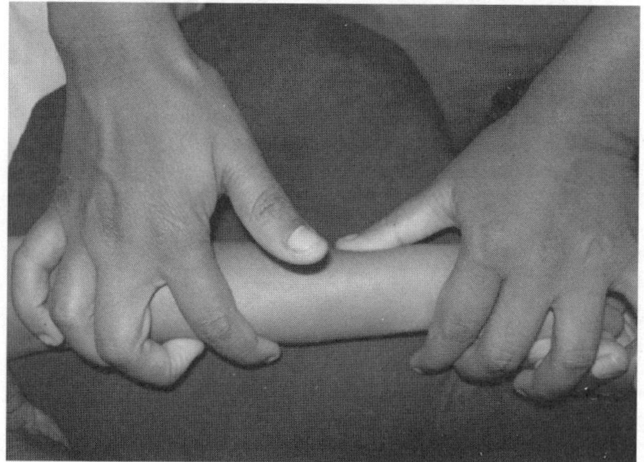

Fig. 35.31: Final manipulation.

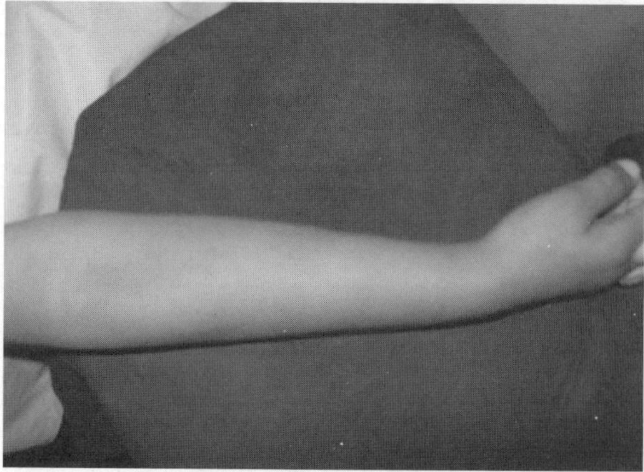

Fig. 35.32: Deformity corrected.

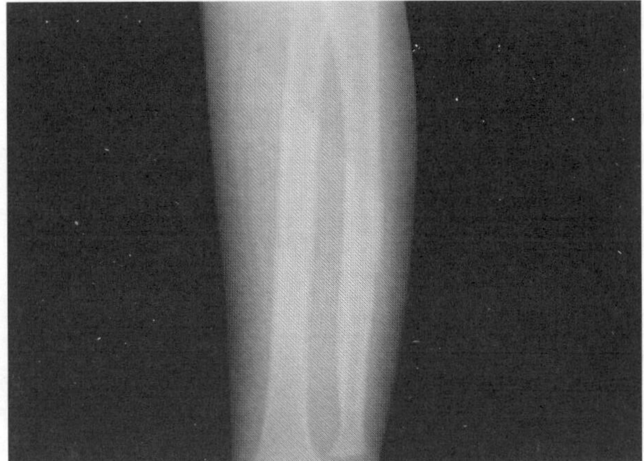

Fig. 35.33: Correction checked over C-arm.

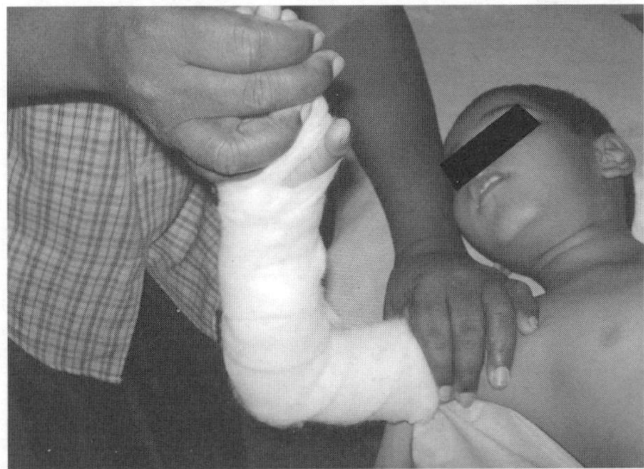

Fig. 35.34: Beginning to plaster—application of soft ban.

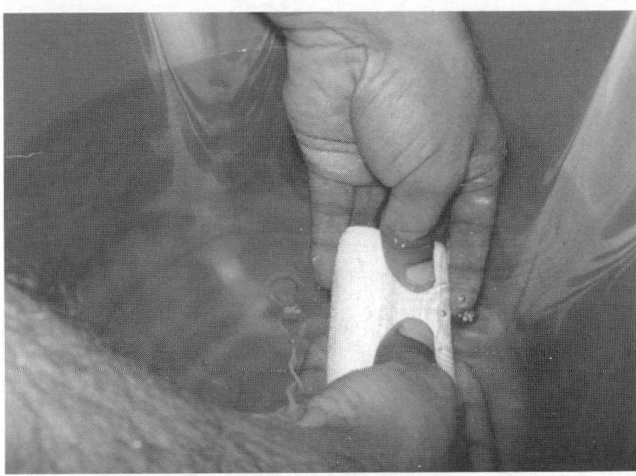

Fig. 35.35: Dipping plaster roll in water.

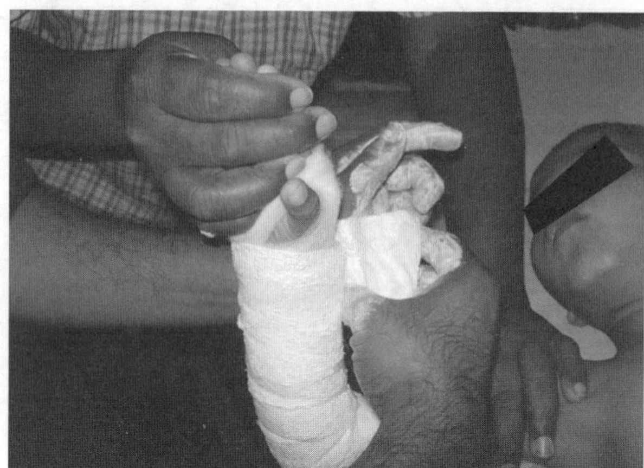

Fig. 35.36: Application of POP.

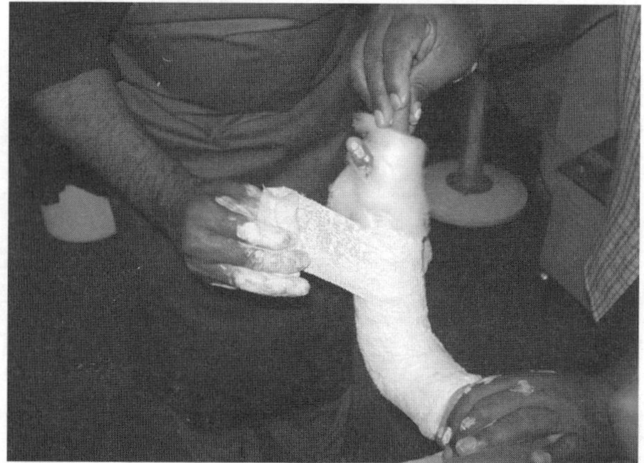

Fig. 35.37: Application continued.

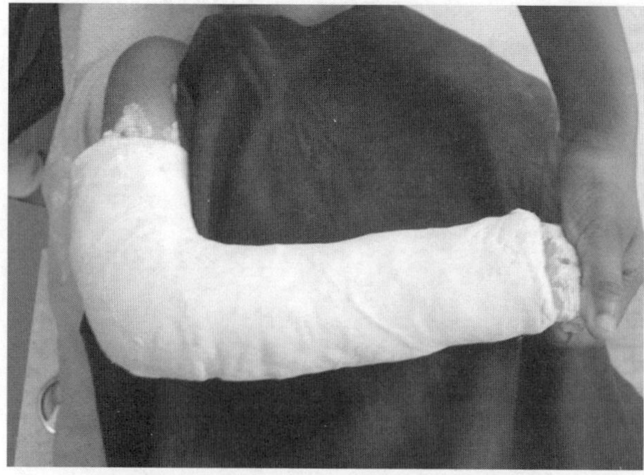

Fig. 35.38: Above elbow plaster applied.

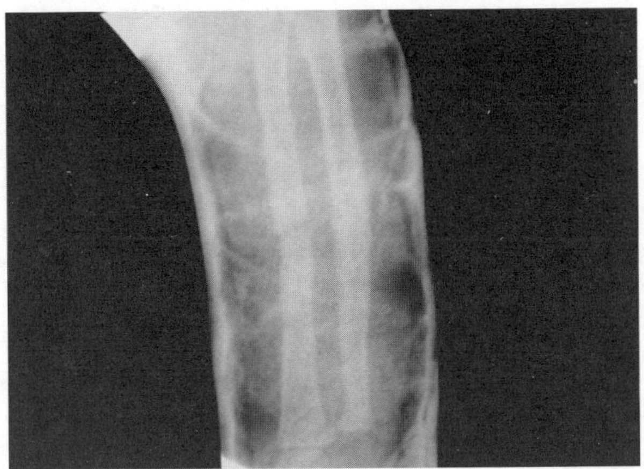

Fig. 35.39: Post-plaster C-arm check.

FRACTURE RADIUS (LOWER END)

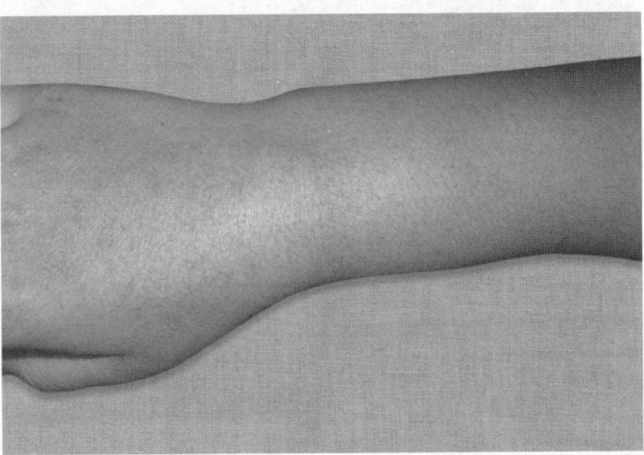

Fig. 35.40: Deformity of the fracture lower end of radius (undisplaced).

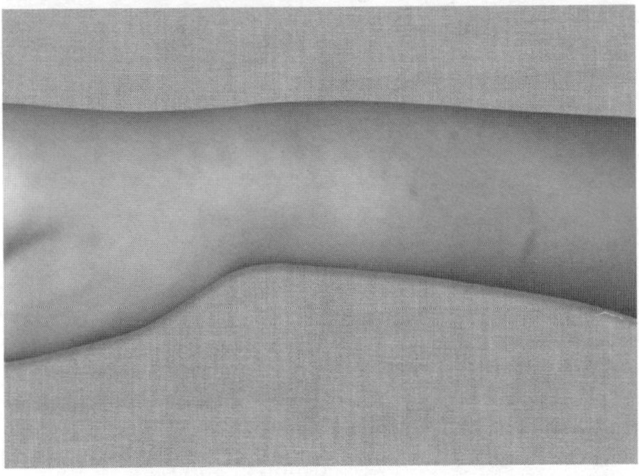

Fig. 35.41: Deformity as seen from the sides.

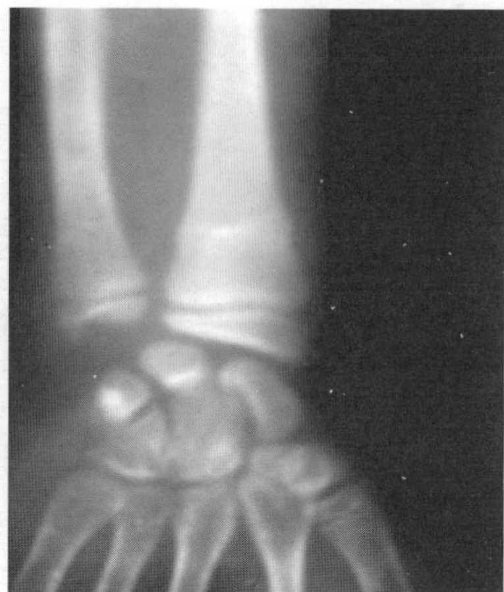

Fig. 35.42: X-ray AP view showing the fracture.

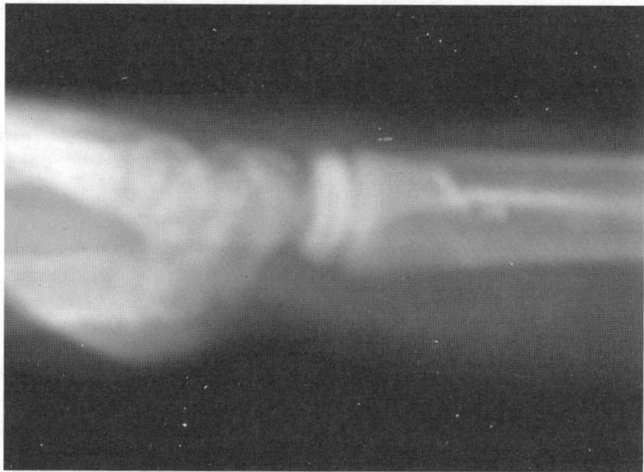

Fig. 35.43: X-ray lateral view.

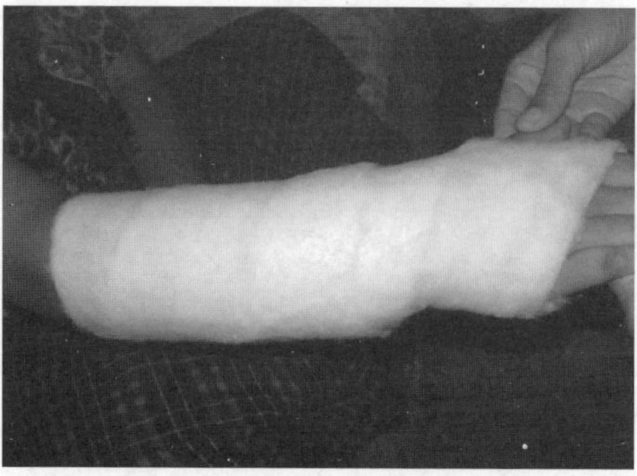

Fig. 35.44: Application of Soft ban.

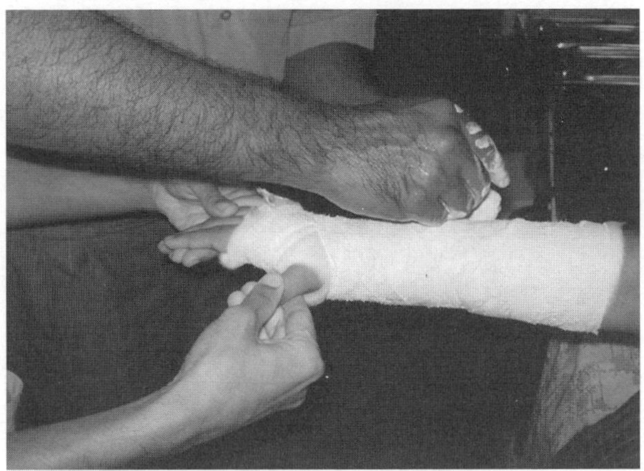

Fig. 35.45: Preparing to apply below elbow cast.

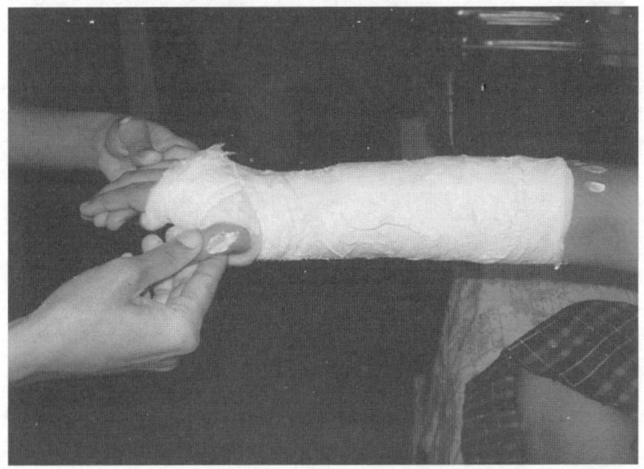

Fig. 35.46: Application of cast continued.

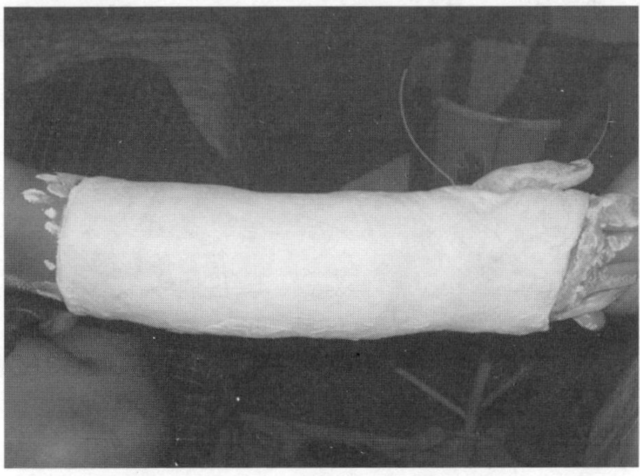

Fig. 35.47: The final finish of the cast.

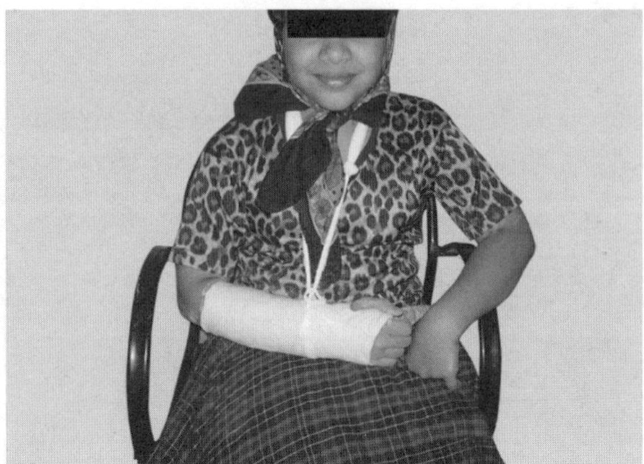

Fig. 35.48: Cast and sling.

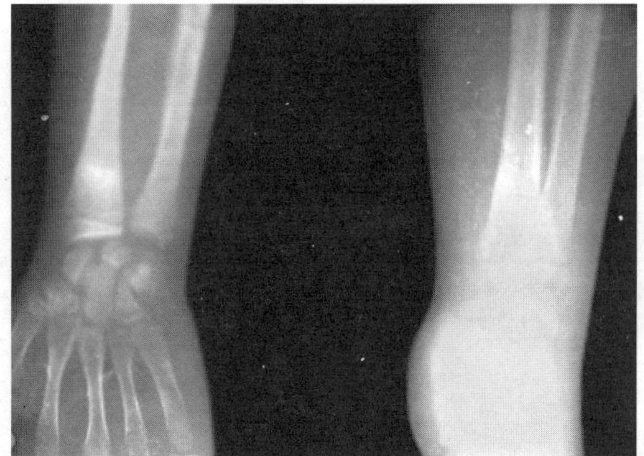

Fig. 35.49: Follow up X-ray after 1 month.

GREENSTICK FRACTURE BOTH BONES FOREARM (TORUS FRACTURE) (BUCKLING OF THE CORTEX)

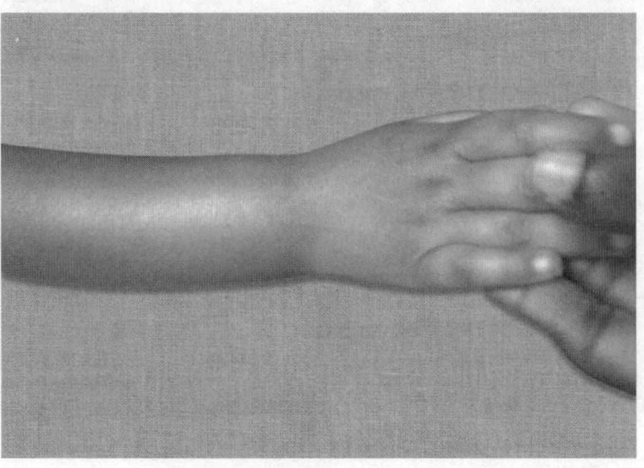

Fig. 35.50: Deformity.

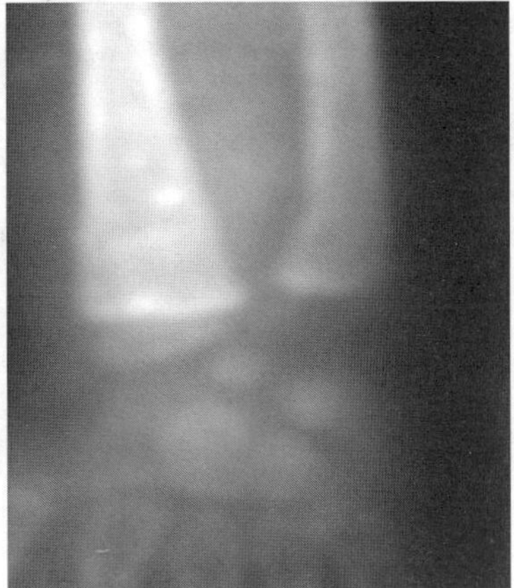

Fig. 35.51: X-ray AP view.

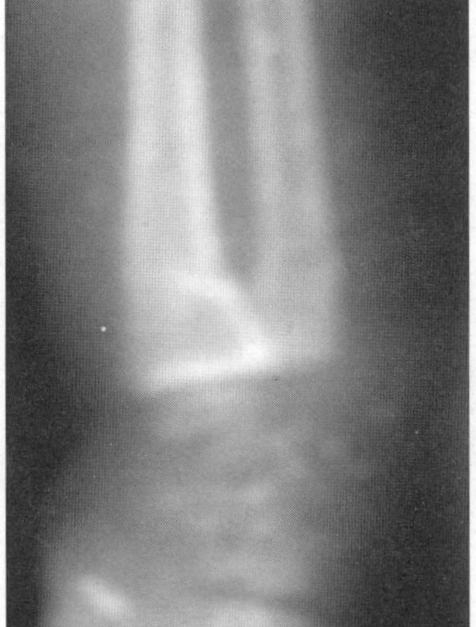

Fig. 35.52: X-ray lateral view.

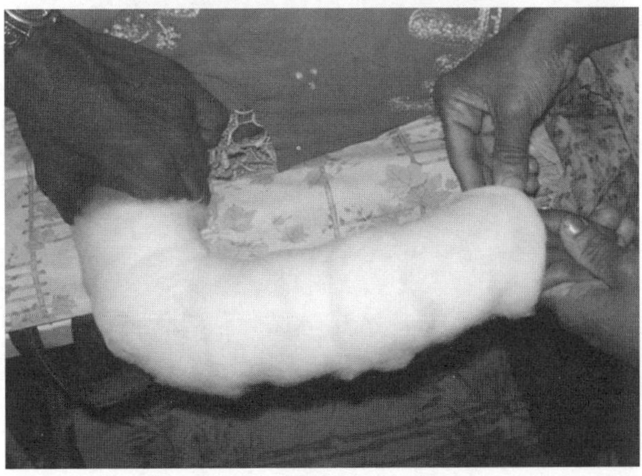

Fig. 35.53: Application of soft ban.

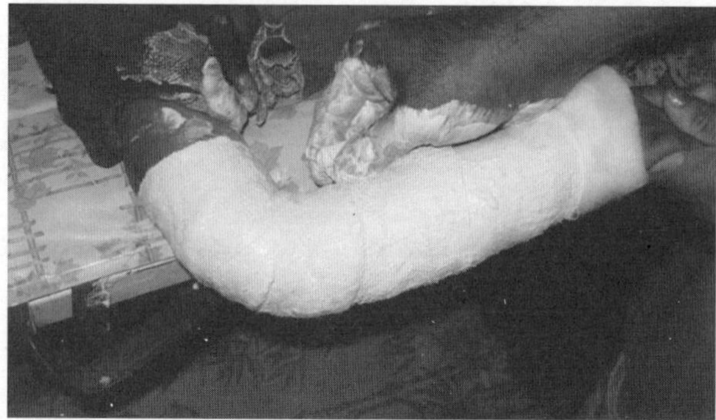

Fig. 35.54: Beginning of plaster application.

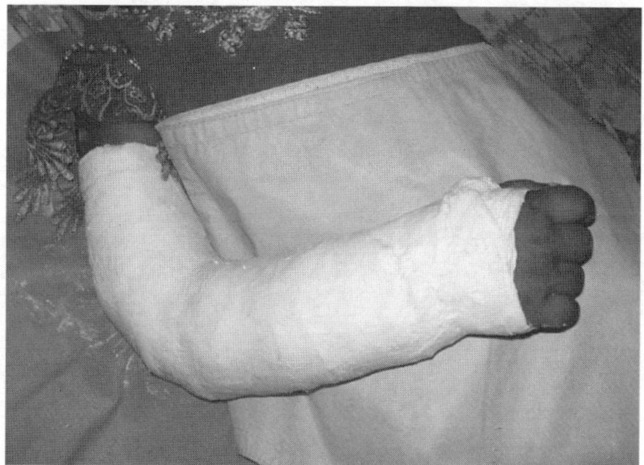

Fig. 35.55: Completion of above elbow cast.

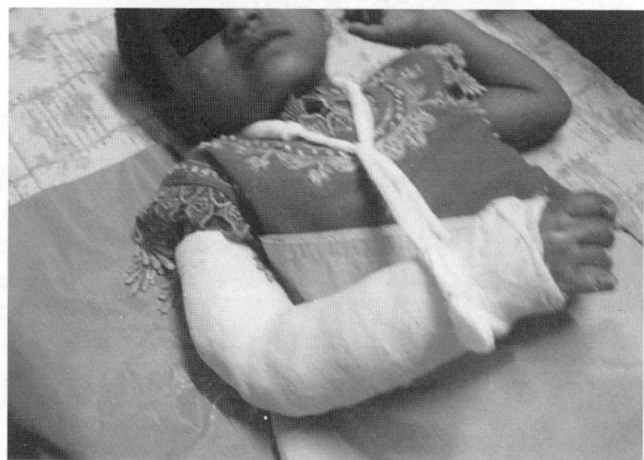

Fig. 35.56: Cast and forearm sling.

OLECRANON FRACTURE (GREENSTICK VARIETY)

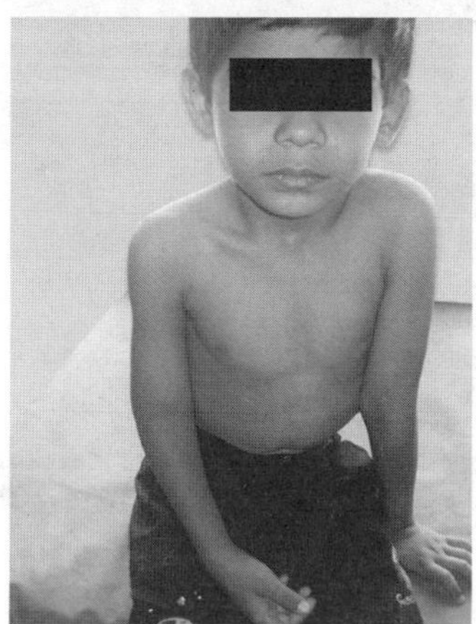

Fig. 35.57: Deformity as seen from the front.

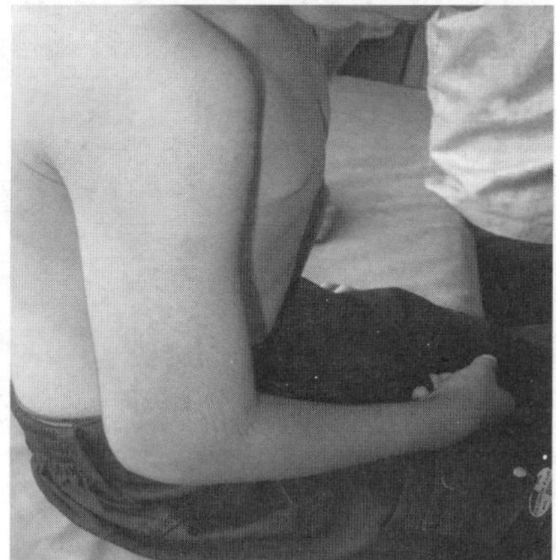

Fig. 35.58: Deformity from the sides.

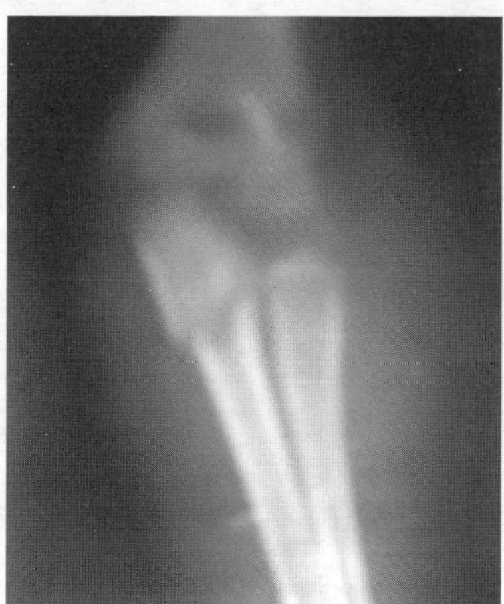

Fig. 35.59: X-ray—AP view.

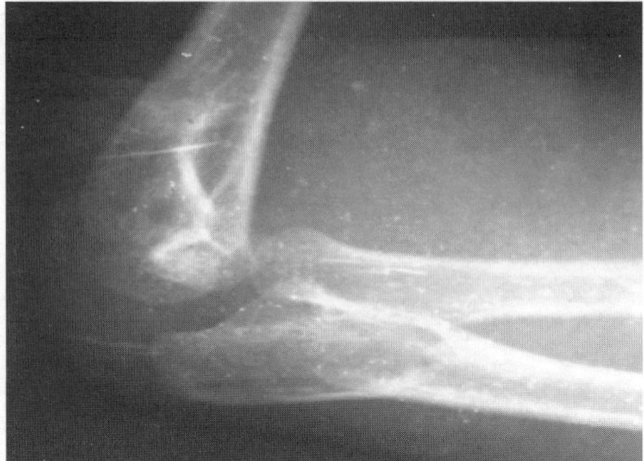

Fig. 35.60: Lateral view.

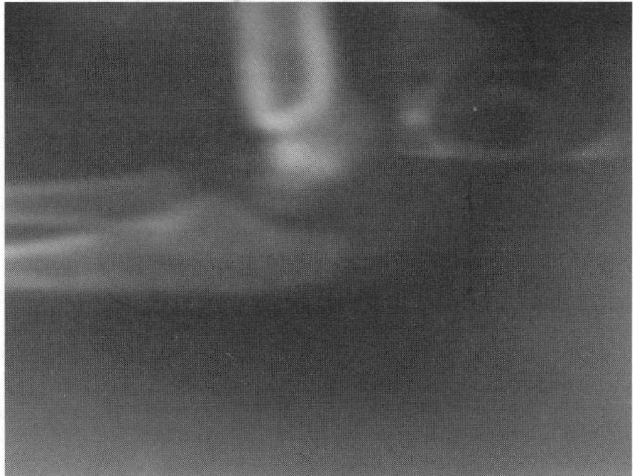

Fig. 35.61: Post-reduction X-ray lateral view.

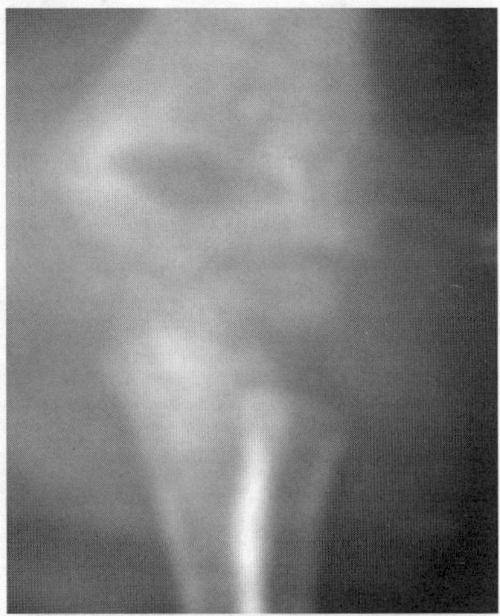

Fig. 35.62: Post-reduction AP—X-ray. Position satisfactory.

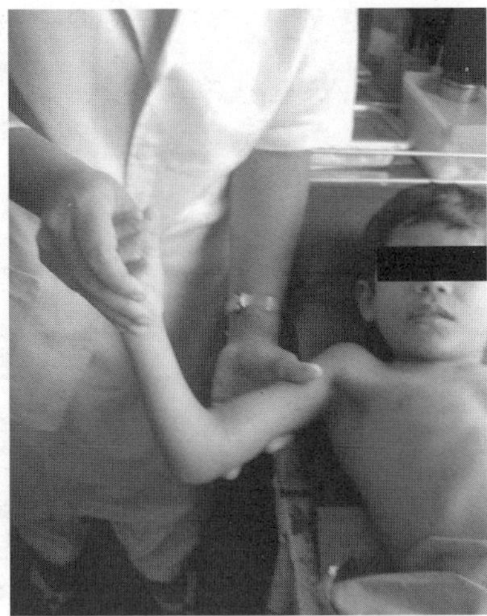

Fig. 35.63: Position of elbow.

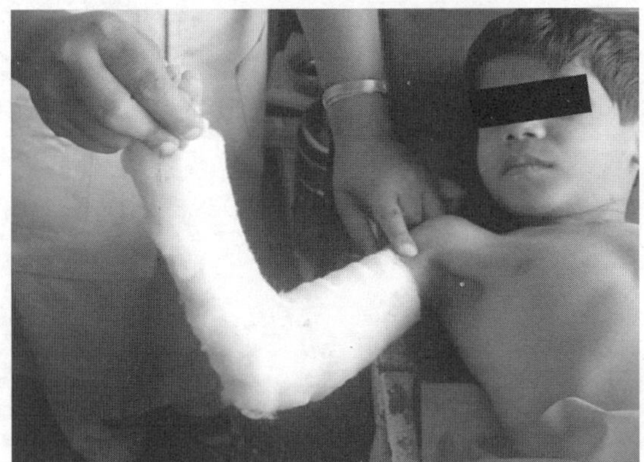

Fig. 35.64: Application of soft ban.

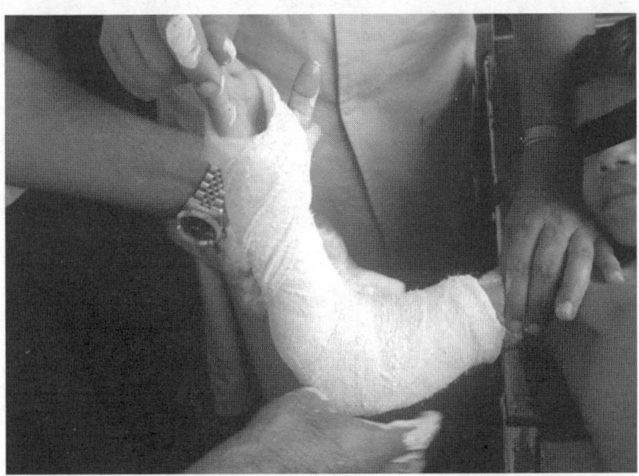

Fig. 35.65: Application of above elbow cast.

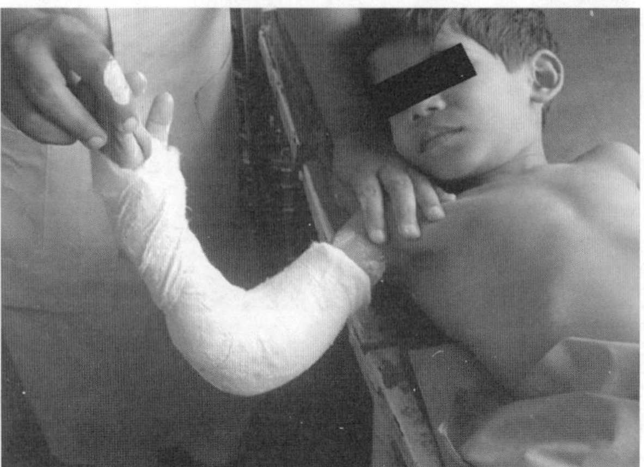

Fig. 35.66: Application of cast completed.

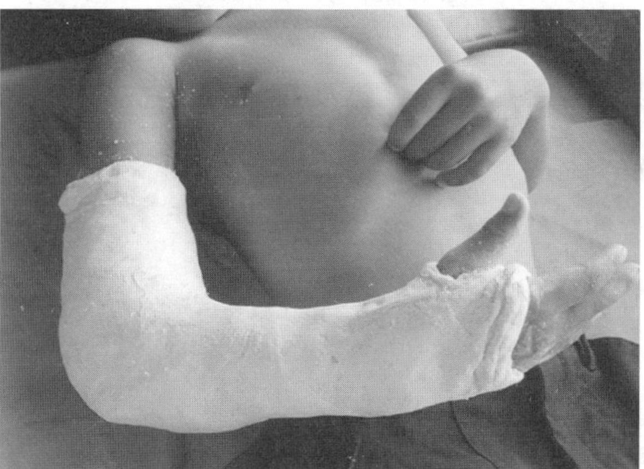

Fig. 35.67: Final picture.

ULNA FRACTURE

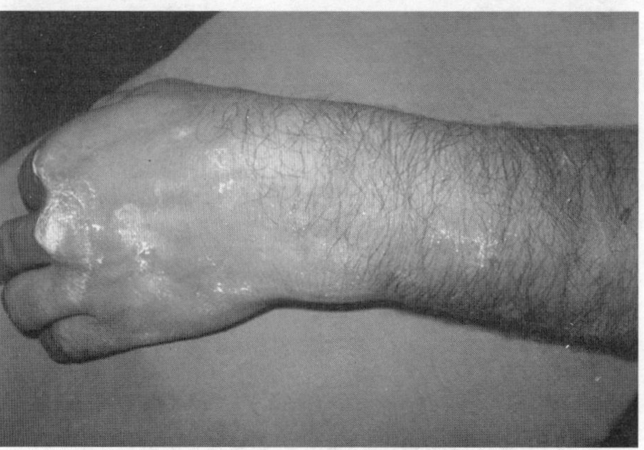

Fig. 35.68: Deformity as seen from the front.

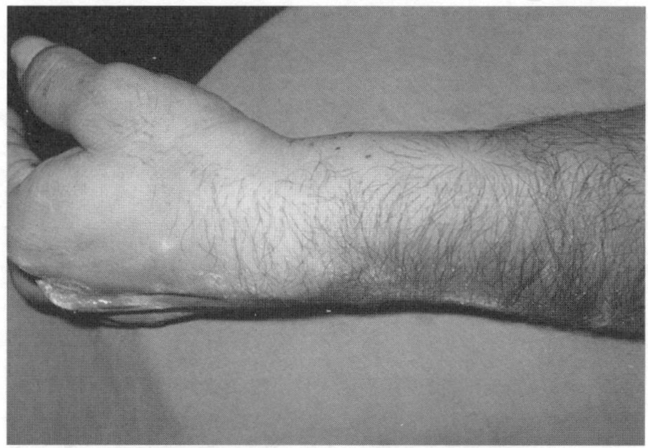

Fig. 35.69: Deformity from the sides.

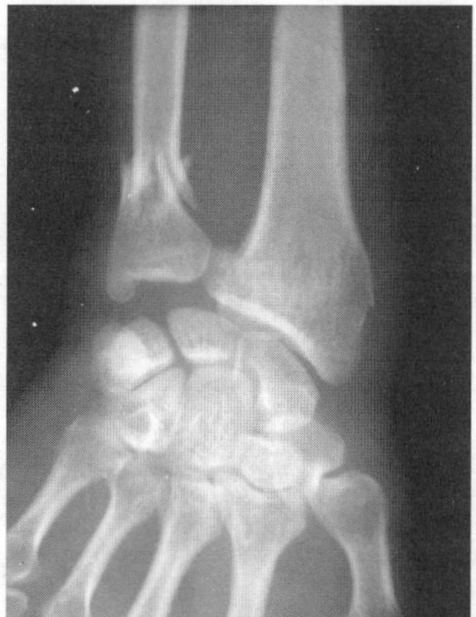

Fig. 35.70: X-ray—AP view.

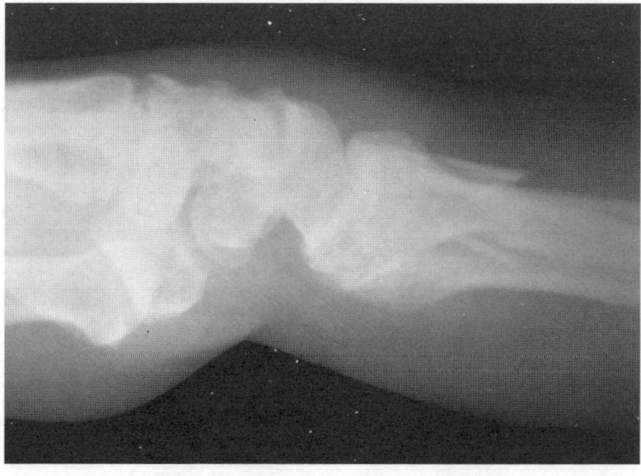

Fig. 35.71: X-ray lateral view.

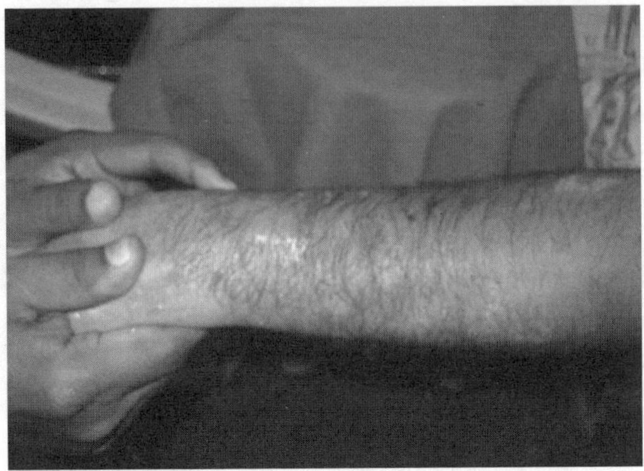

Fig. 35.72: Reduction method.

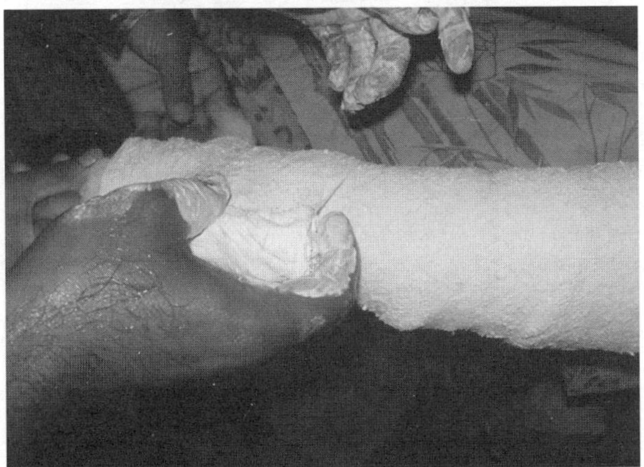

Fig. 35.73: Application of below elbow cast.

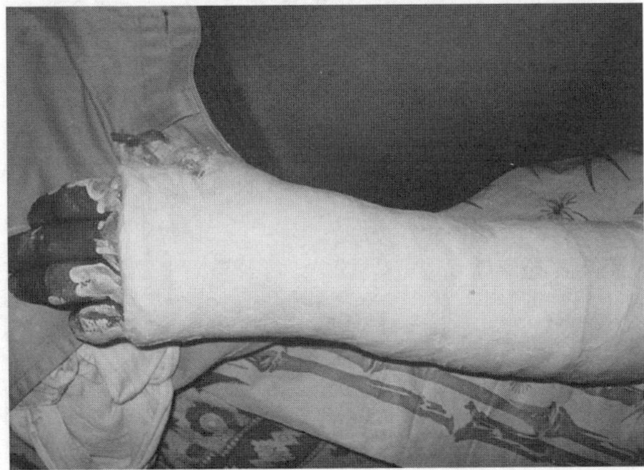

Fig. 35.74: Cast completed.

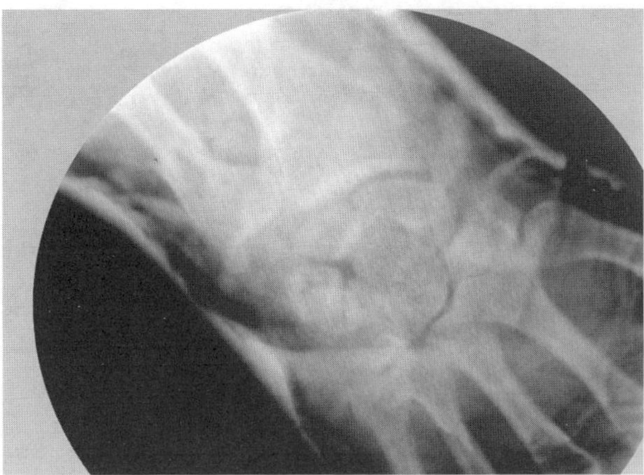

Fig. 35.75: Post-reduction X-ray AP view.

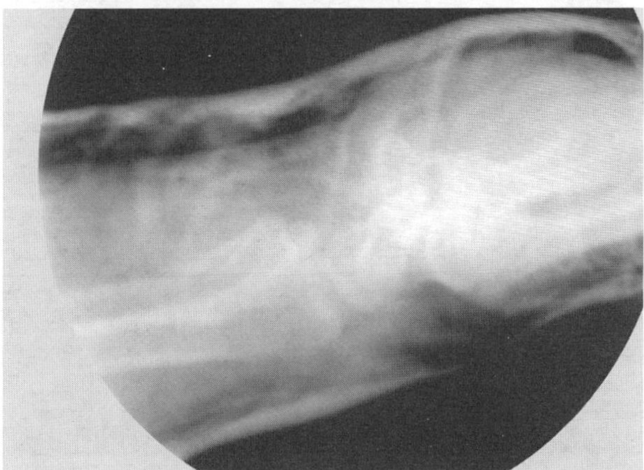

Fig. 35.76: Post-reduction lateral view.

POSTEROLATERAL DISLOCATION ELBOW

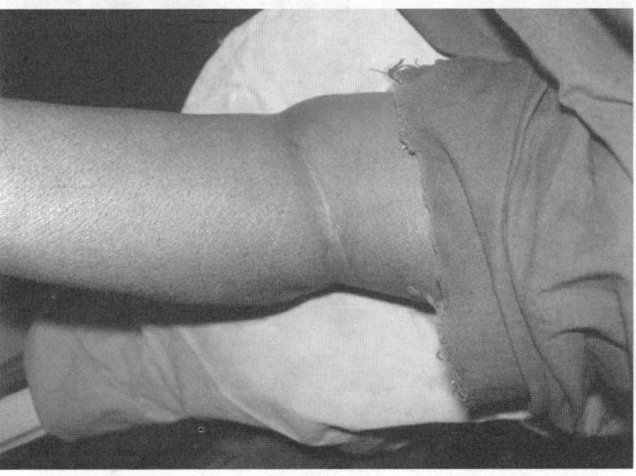

Fig. 35.77: Deformity from the front.

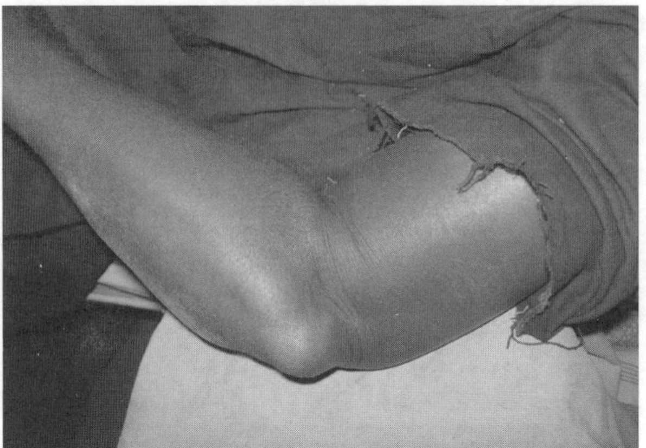

Fig. 35.78: Deformity from the sides.

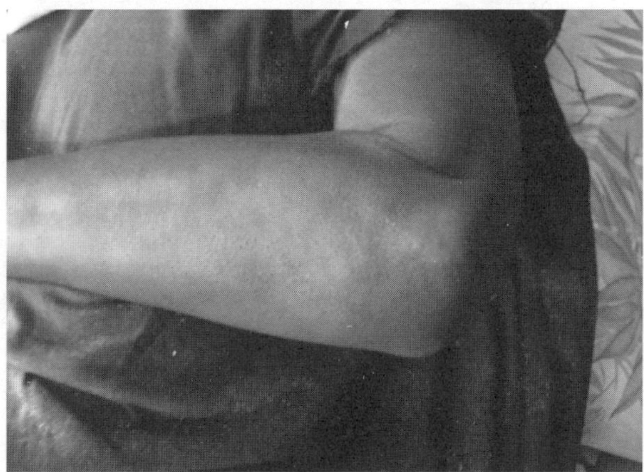

Fig. 35.79: Deformity from the closer view.

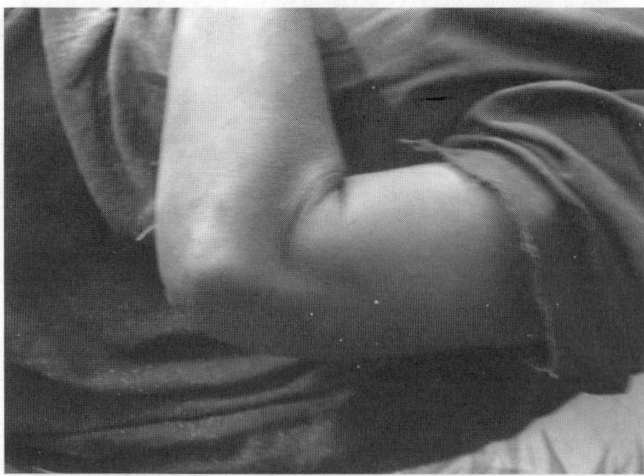

Fig. 35.80: Deformity lateral closer view.

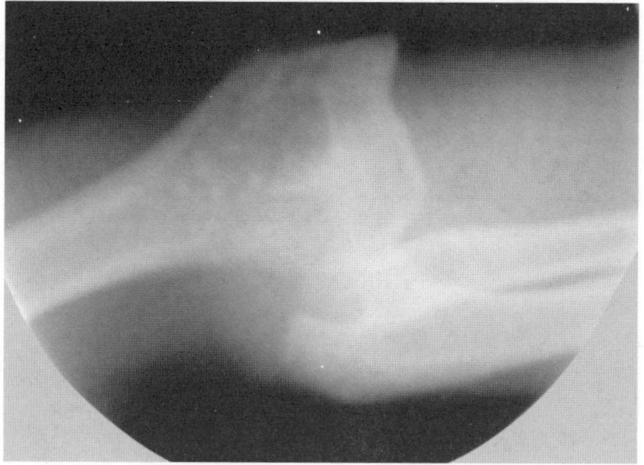

Fig. 35.81: X-ray lateral view.

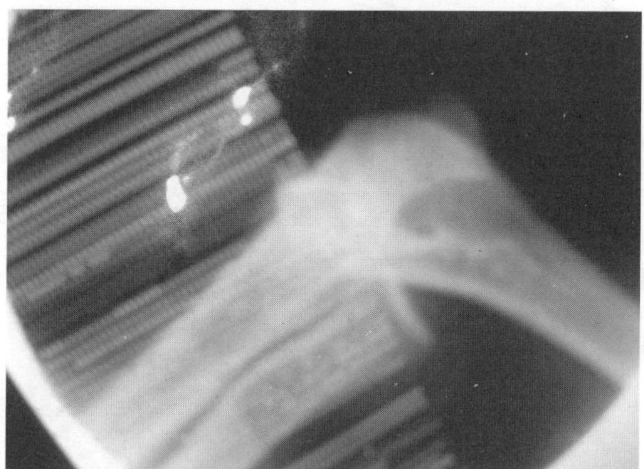

Fig. 35.82: X-ray lateral view (another view).

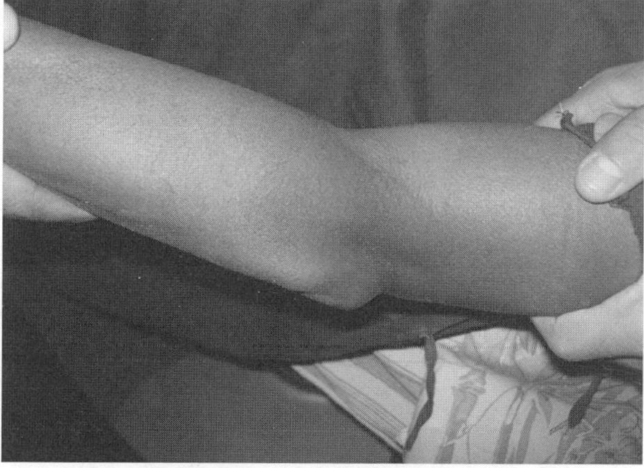

Fig. 35.83: Method of reduction—traction.

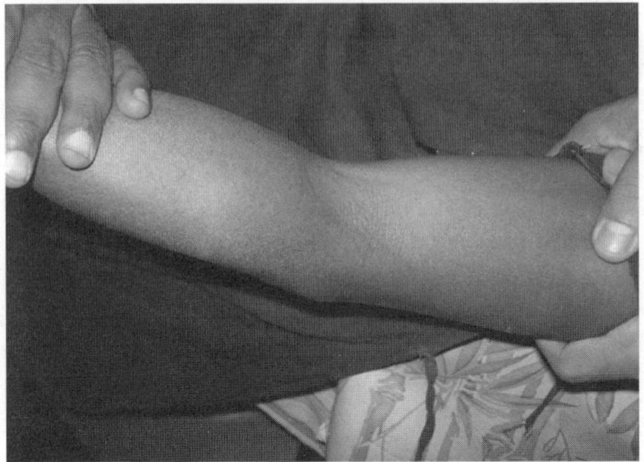

Fig. 35.84: Traction and counter traction.

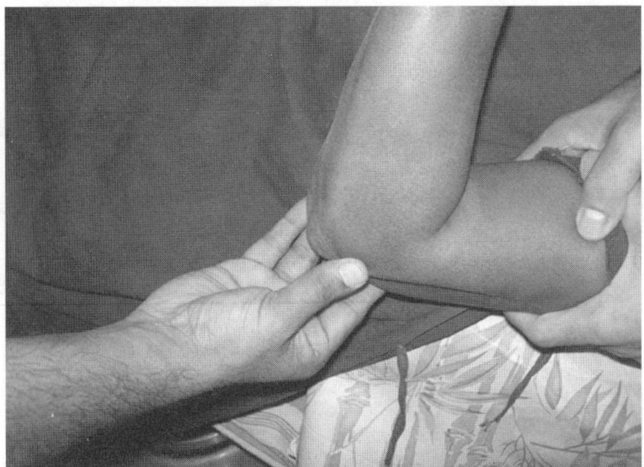

Fig. 35.85: Reduction successful.

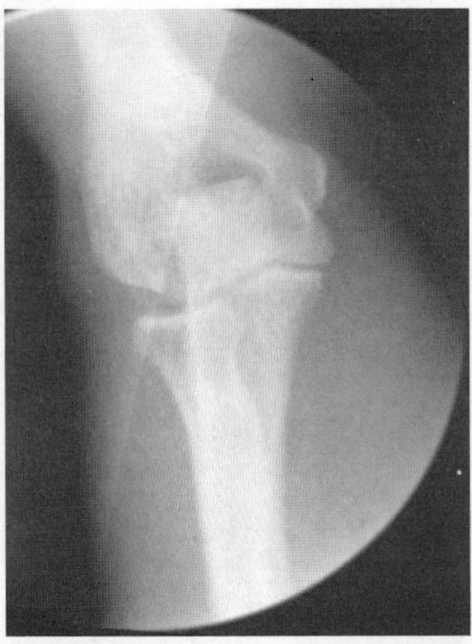

Fig. 35.86: Post-reduction C-arm picture AP view.

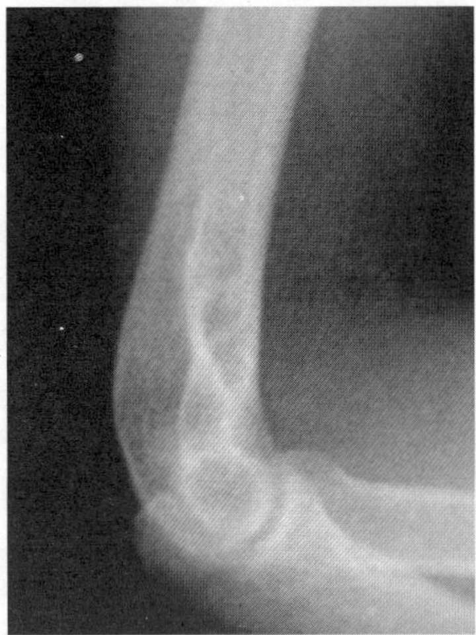

Fig. 35.87: Post-reduction C-arm picture—lateral view.

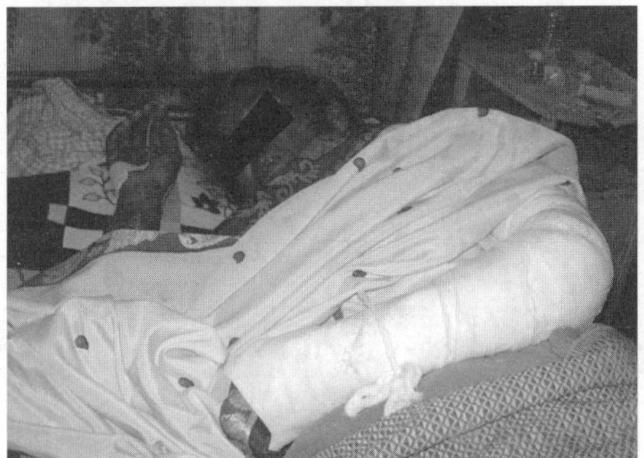

Fig. 35.88: Immobilization in above elbow slab.

Wrist Injuries

This chapter deals with the practical techniques of managing the common wrist injuries.

COLLES FRACTURE

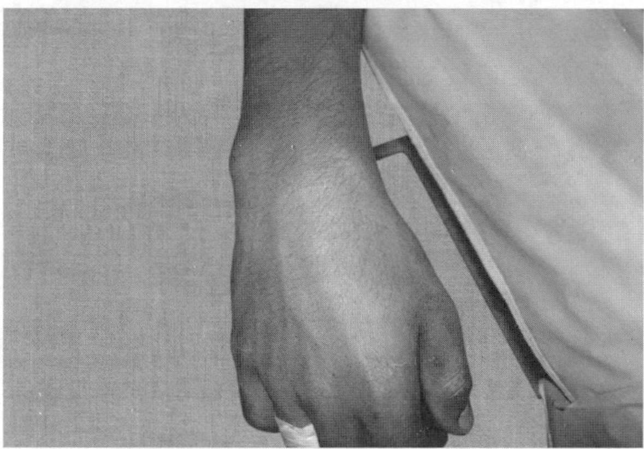

Fig. 36.1: Dinner fork deformity.

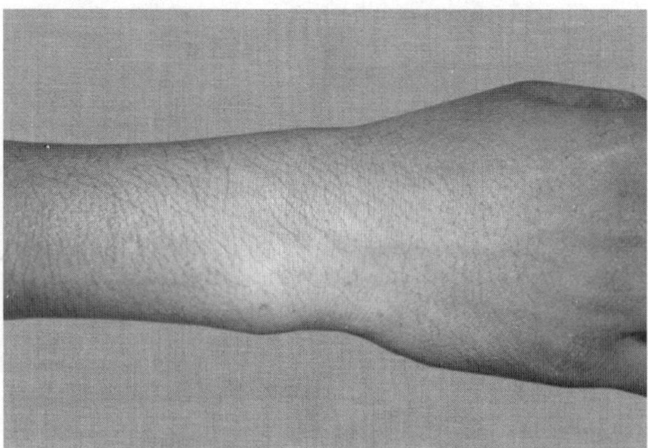

Fig. 36.2: Other view of the deformity.

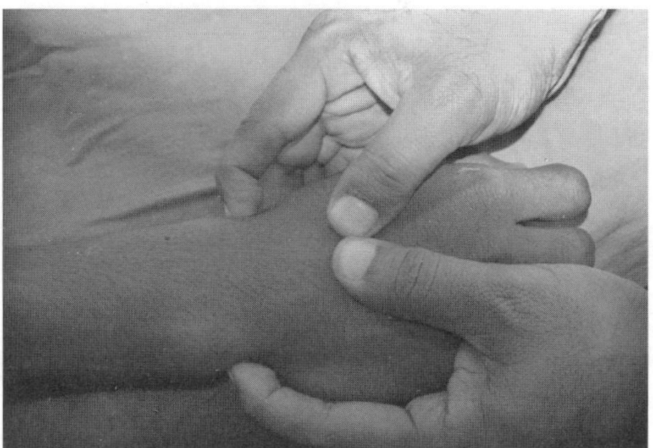

Fig. 36.3: The styloid process test.

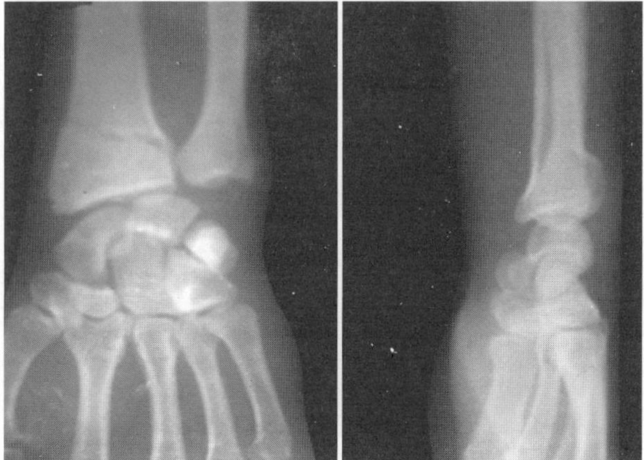

Fig. 36.4: X-ray AP and lateral views.

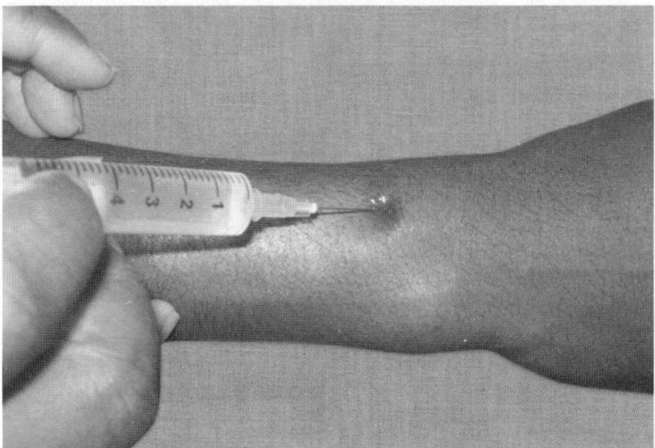

Fig. 36.5: Injecting local anesthetic into the fracture site.

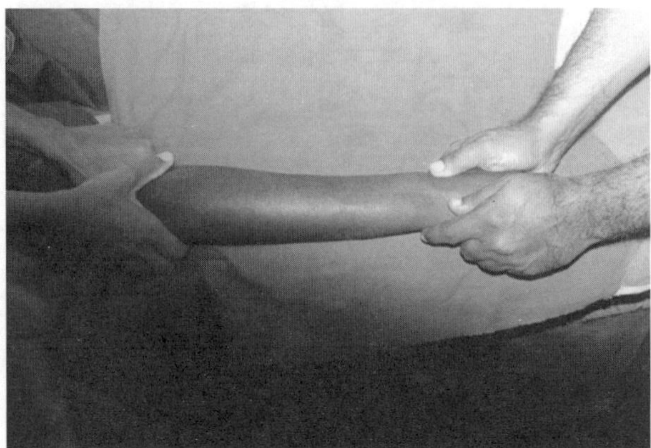

Fig. 36.6: Reduction by traction and counter traction.

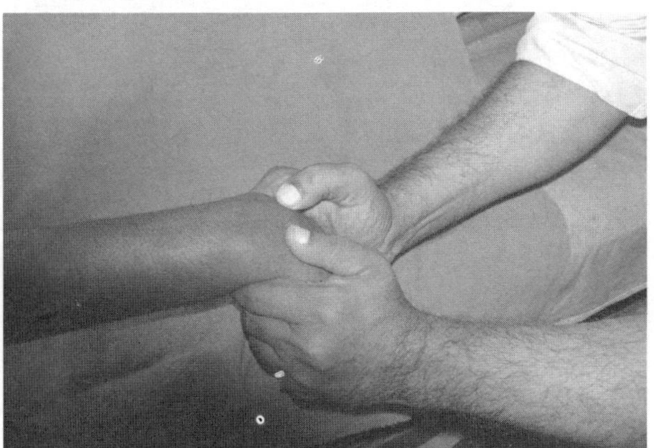

Fig. 36.7: Manipulation of the fracture.

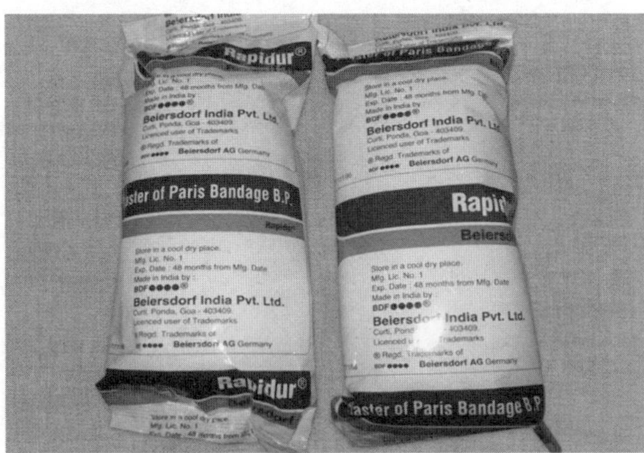

Fig. 36.8: POP rolls.

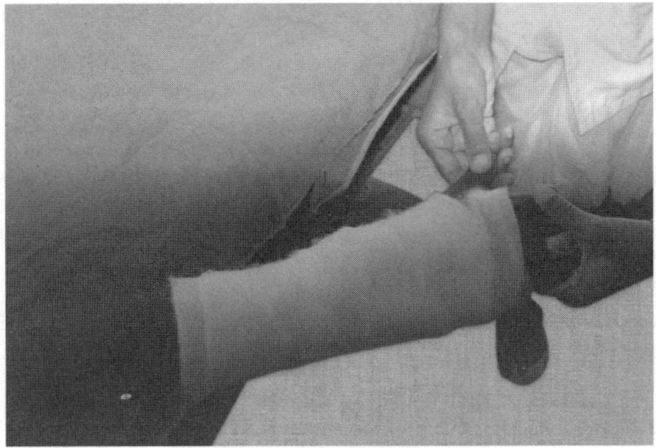

Fig. 36.9: Application of soft ban.

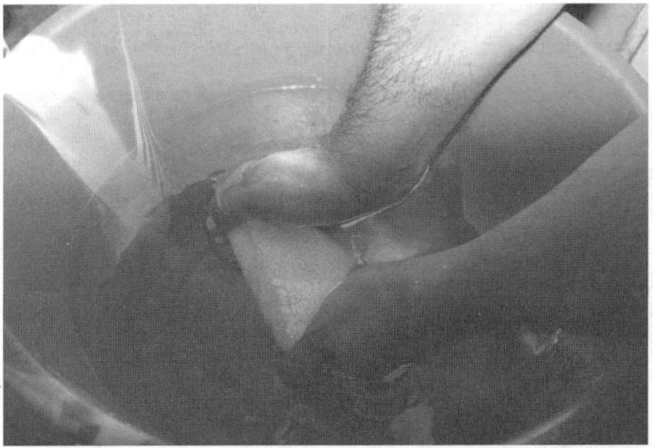

Fig. 36.10: Immersion of plaster roll in water.

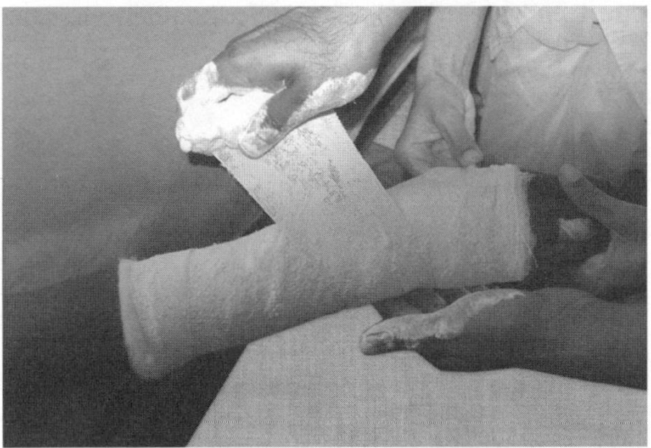

Fig. 36.11: Application of the cast.

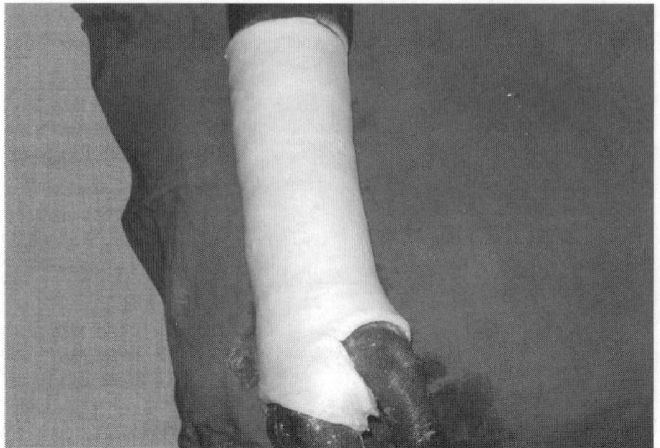

Fig. 36.12: Colles cast final presentation.

RADIAL STYLOID PROCESS FRACTURE—PINS AND PLASTER

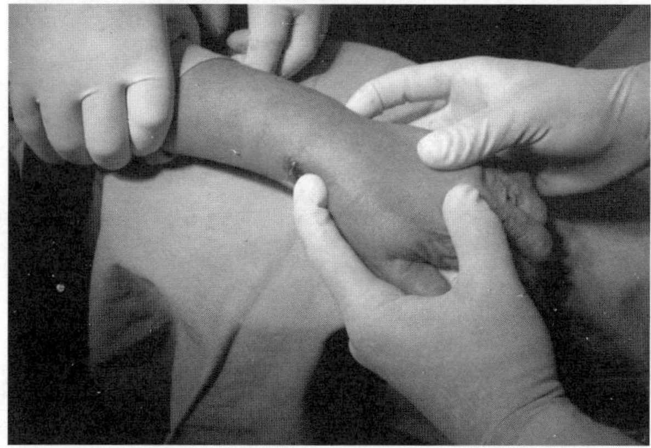

Fig. 36.13: Checking the reduction by the styloid process test.

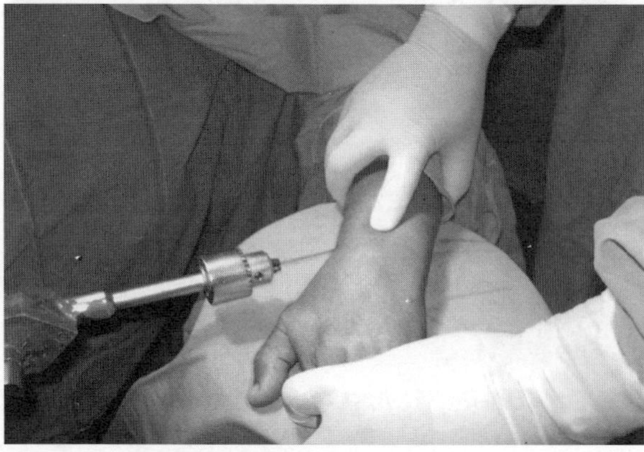

Fig. 36.14: K-wire being passed.

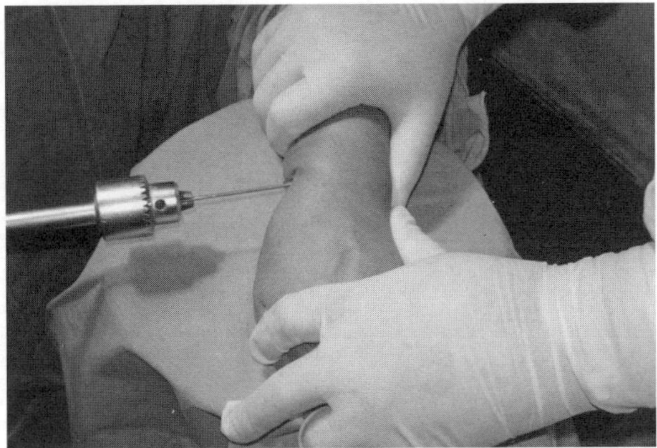

Fig. 36.15: Placement of second K-wire.

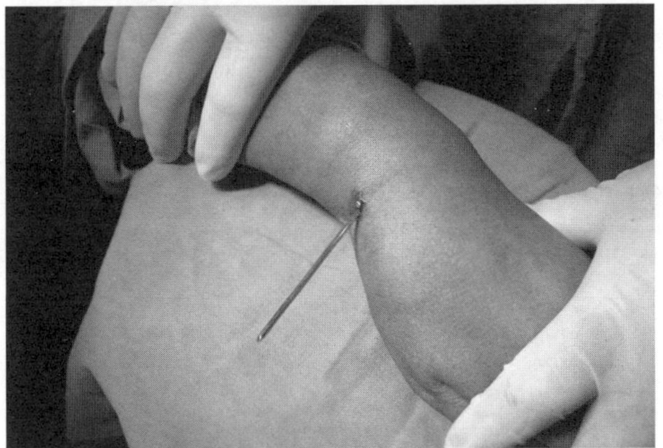

Fig. 36.16: Second K-wire before cutting.

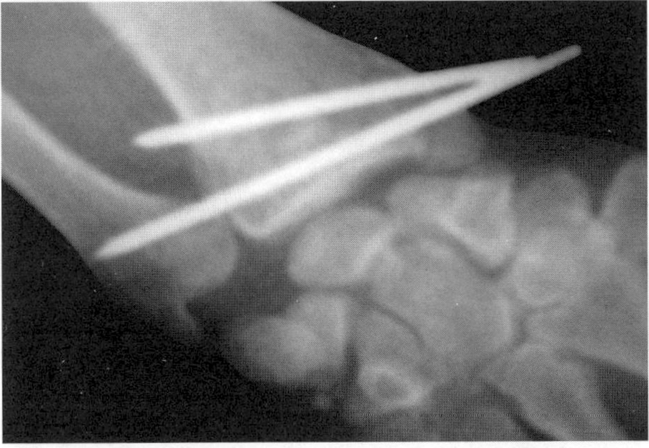

Fig. 36.17: Close up view of the final fixation.

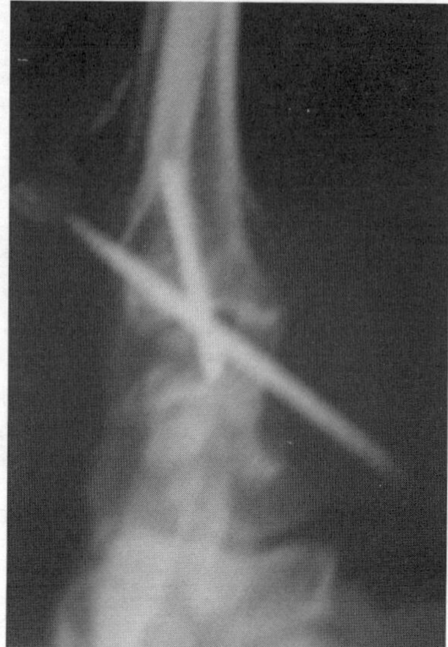

Fig. 36.18: Lateral view.

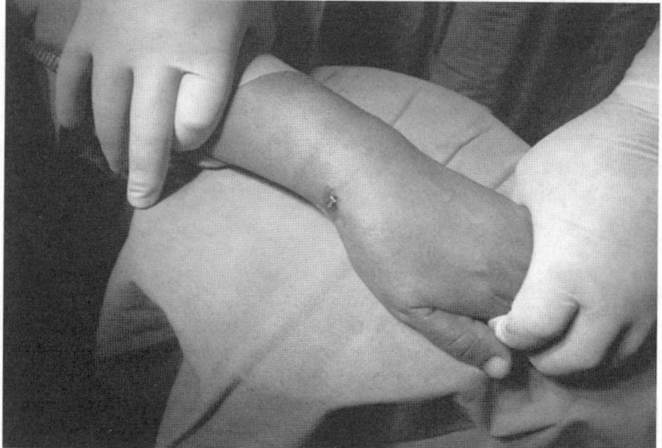

Fig. 36.19: Both K-wires cut to the level of the skin.

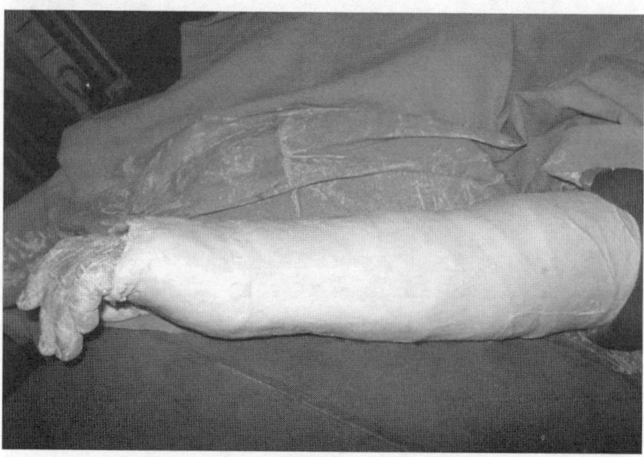

Fig. 36.20: Below elbow plaster reinforcement.

ULNAR HEAD FRACTURE

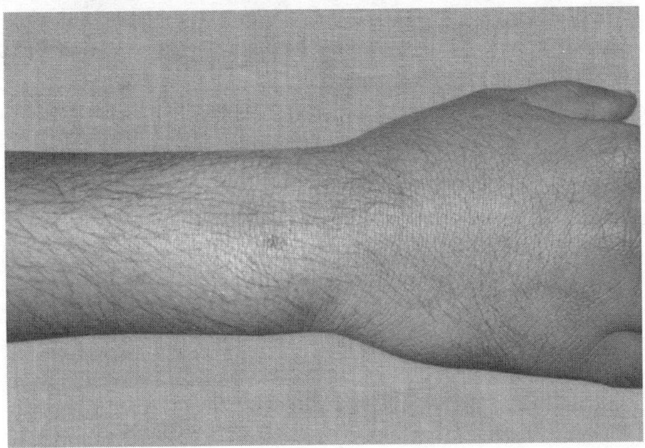

Fig. 36.21: Deformity due to ulnar prominence.

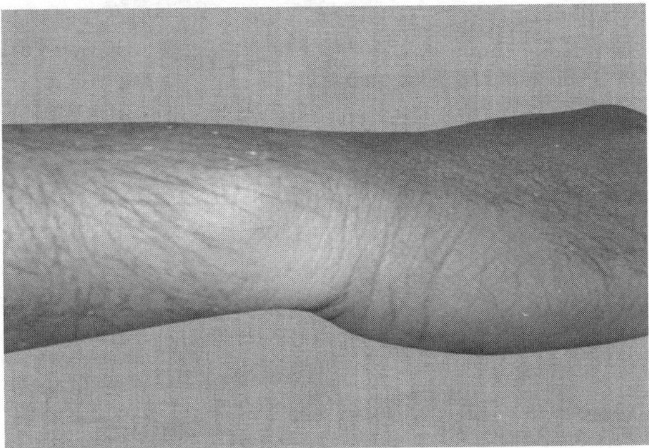

Fig. 36.22: Side view.

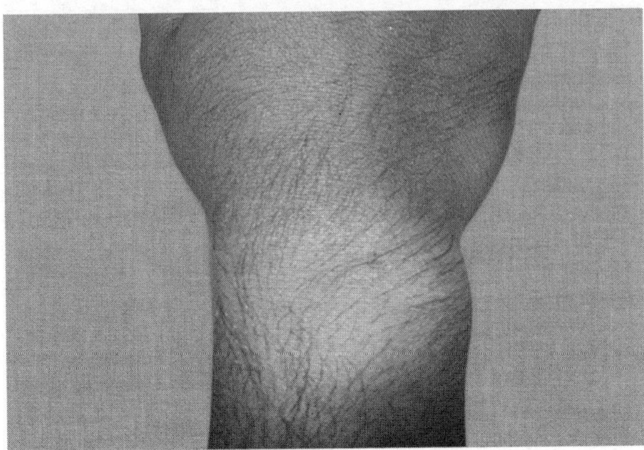

Fig. 36.23: Deformity corrected.

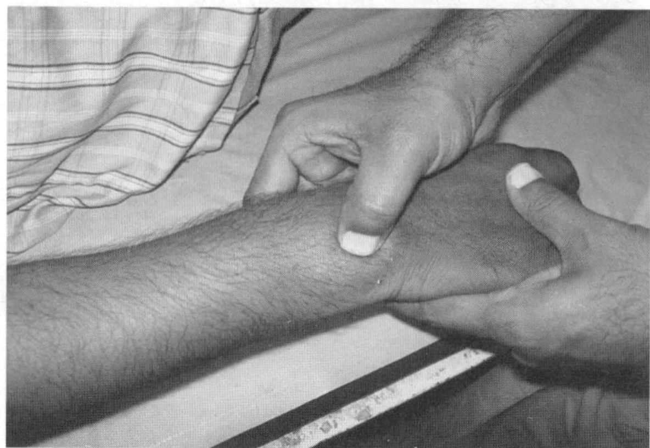

Fig. 36.24: Manipulation and reduction.

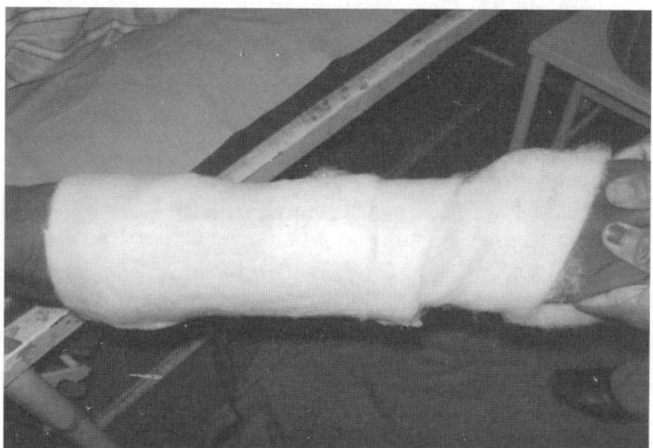

Fig. 36.25: Application of soft ban.

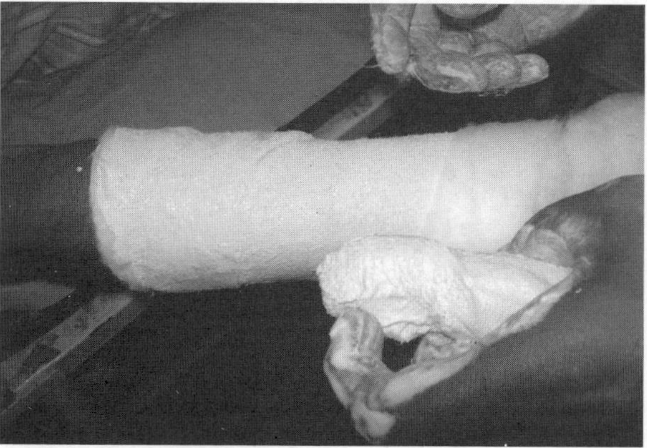

Fig. 36.26: Application of plaster.

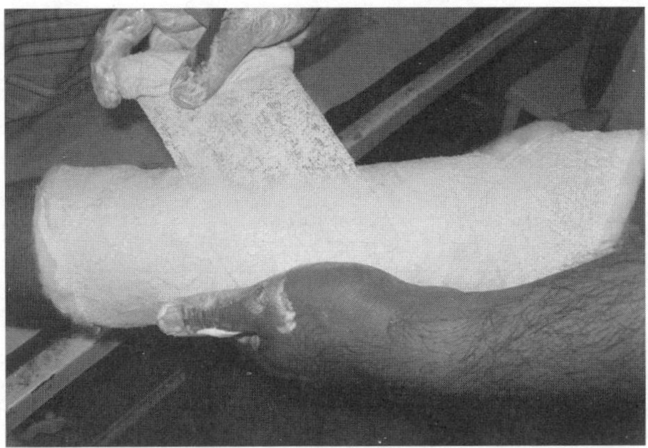

Fig. 36.27: Application continued.

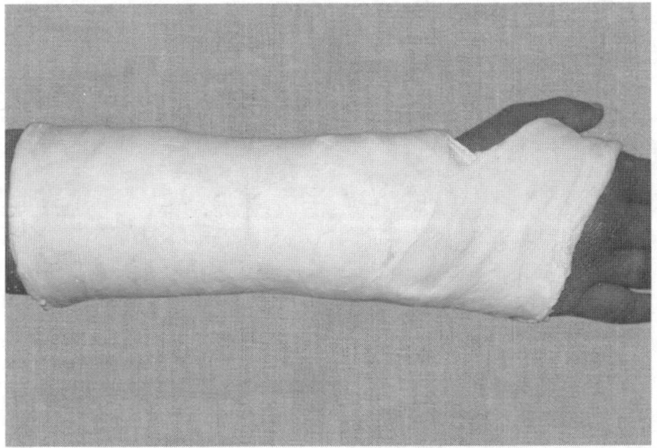

Fig. 36.28: Application completed.

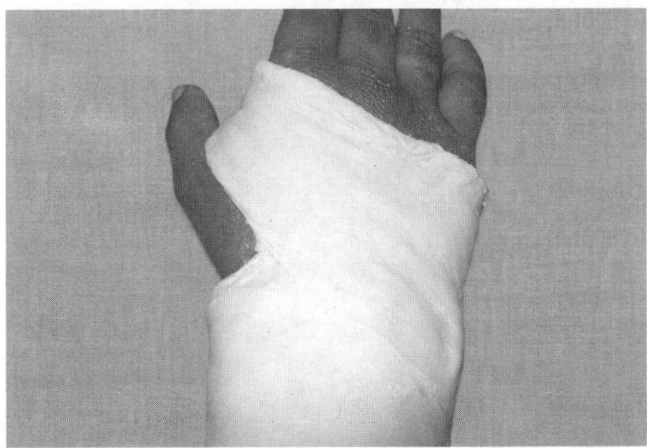

Fig. 36.29: Final cast.

Hand Injuries

This chapter deals with the practical techniques of managing the common hand injuries.

FRACTURE BASE PHALANX

Buddy Taping

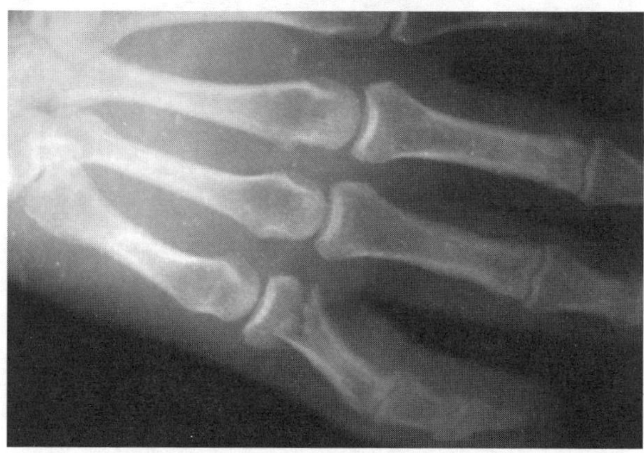

Fig. 37.1: Plain X-ray (1).

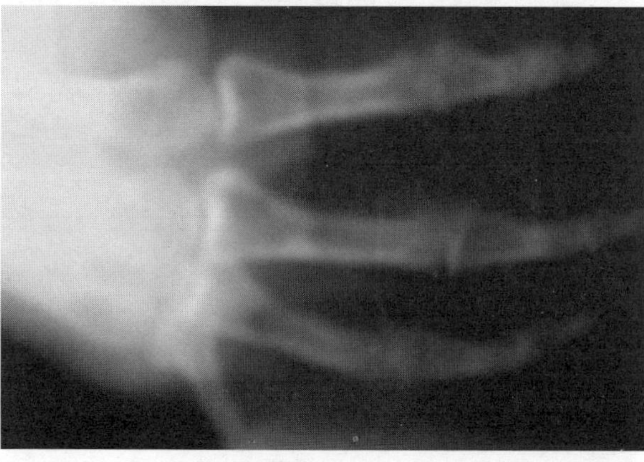

Fig. 37.2: Plain X-ray (2).

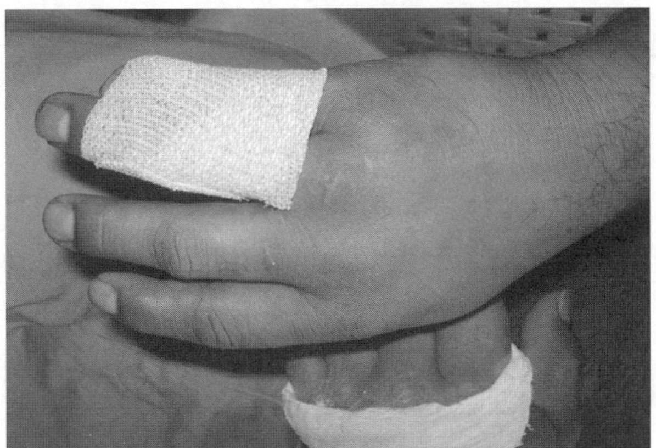

Fig. 37.3: Buddy Taping.

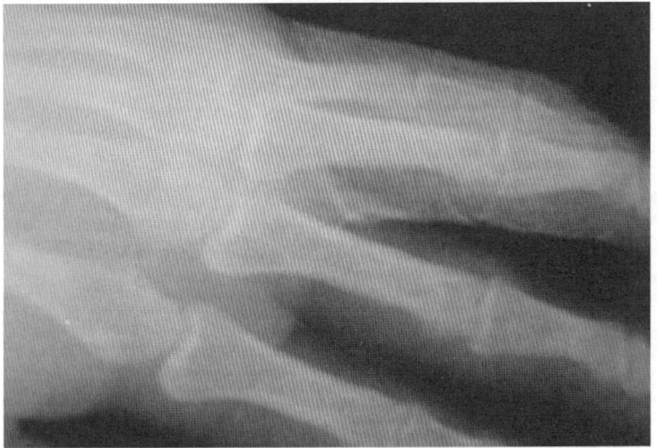

Fig. 37.4: Post-strapping X-ray (1).

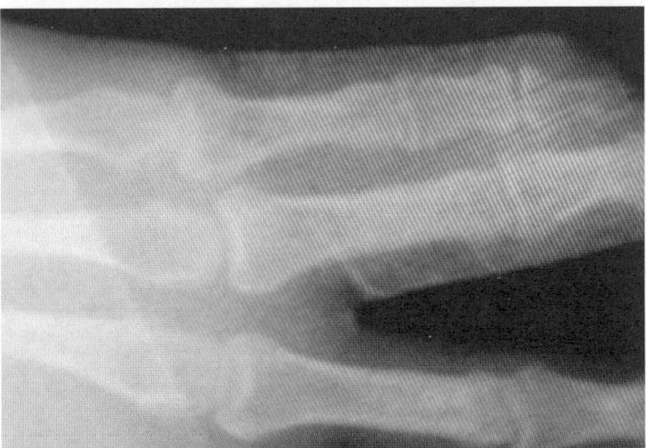

Fig. 37.5: Post-strapping X-ray (2).

FINGER FRACTURE

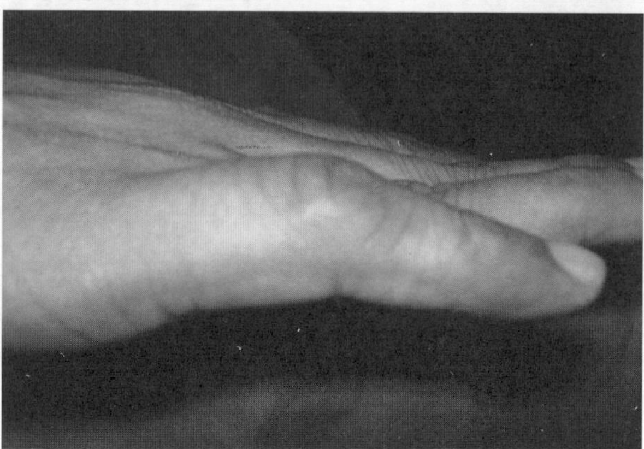

Fig. 37.6: Deformity.

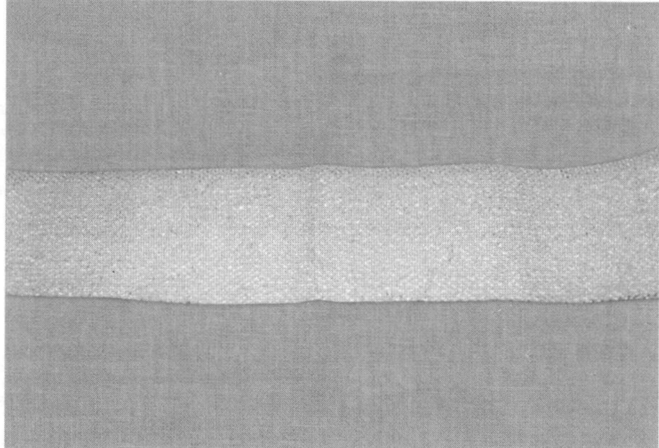

Fig. 37.7: Preparation of the Buddy Tape.

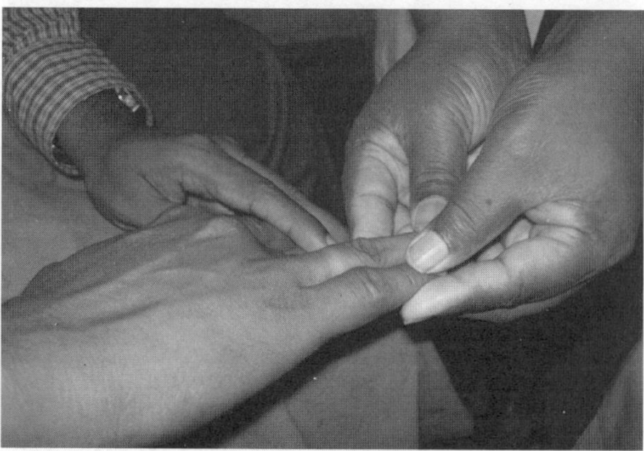

Fig. 37.8: Reduction of the deformity.

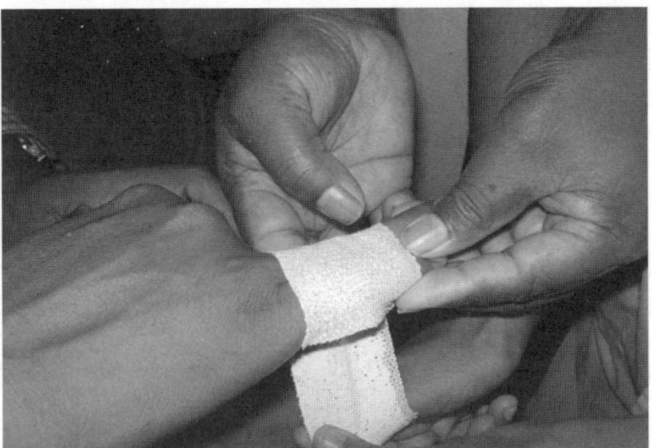

Fig. 37.9: Technique of applying the Buddy Tape (1).

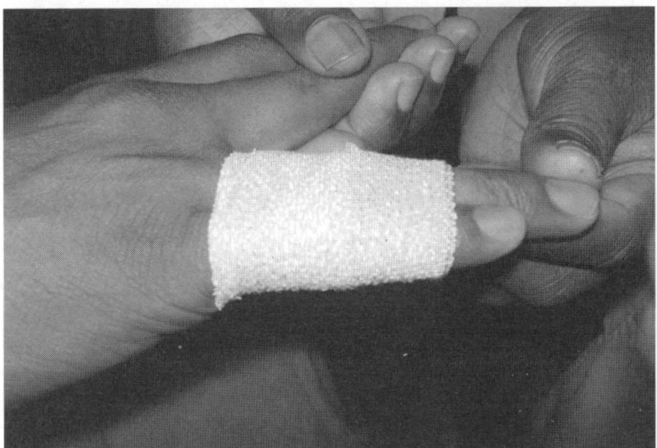

Fig. 37.10: Technique of applying the Buddy Tape (2).

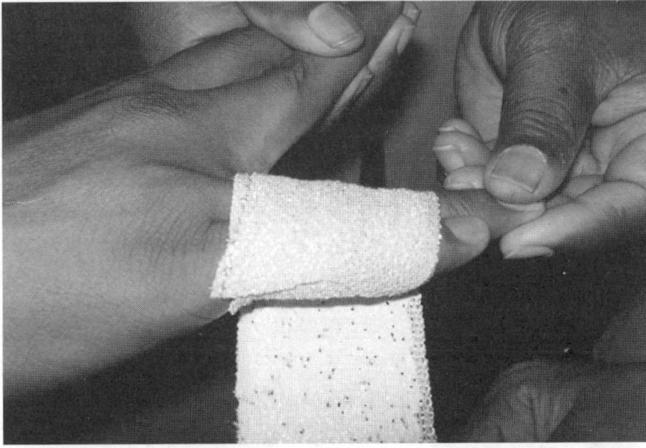

Fig. 37.11: Technique of applying the Buddy Tape (3).

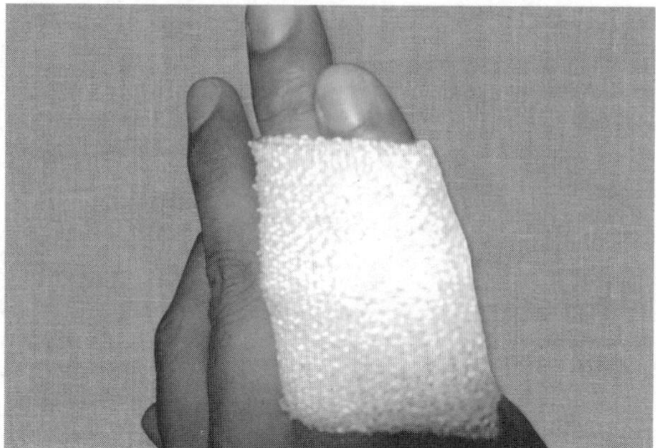

Fig. 37.12: Technique of applying the Buddy Tape (4).

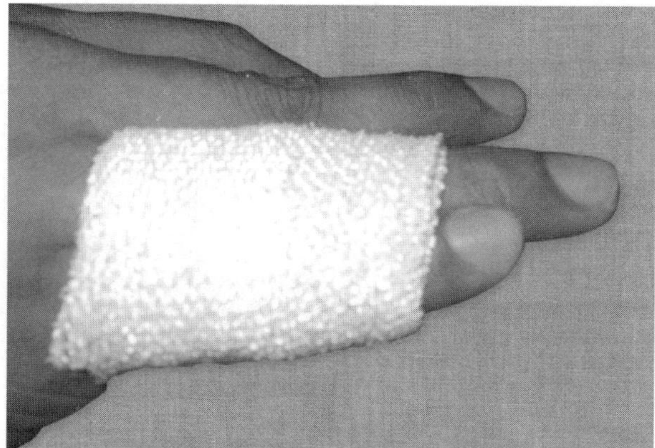

Fig. 37.13: Technique of applying the Buddy Tape (5).

KAPLAN'S LESION

Dislocation of First Metacarpophalangeal Joint

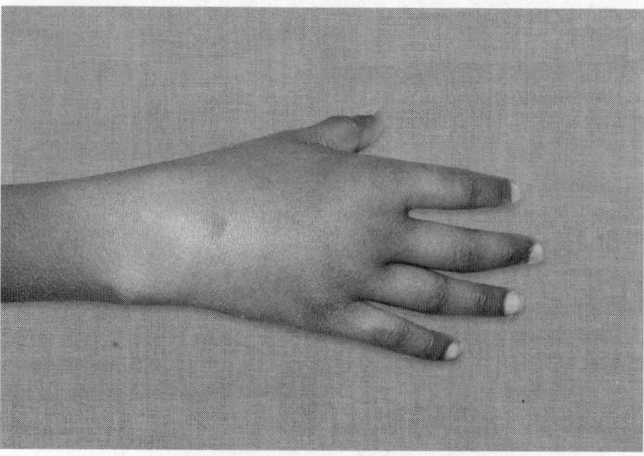

Fig. 37.14: Deformity (1).

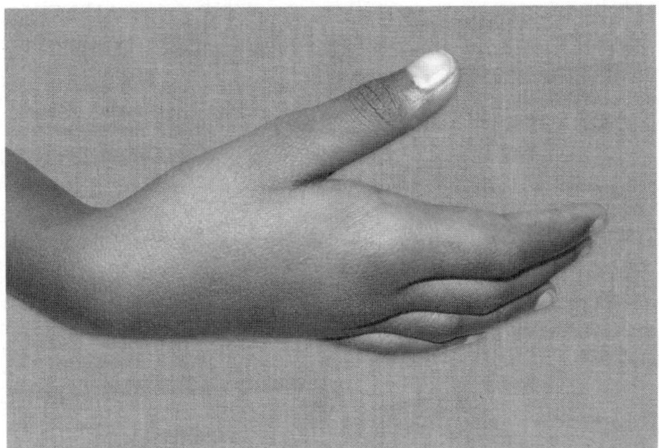

Fig. 37.15: Deformity (2).

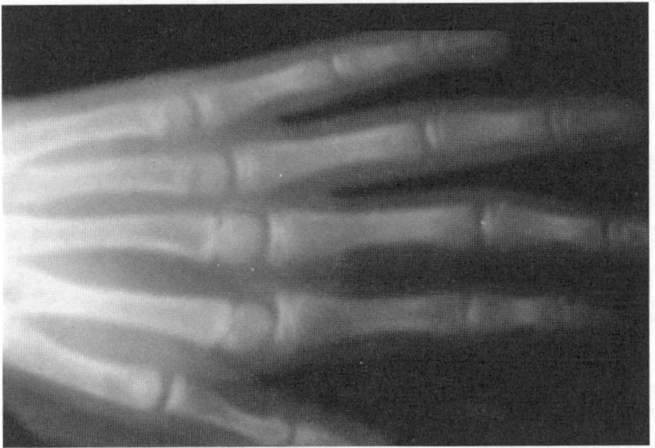

Fig. 37.16: Plain X-ray (1).

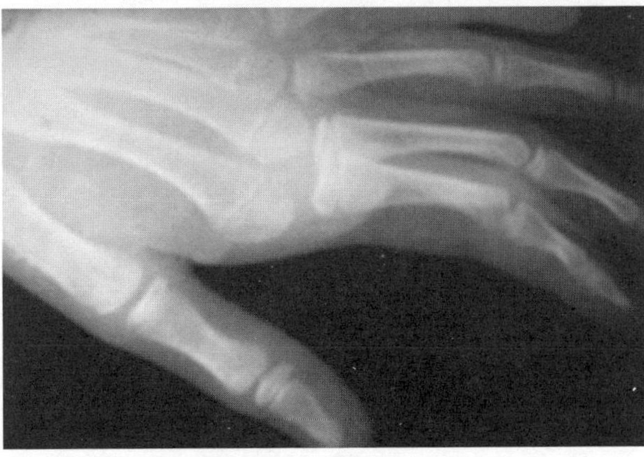

Fig. 37.17: Plain X-ray (2).

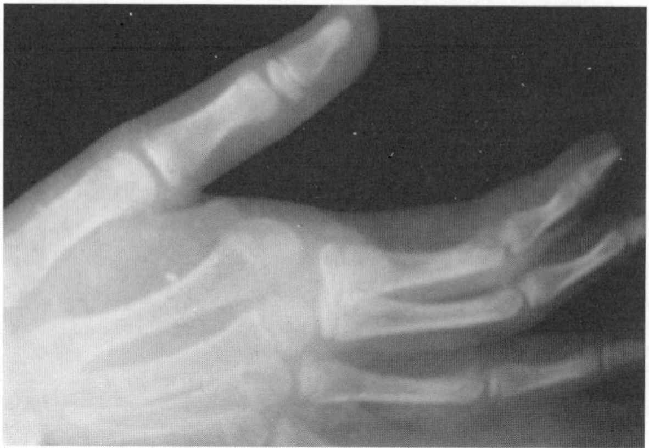

Fig. 37.18: Plain X-ray (3).

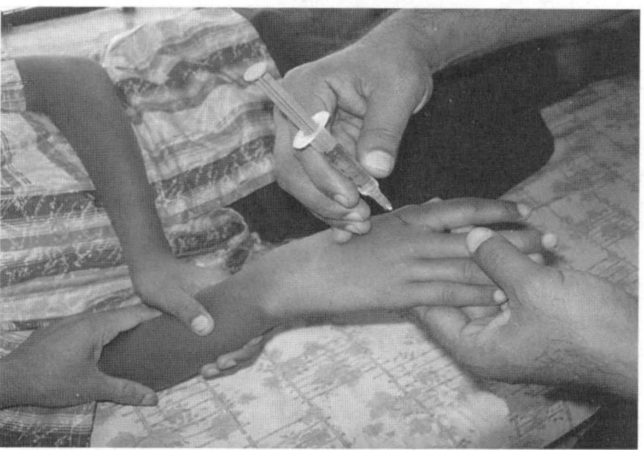

Fig. 37.19: Finger block (1).

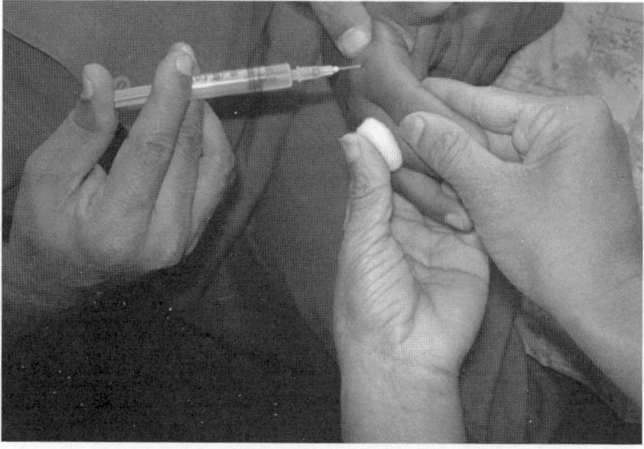

Fig. 37.20: Finger block (2).

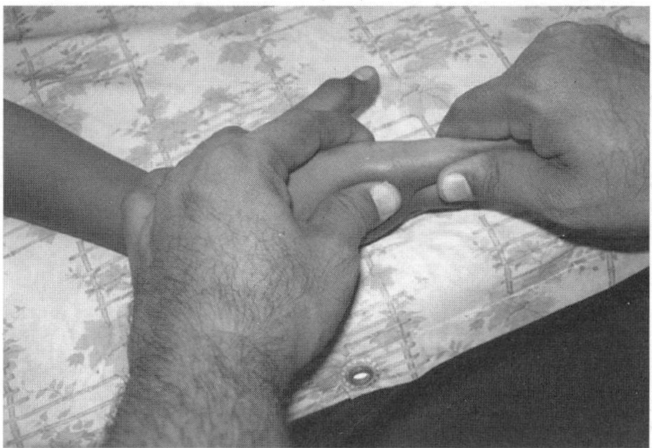

Fig. 37.21: Technique of reduction (1).

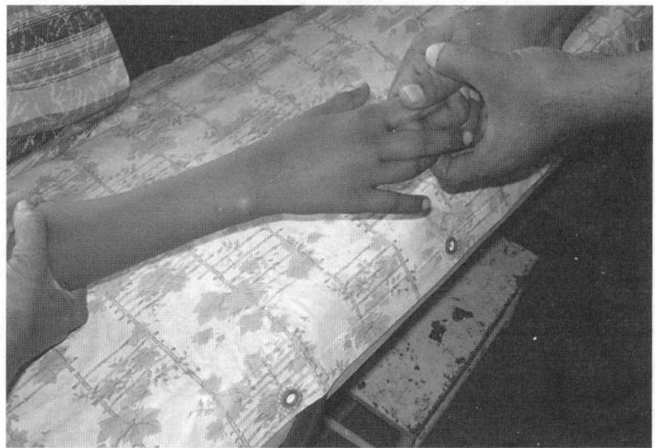

Fig. 37.22: Technique of reduction (2).

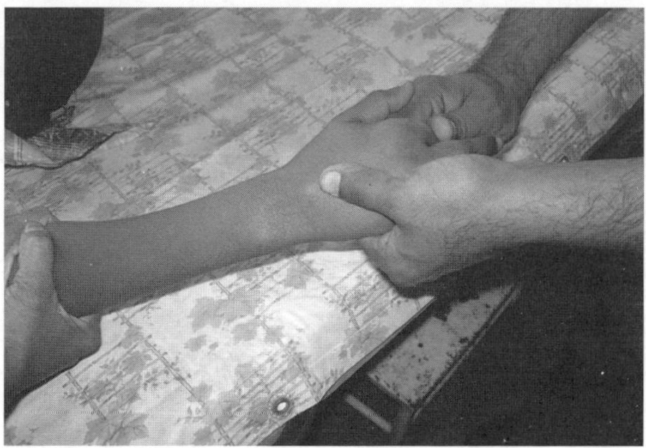

Fig. 37.23: Technique of reduction (3).

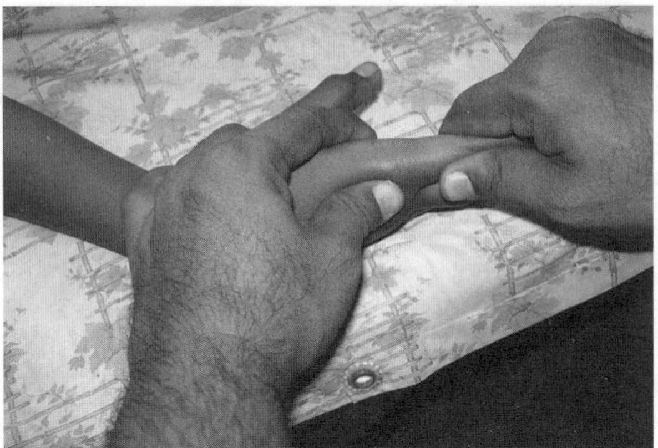

Fig. 37.24: Technique of reduction (4).

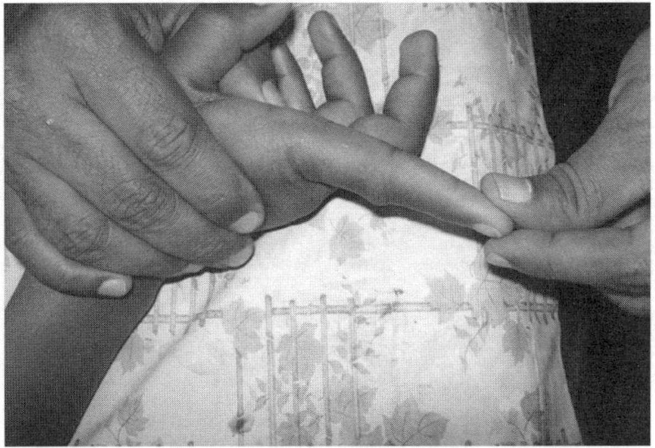

Fig. 37.25: Technique of reduction (hyperextension) (5).

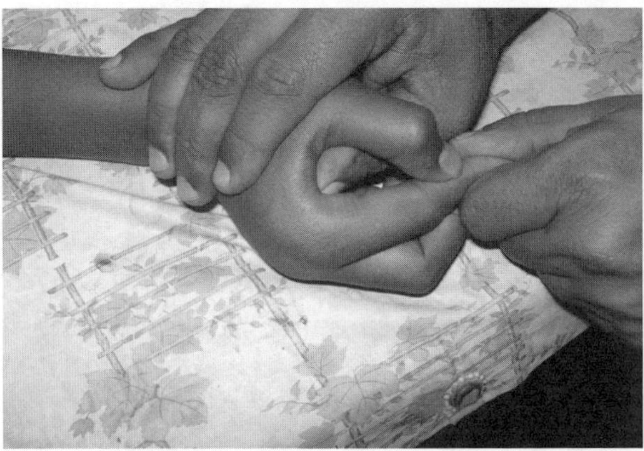

Fig. 37.26: Technique of reduction (flexion) (6).

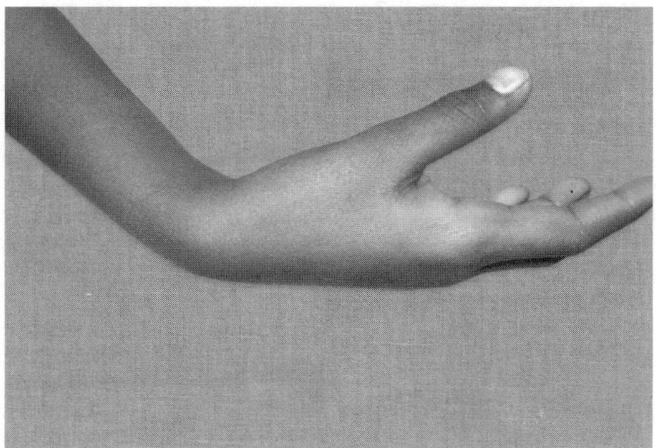

Fig. 37.27: Post-reduction (1).

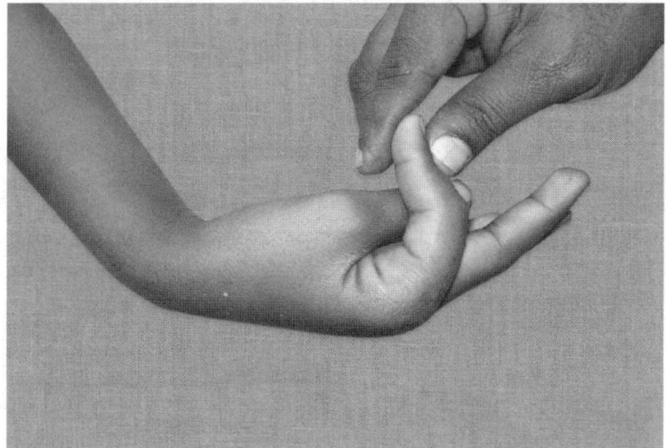

Fig. 37.28: Post-reduction (2).

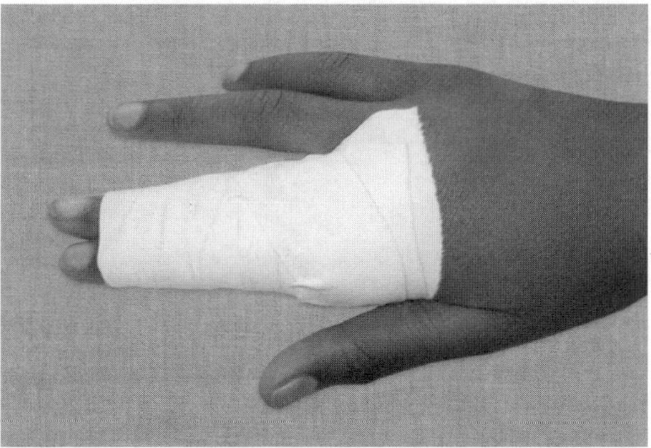

Fig. 37.29: Splinting (1).

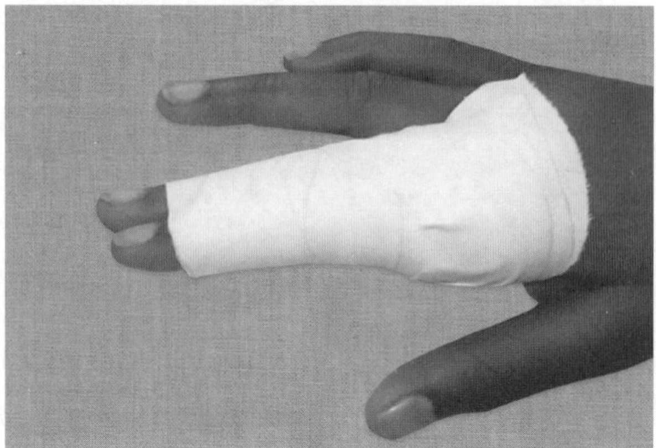

Fig. 37.30: Splinting (2).

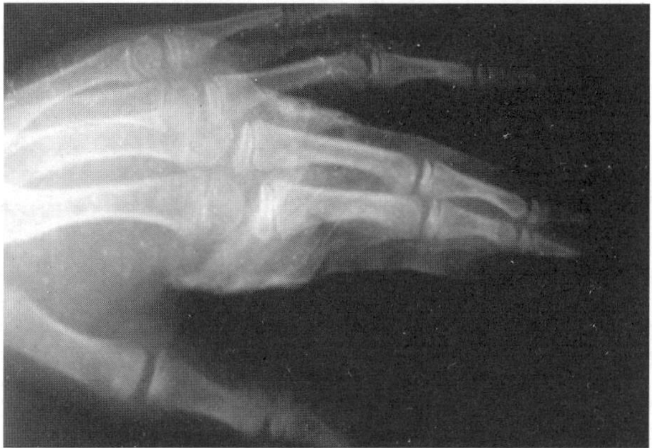

Fig. 37.31: Post-reduction X-ray.

METACARPAL AND PHALANGES FRACTURE GREENSTICK

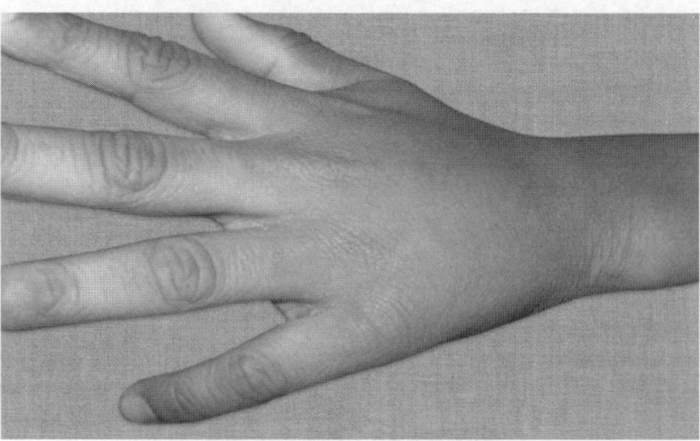

Fig. 37.32: Deformity.

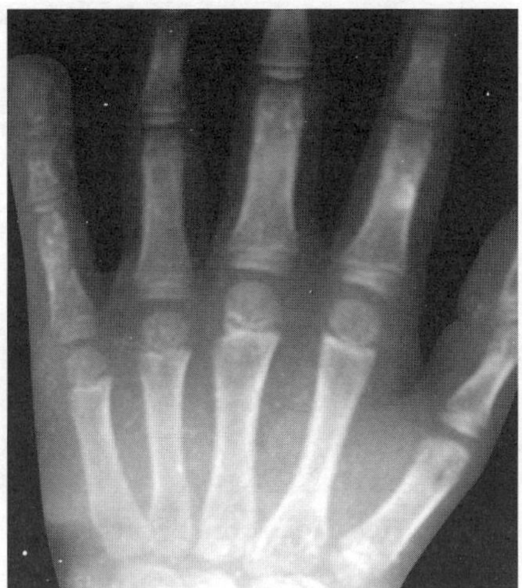

Fig. 37.33: X-ray showing fracture (1).

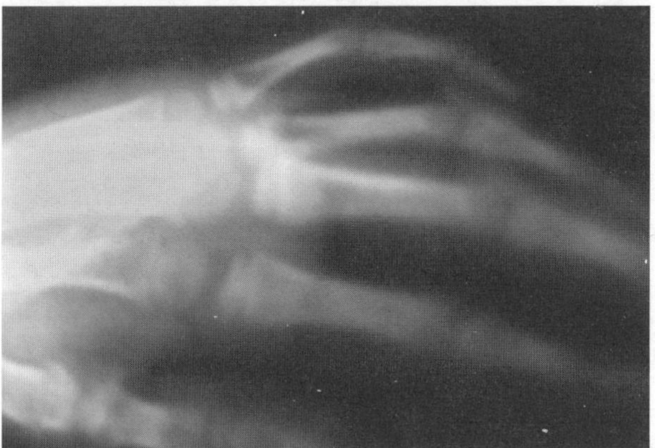

Fig. 37.34: X-ray showing fracture (2).

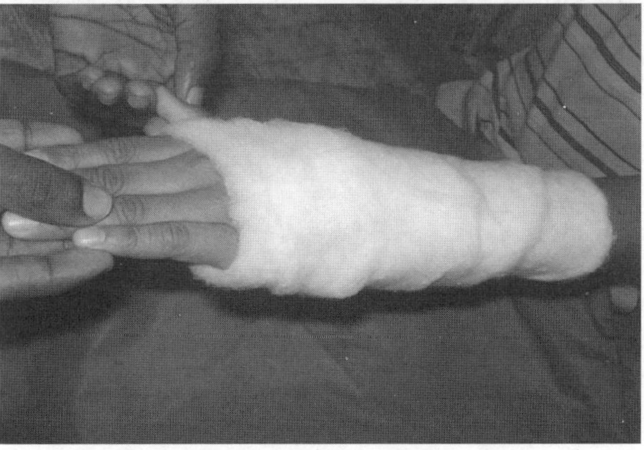

Fig. 37.35: Technique of applying plaster (1).

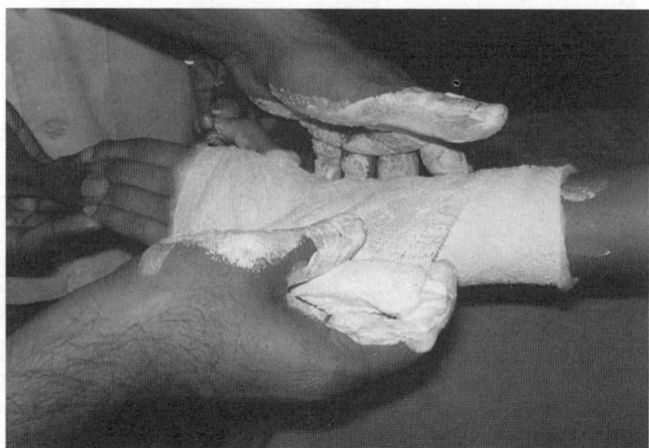

Fig. 37.36: Technique of applying plaster (2).

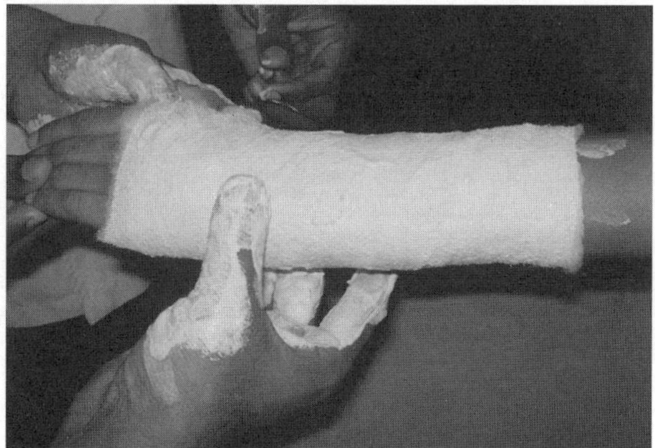

Fig. 37.37: Technique of applying plaster (3).

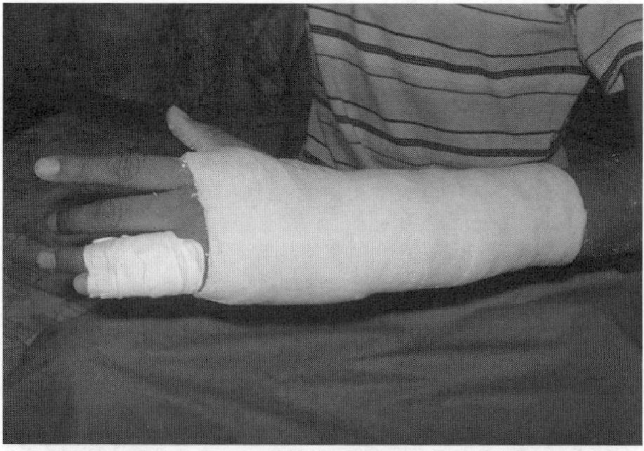

Fig. 37.38: Technique of applying plaster (4).

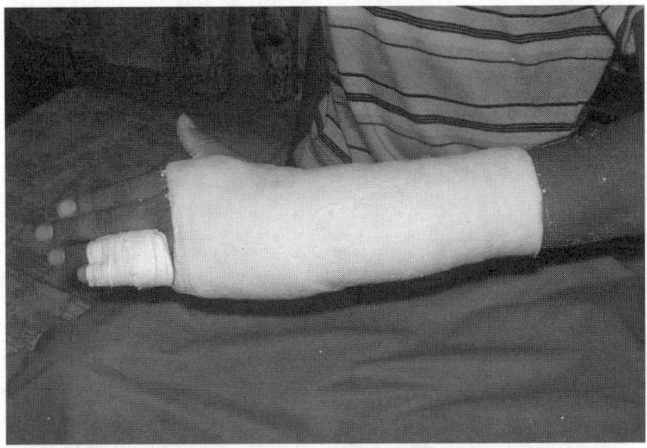

Fig. 37.39: Technique of applying plaster (5).

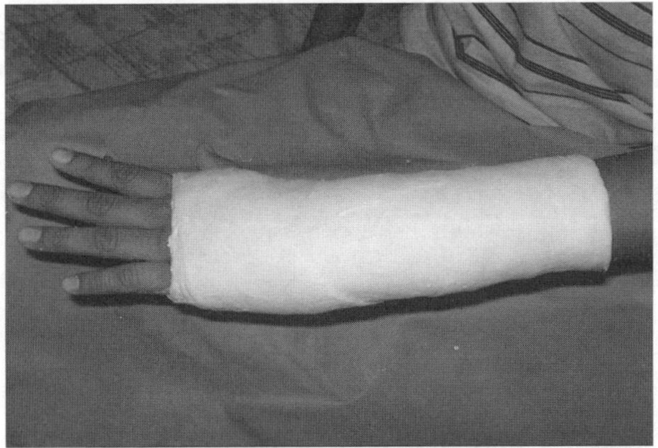

Fig. 37.40: Technique of applying plaster (6).

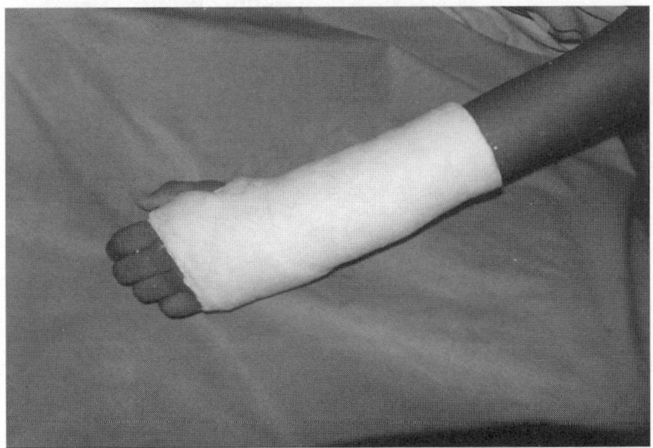

Fig. 37.41: Technique of applying plaster (7).

SESAMOID BONE FRACTURE

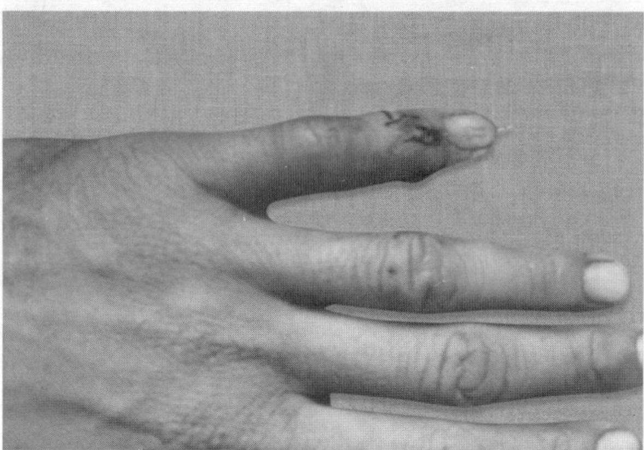

Fig. 37.42: Deformity (1).

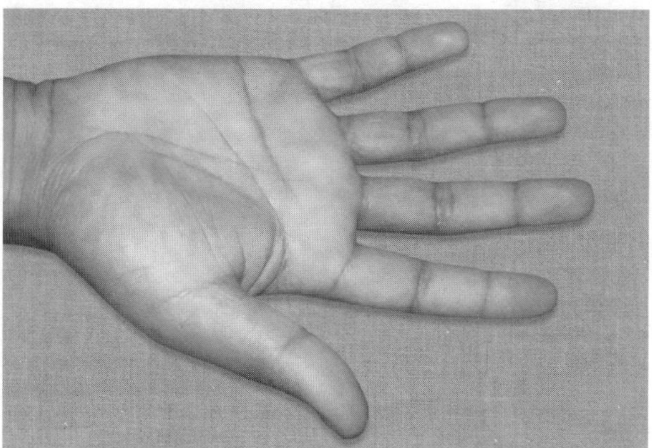

Fig. 37.43: Deformity (2).

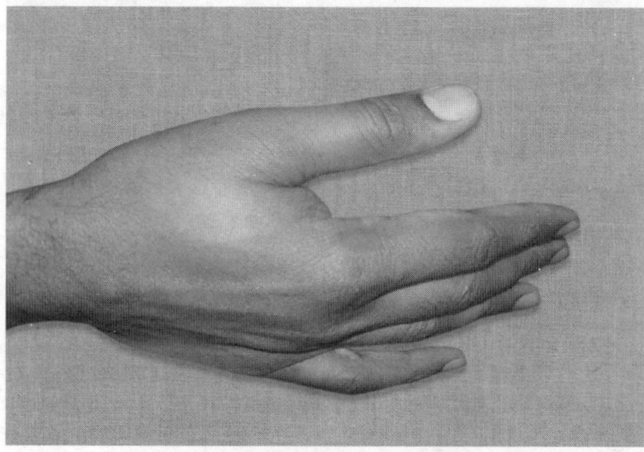

Fig. 37.44: Deformity (3).

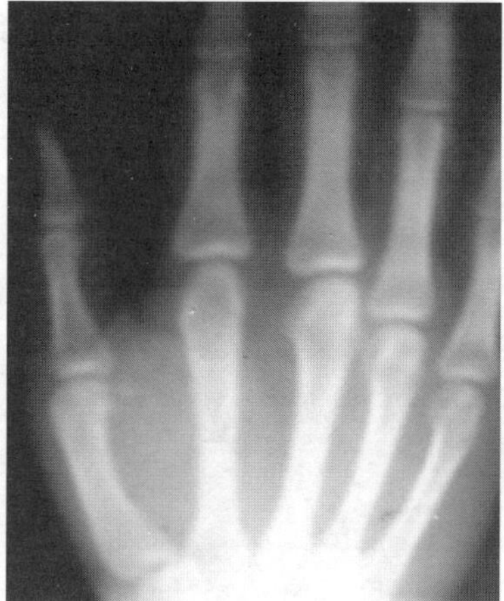

Fig. 37.45: Plain X-ray (1).

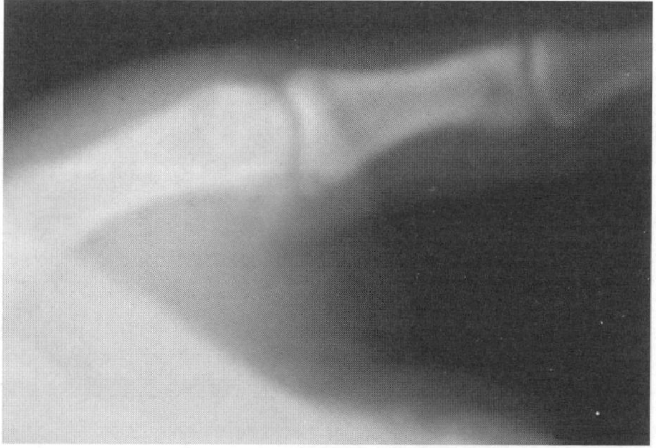

Fig. 37.46: Plain X-ray (2).

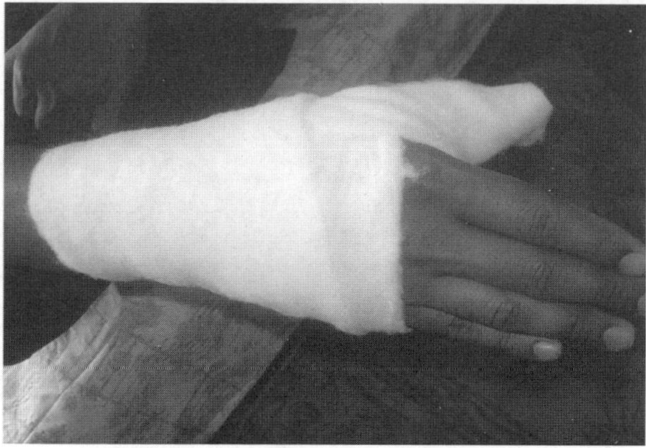

Fig. 37.47: Plaster cast technique (1).

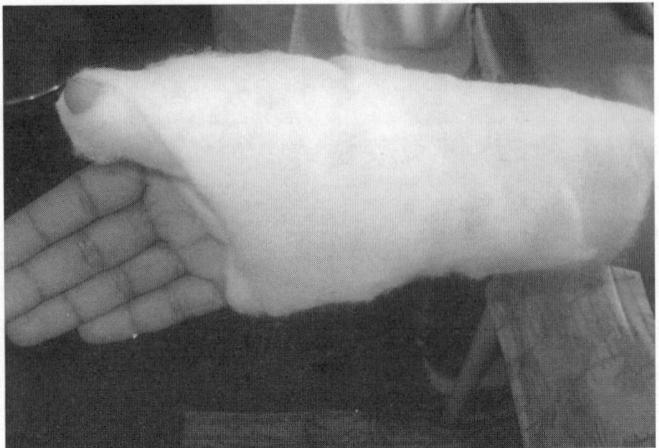

Fig. 37.48: Plaster cast technique (2).

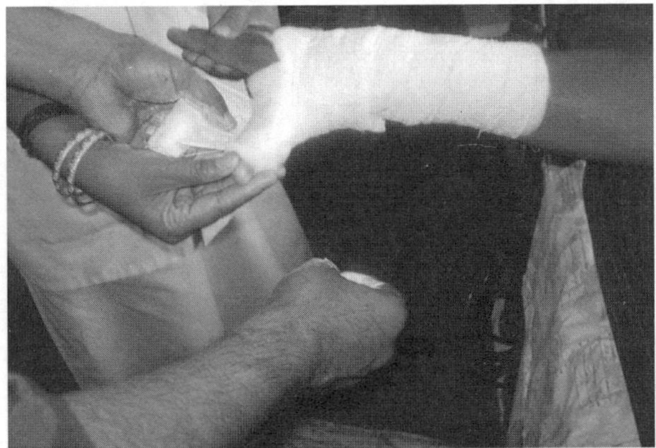

Fig. 37.49: Plaster cast technique (3).

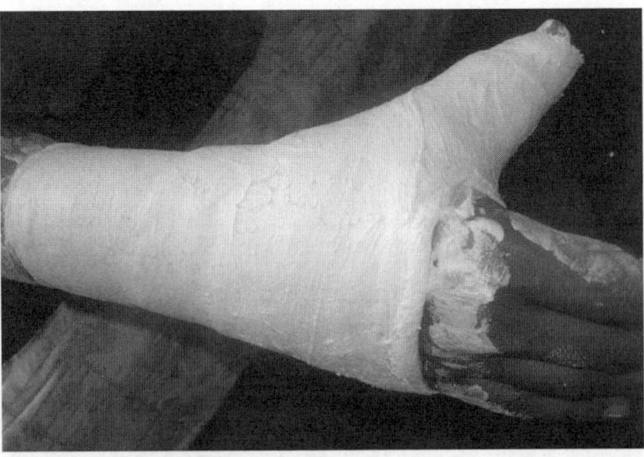

Fig. 37.50: Plaster cast technique (4).

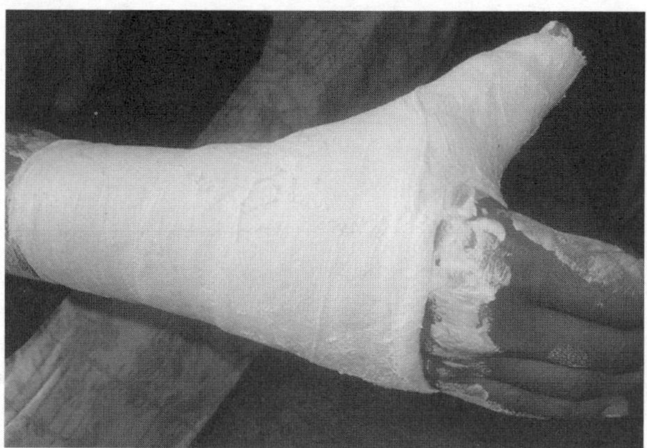

Fig. 37.51: Plaster cast technique (5).

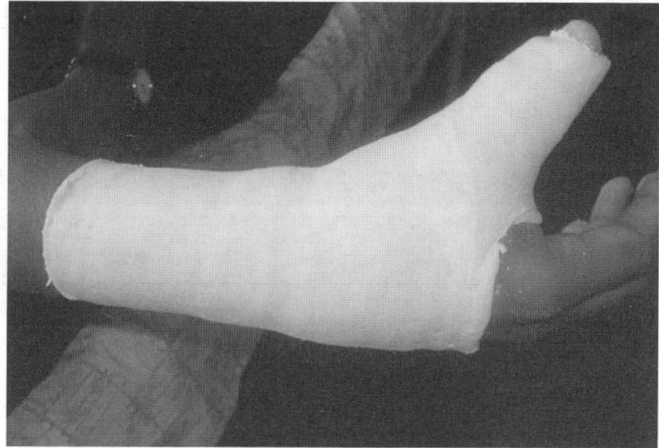

Fig. 37.52: Plaster cast technique (6).

Lower Limbs

Hip Injuries

This chapter deals with the practical techniques of managing the common hip injuries.

HIP SPICA APPLICATION FOR GREATER TROCHANTER FRACTURE

This technique is used in children.

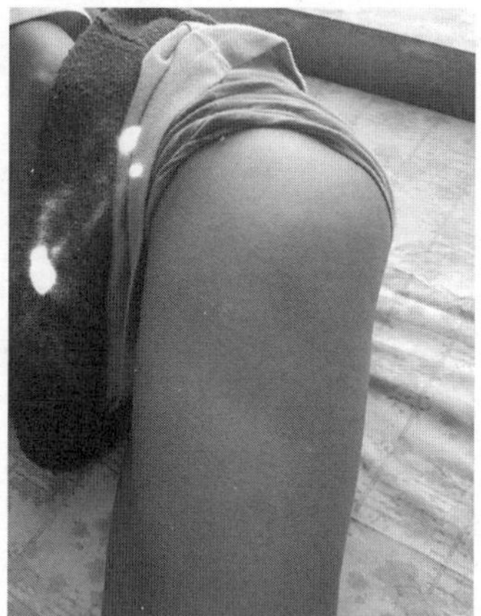

Fig. 38.1: Clinical picture.

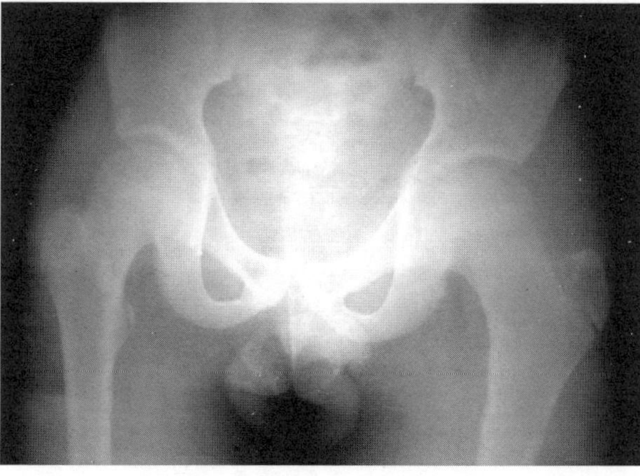

Fig. 38.2: Plain X-ray.

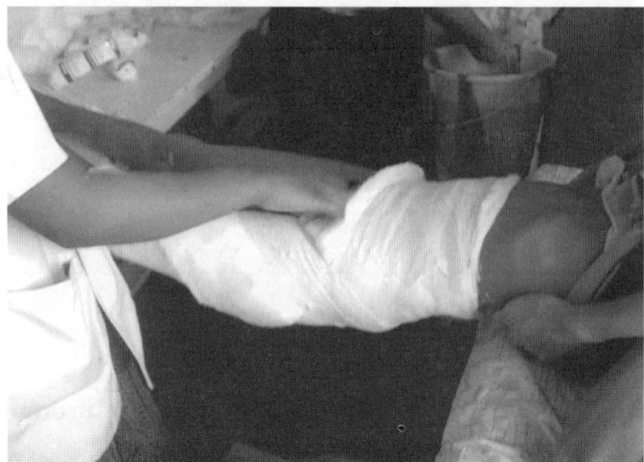

Fig. 38.3: Method of hip spica application (1).

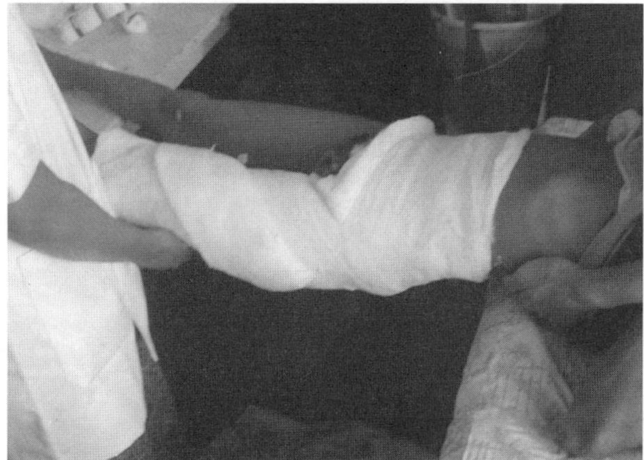

Fig. 38.4: Method of hip spica application (2).

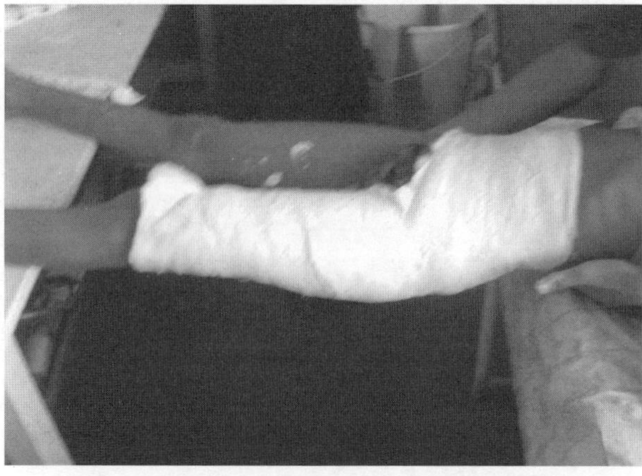

Fig. 38.5: Method of hip spica application (3).

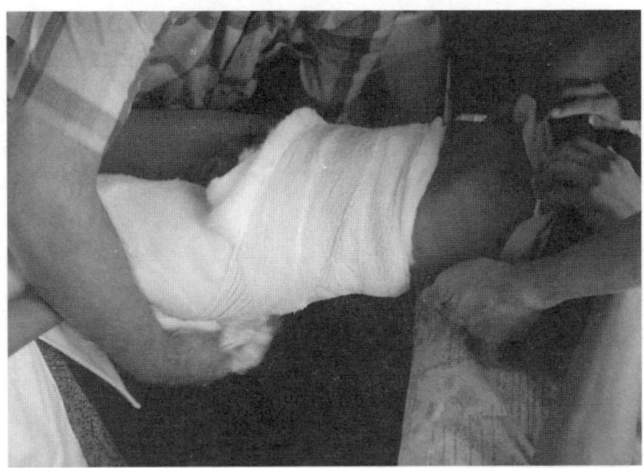

Fig. 38.6: Method of hip spica application (4).

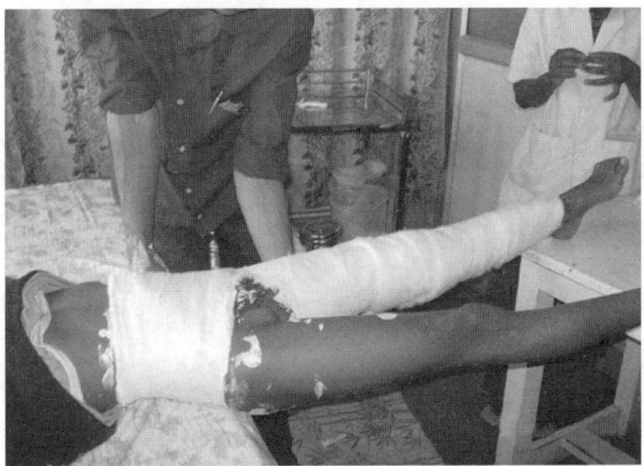

Fig. 38.7: Method of hip spica application (5).

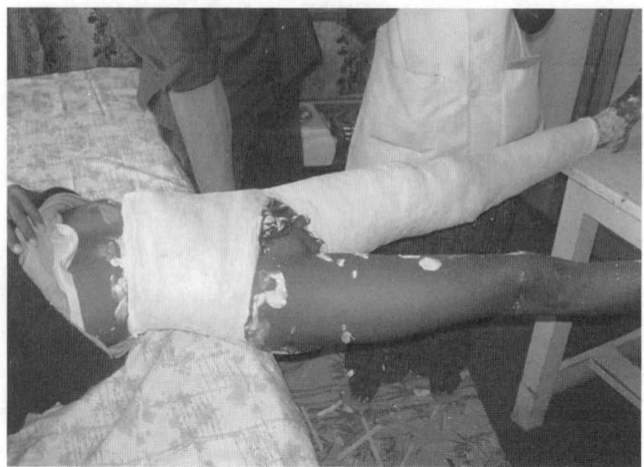

Fig. 38.8: Method of hip spica application (6).

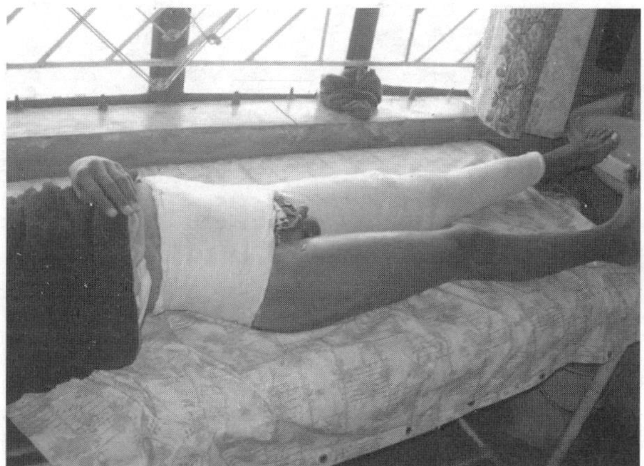

Fig. 38.9: Final picture.

Knee Aspiration

This chapter deals with the practical techniques of managing the common knee injuries.

After Sterile Draping

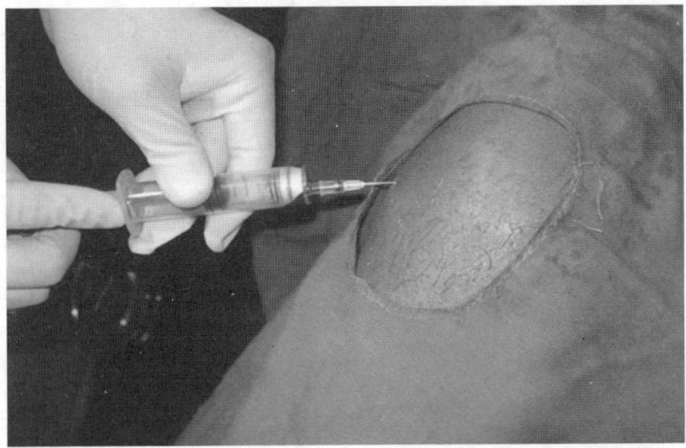

Fig. 39.1: Technique of knee aspiration (Giving local anesthesia) (1).

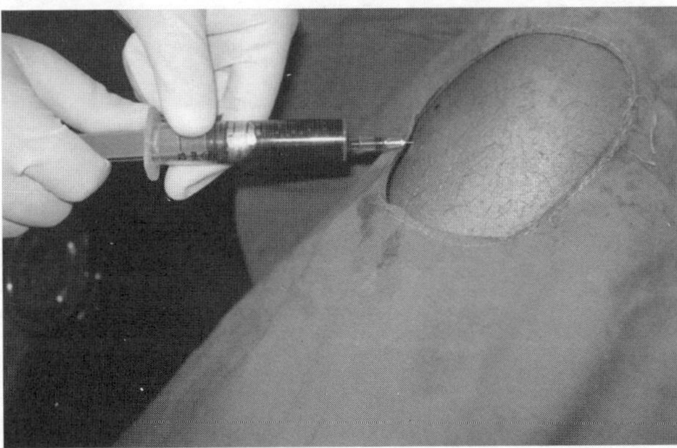

Fig. 39.2: Technique of knee aspiration (Drawing cloud from the knee through a thick bore needle) (2).

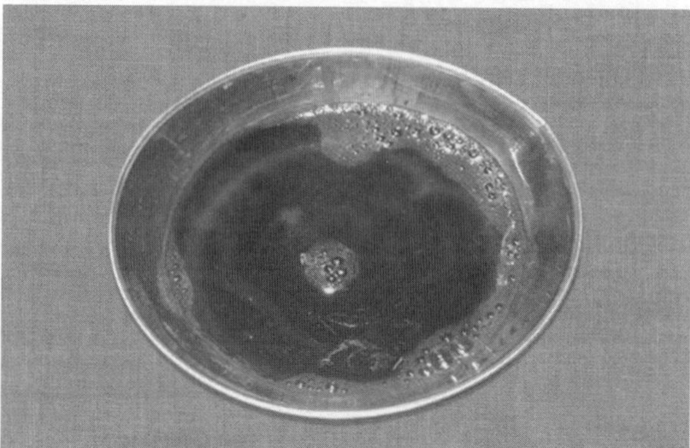

Fig. 39.3: Technique of knee aspiration (3).

Leg Injuries

This chapter deals with the practical techniques of managing the common leg injuries.

FIBULA FRACTURE

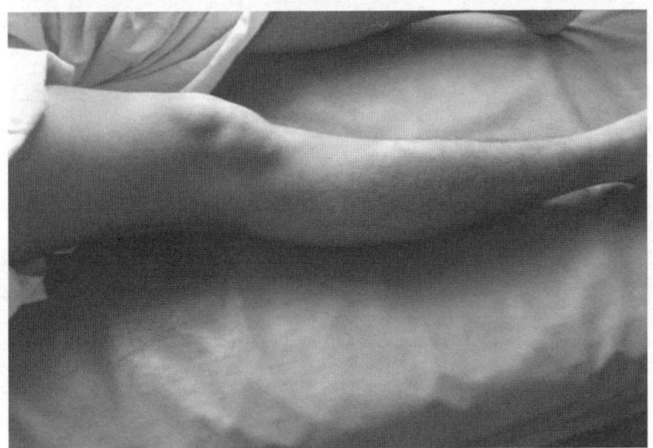

Fig. 40.1: Clinical deformity.

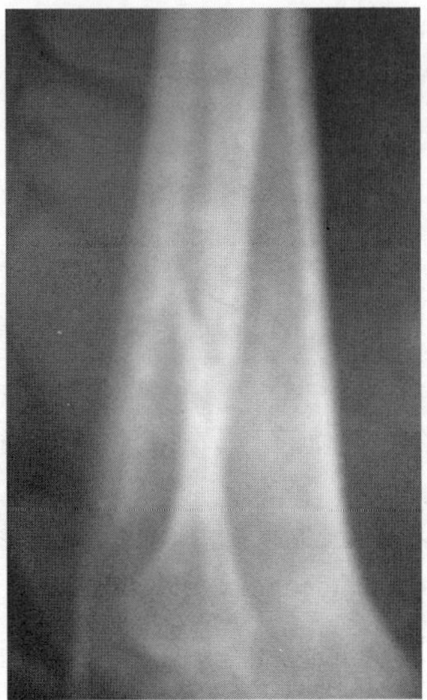

Fig. 40.2: Plain X-ray.

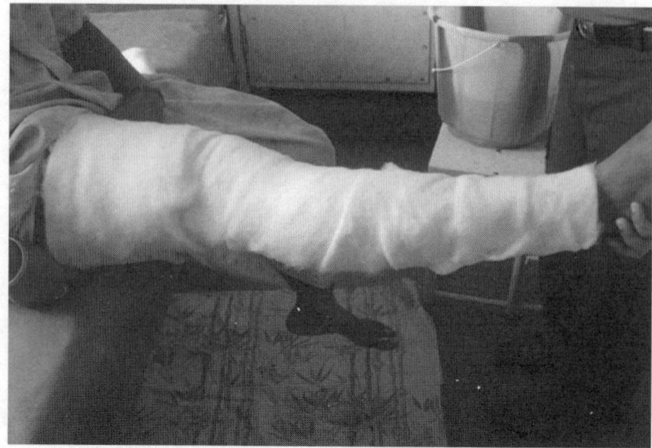

Fig. 40.3: Technique of AK POP cast (1).

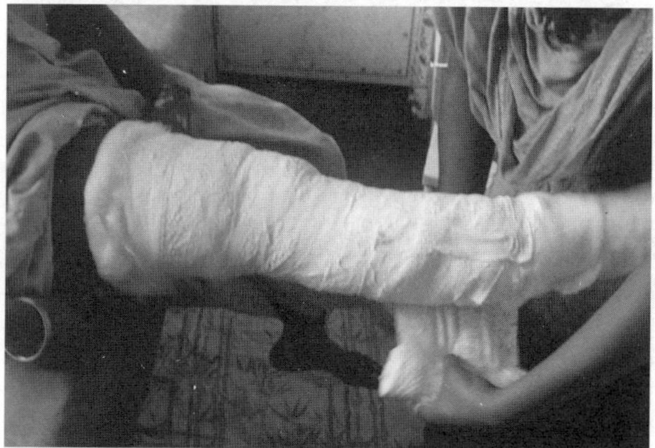

Fig. 40.4: Technique of AK POP cast (2).

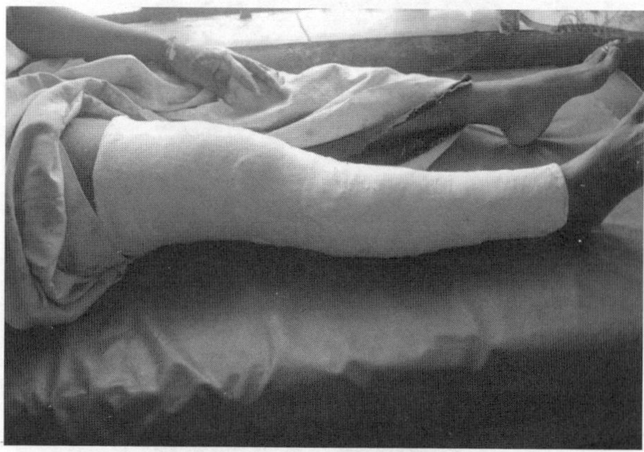

Fig. 40.5: Technique of AK POP cast (3).

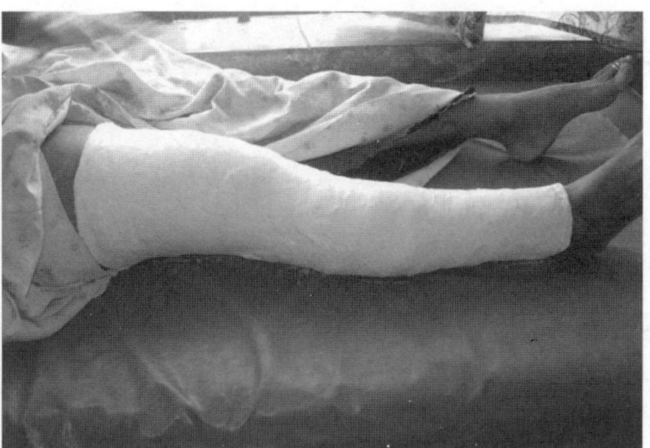

Fig. 40.6: Final appearance.

TIBIA FRACTURE

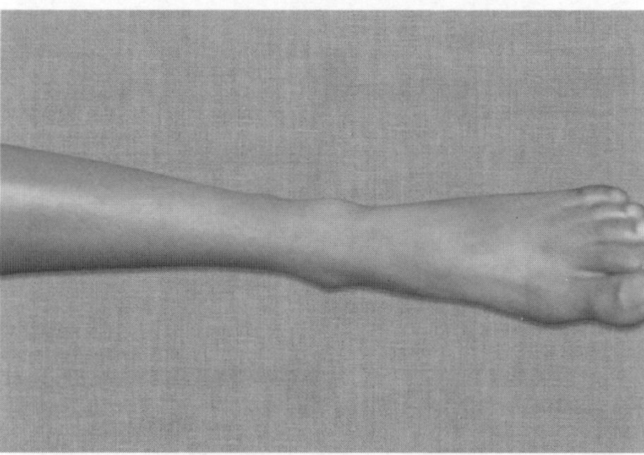

Fig. 40.7: Clinical deformity (1).

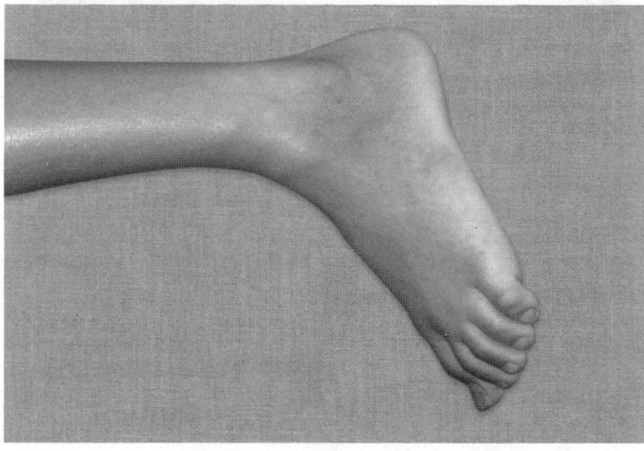

Fig. 40.8: Clinical deformity (2).

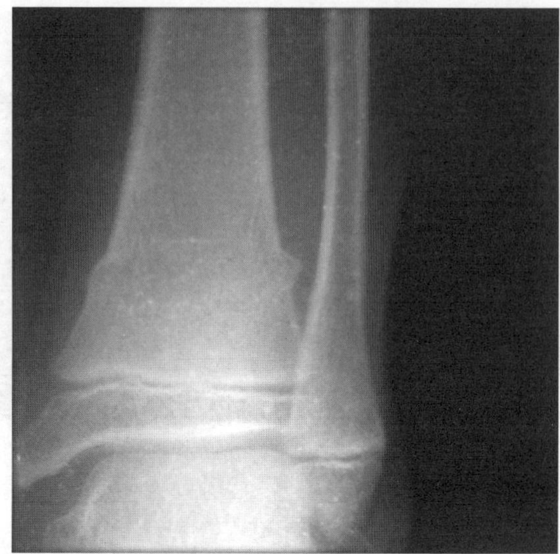

Fig. 40.9: Plain X-ray (1).

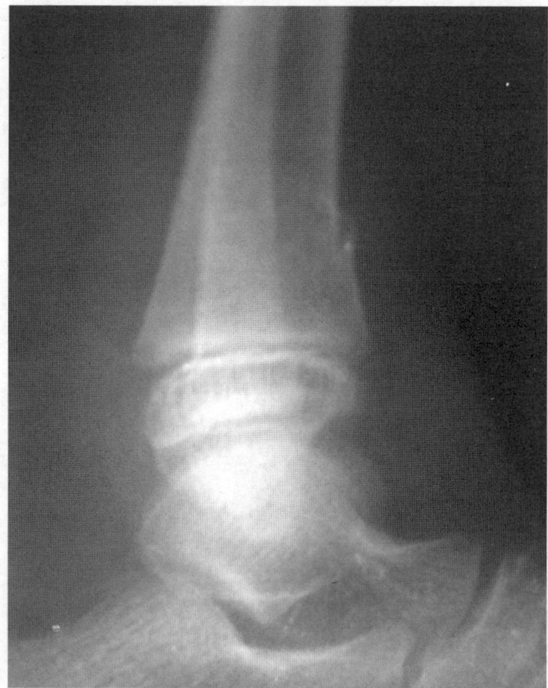

Fig. 40.10: Plain X-ray (2).

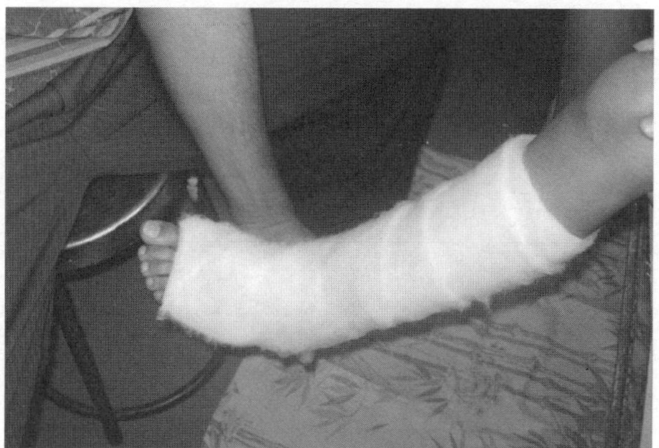

Fig. 40.11: Technique of plaster application (1).

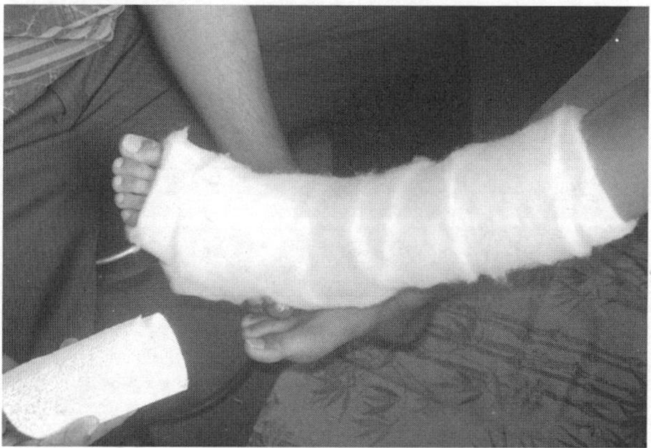

Fig. 40.12: Technique of plaster application (2).

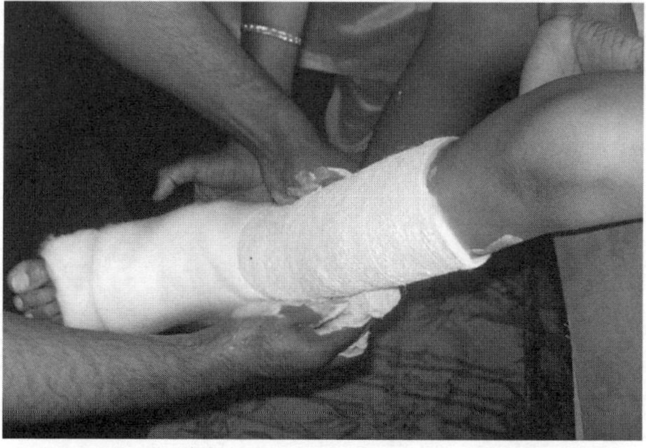

Fig. 40.13: Technique of plaster application (3).

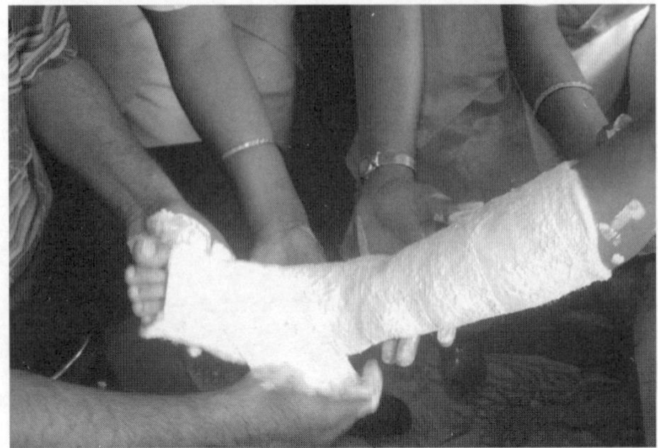

Fig. 40.14: Technique of plaster application (4).

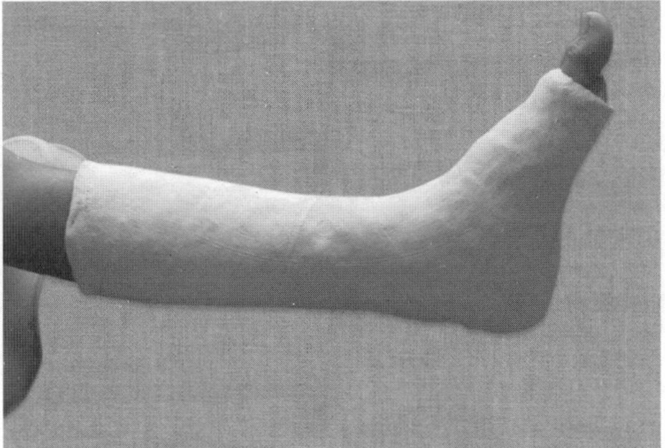

Fig. 40.15: Technique of plaster application (5).

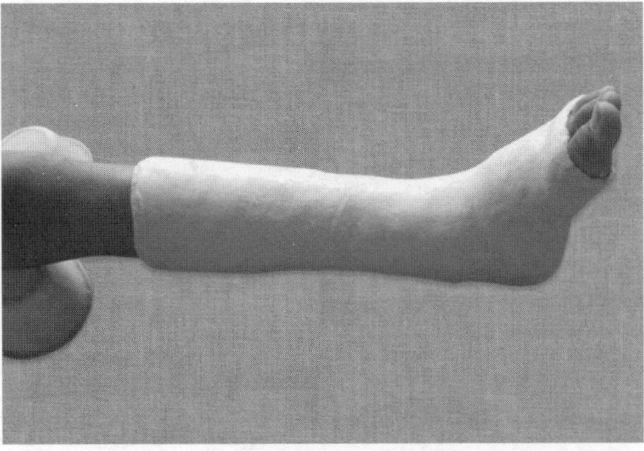

Fig. 40.16: Final appearance.

PINPOINT COMPOUND FRACTURE TIBIA

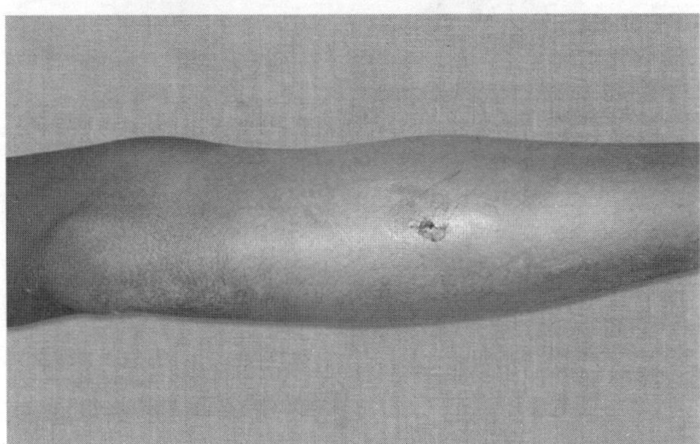

Fig. 40.17: Clinical picture.

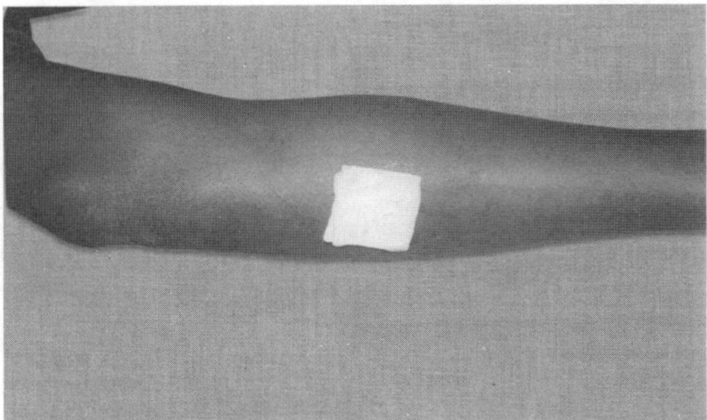

Fig. 40.18: Closing the wound, after cleaning with antiseptic solution.

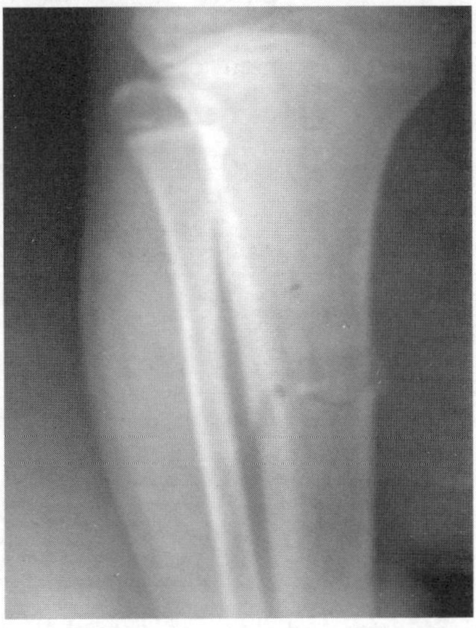

Fig. 40.19: Plain X-ray (1).

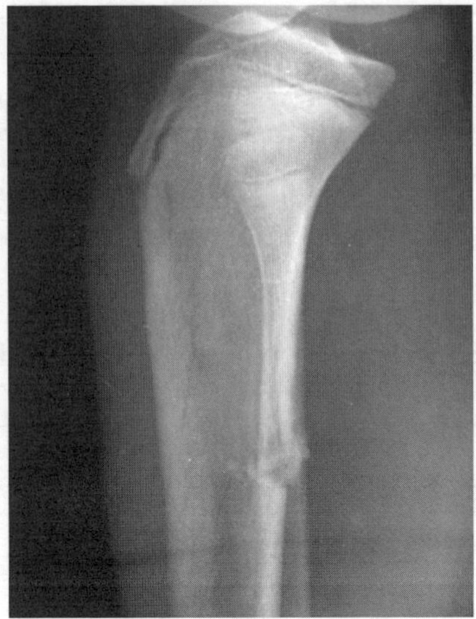

Fig. 40.20: Plain X-ray (2).

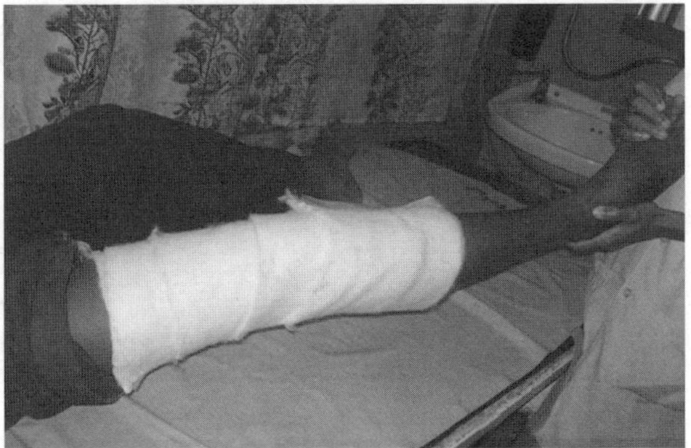

Fig. 40.21: Technique of POP casting (1).

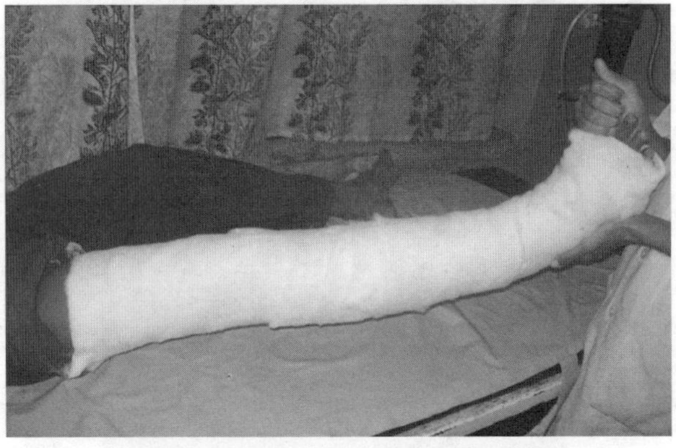

Fig. 40.22: Technique of POP casting (2).

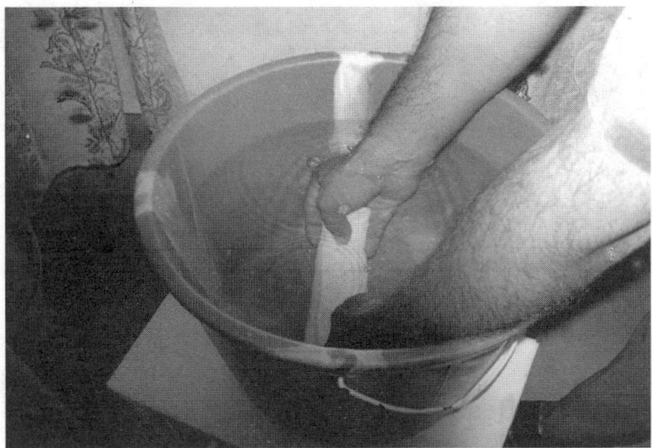

Fig. 40.23: Technique of POP casting (3).

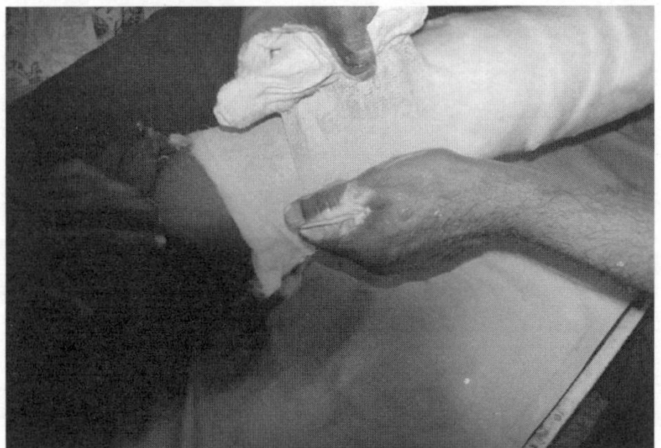

Fig. 40.24: Technique of POP casting (4).

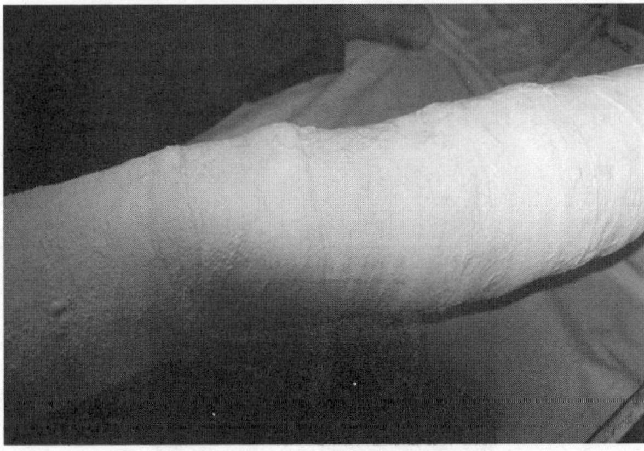

Fig. 40.25: Technique of POP casting (5).

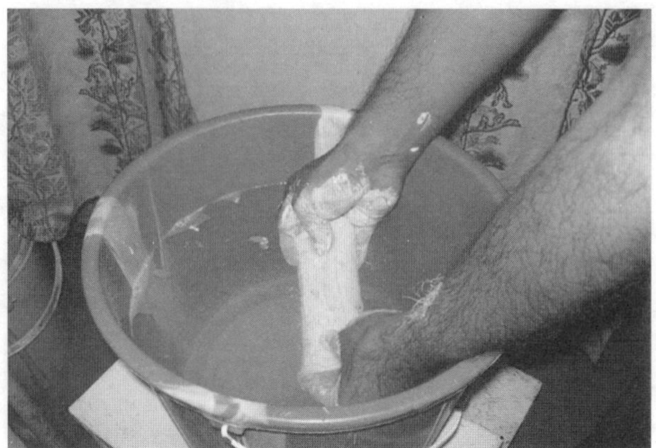

Fig. 40.26: Technique of POP casting (6).

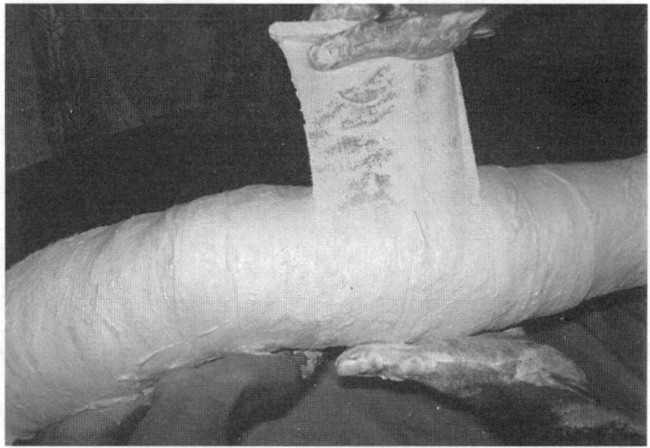

Fig. 40.27: Technique of POP casting (7).

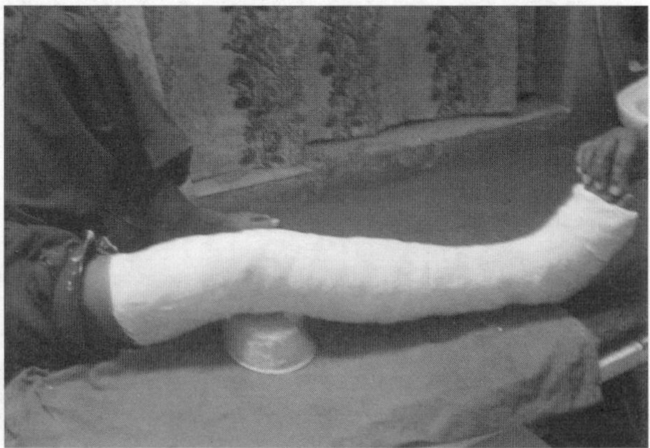

Fig. 40.28: Final appearance.

PROXIMAL TIBIA FRACTURE

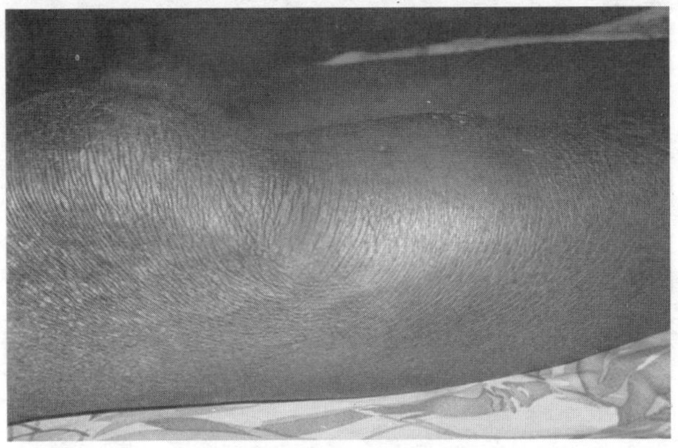

Fig. 40.29: Clinical deformity.

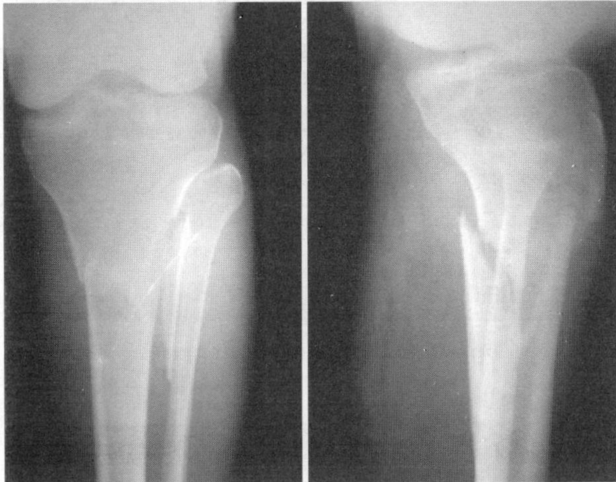

Fig. 40.30: Plain X-ray (1).

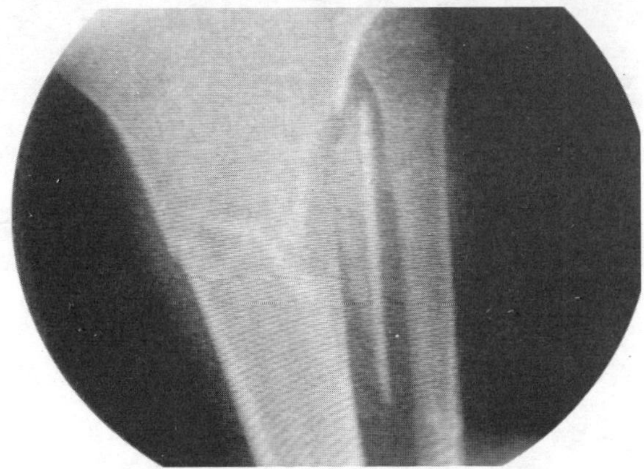

Fig. 40.31: Plain X-ray (2).

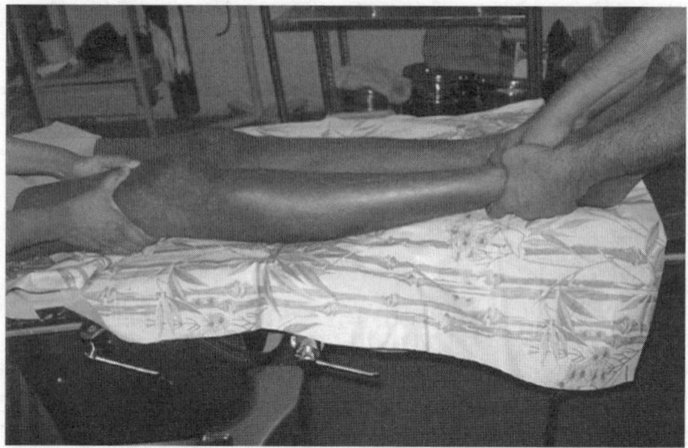

Fig. 40.32: Reduction technique (1).

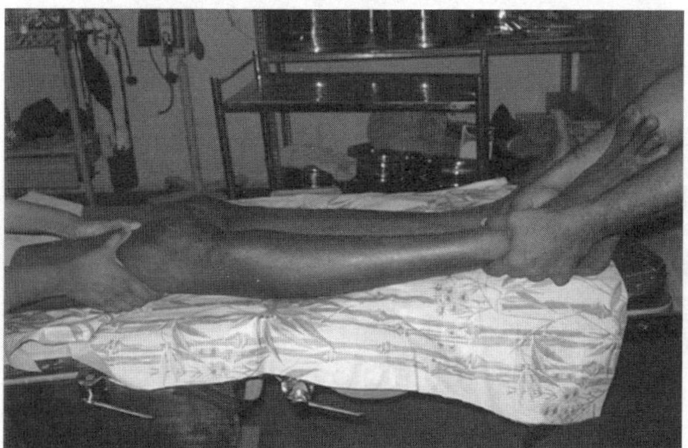

Fig. 40.33: Reduction technique (2).

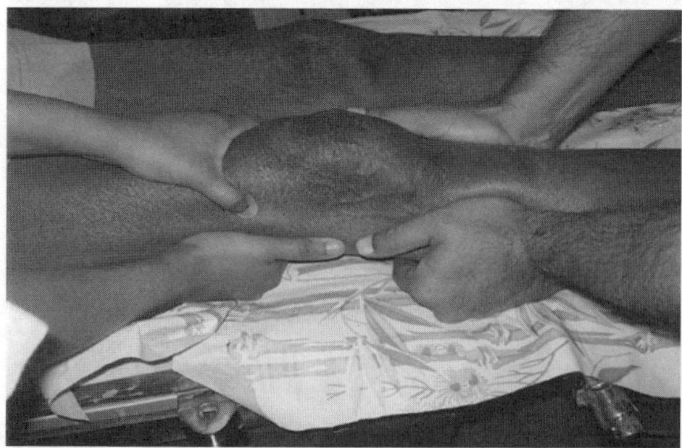

Fig. 40.34: Reduction technique (3).

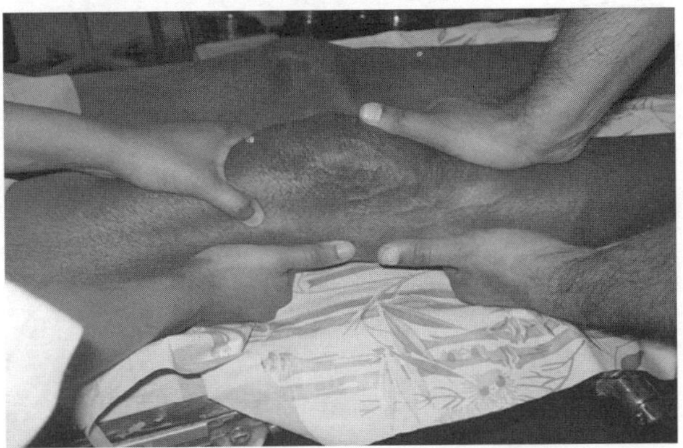

Fig. 40.35: Reduction technique (4).

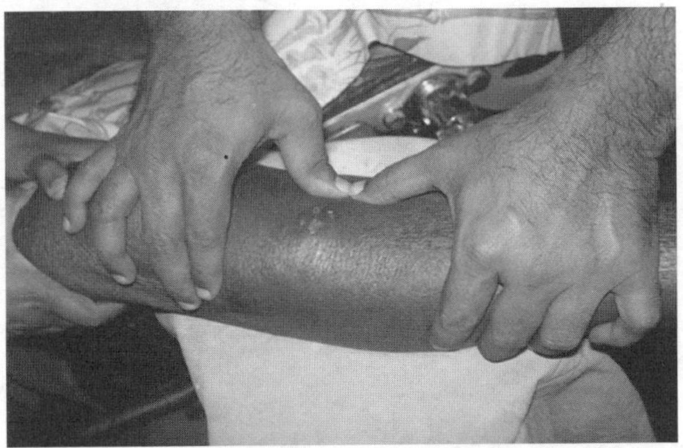

Fig. 40.36: Reduction technique (5).

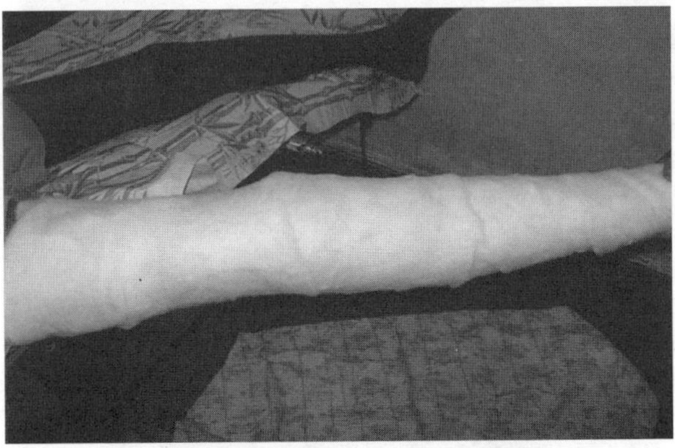

Fig. 40.37: Technique of AK POP cast (1).

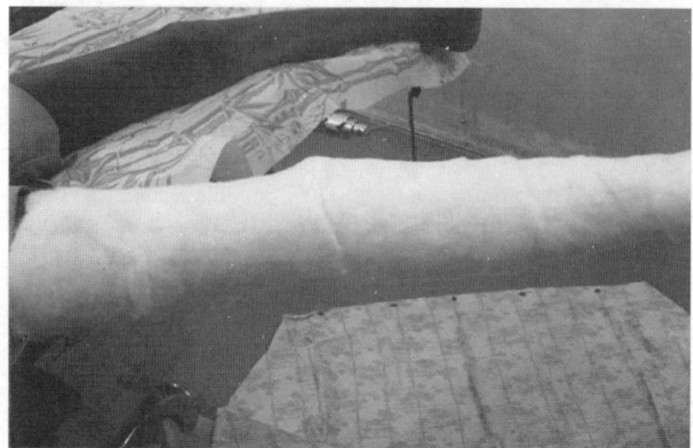

Fig. 40.38: Technique of AK POP cast (2).

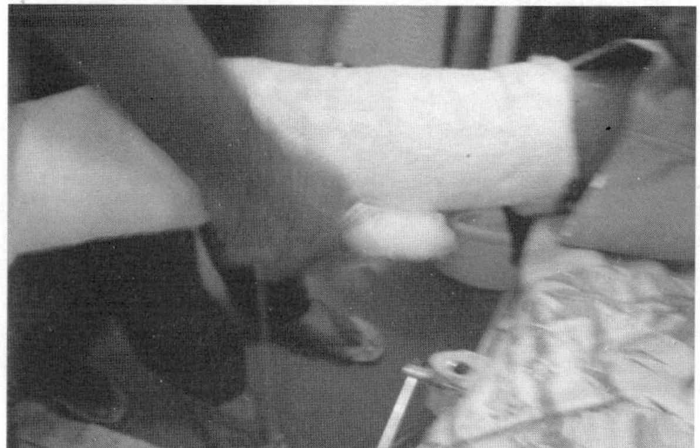

Fig. 40.39: Technique of AK POP cast (3).

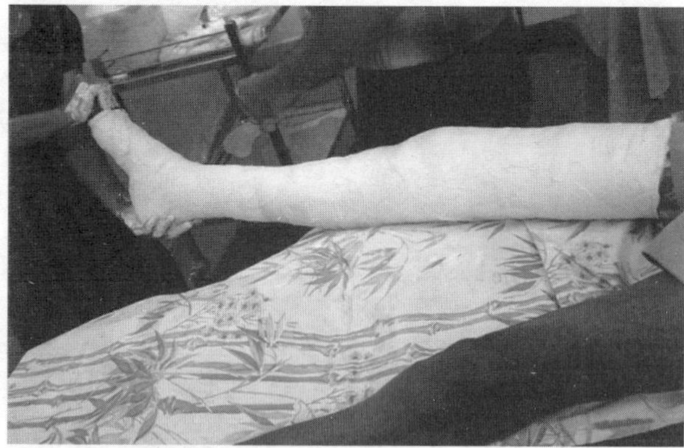

Fig. 40.40: Technique of AK POP cast (4).

TIBIA FRACTURE (GREENSTICK)

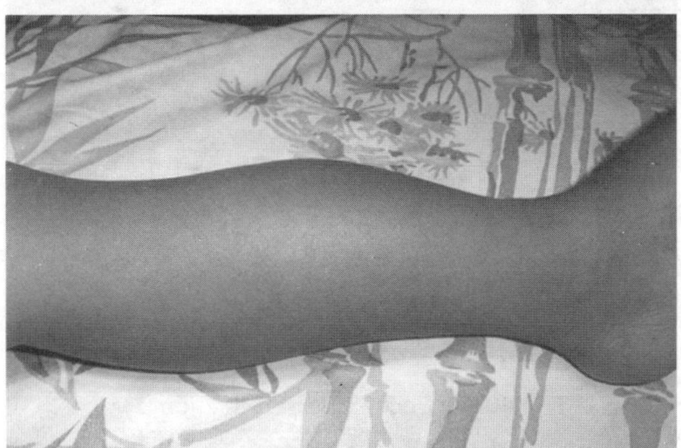

Fig. 40.41: Clinical deformity (1).

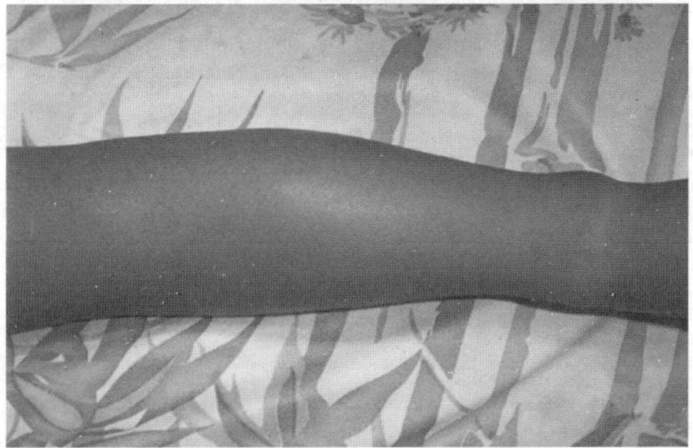

Fig. 40.42: Clinical deformity (2).

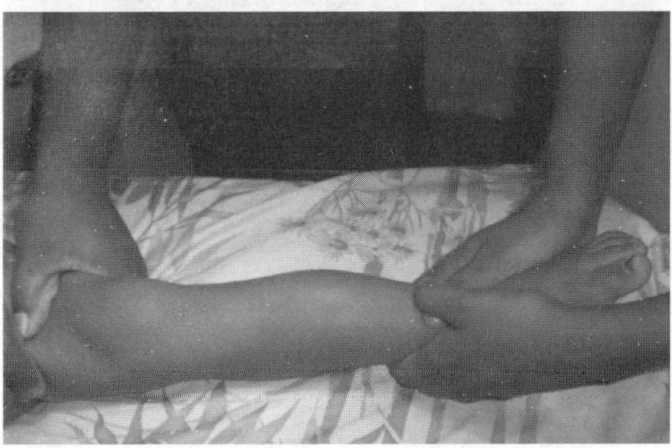

Fig. 40.43: Technique of reduction (1).

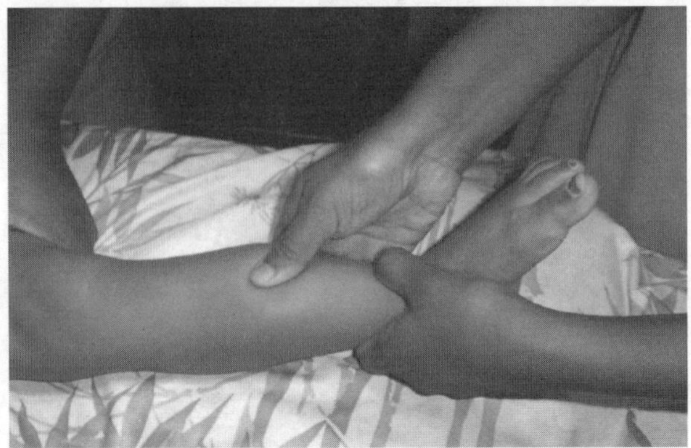

Fig. 40.44: Technique of reduction (2).

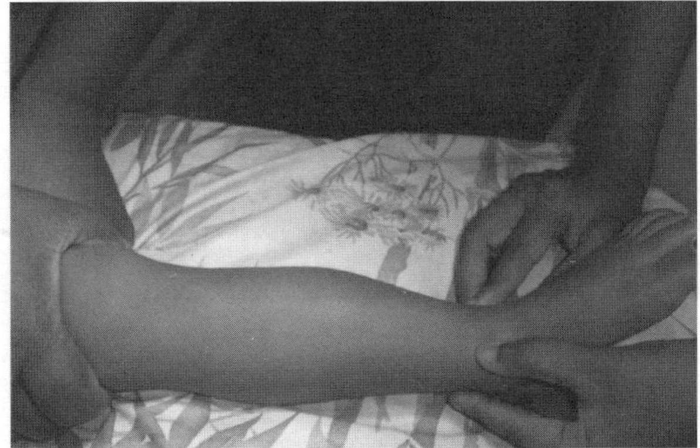

Fig. 40.45: Technique of reduction (3).

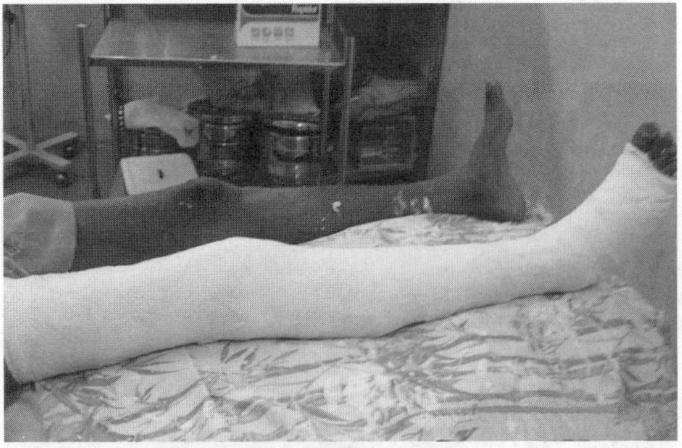

Fig. 40.46: Above knee POP cast.

PLASTER REMOVAL

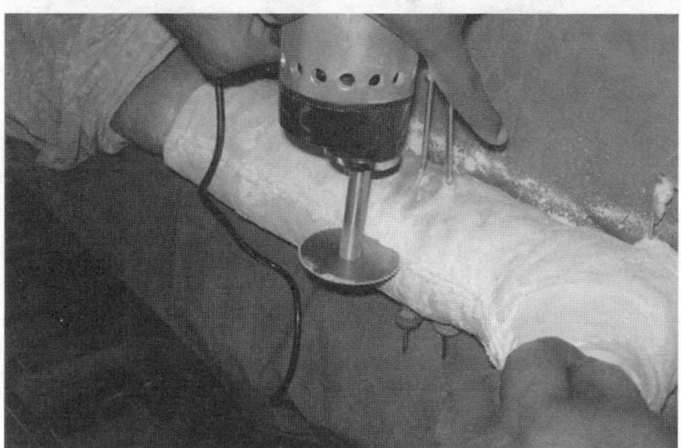

Fig. 40.47: Technique of electric plaster cutting.

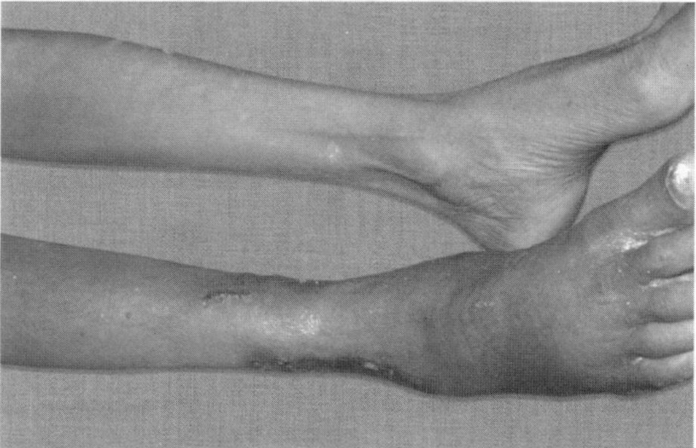

Fig. 40.48: Clinical appearance after plaster removal (1).

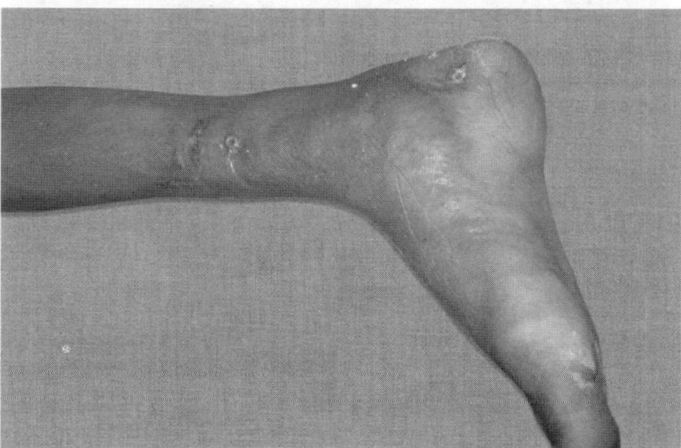

Fig. 40.49: Clinical appearance after plaster removal (2).

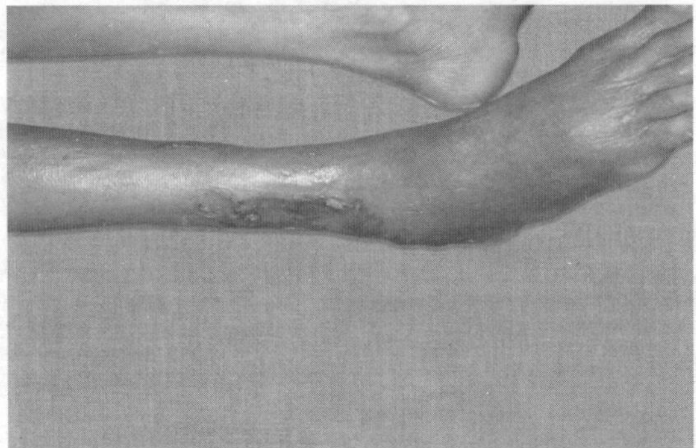

Fig. 40.50: Clinical appearance after plaster removal (3).

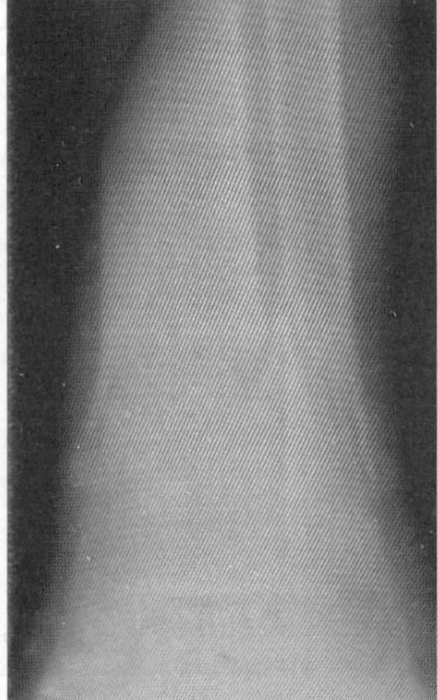

Fig. 40.51: Post-reduction X-ray (1).

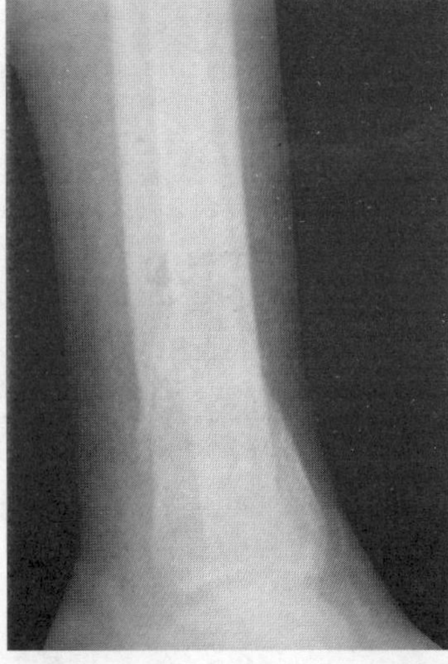

Fig. 40.52: Post-reduction X-ray (2).

Foot Injuries

This chapter deals with the practical techniques of managing the common heel injuries.

CALCANEAL FRACTURE

Undisplaced Calcaneal Fracture

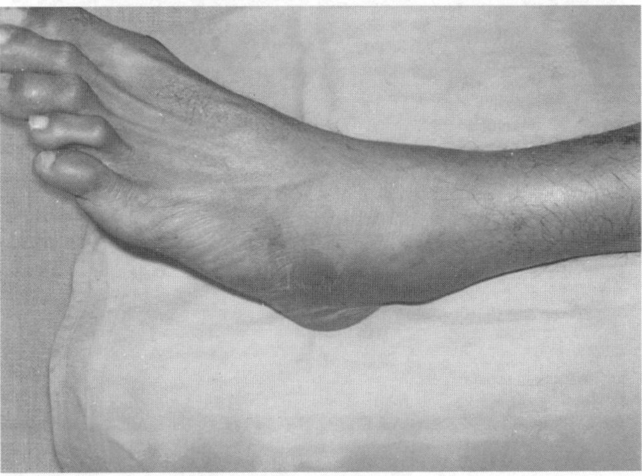

Fig. 41.1: Clinical deformity.

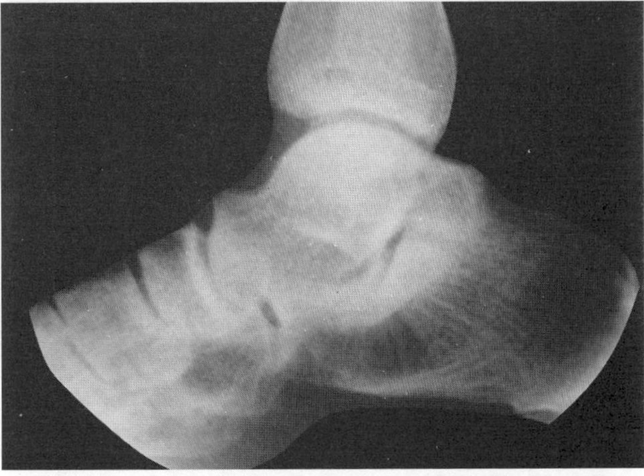

Fig. 41.2: Plain X-ray of the calcaneum—lateral view.

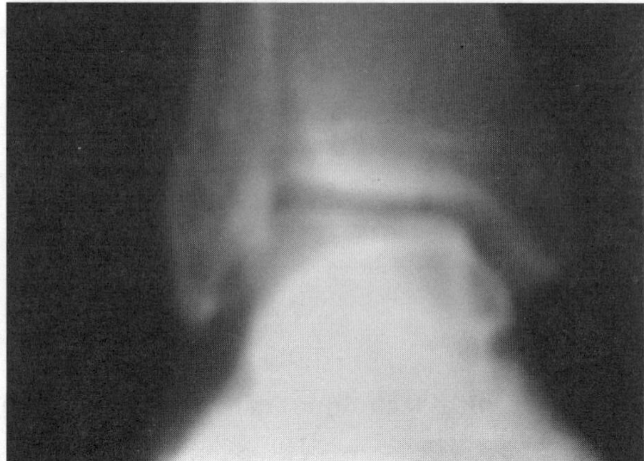

Fig. 41.3: Plain X-ray of the calcaneum—AP view.

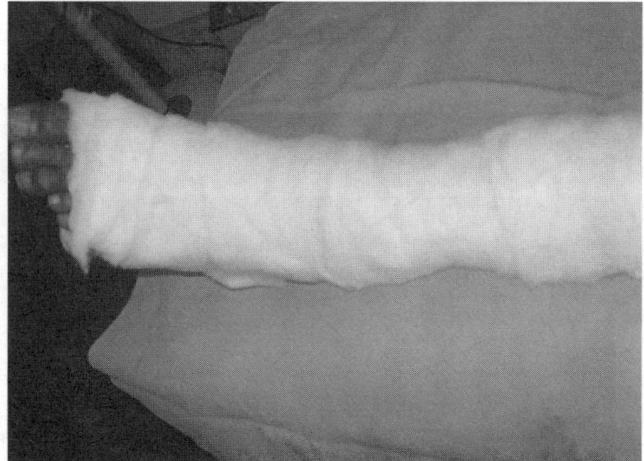

Fig. 41.4: Preparation for the cast application.

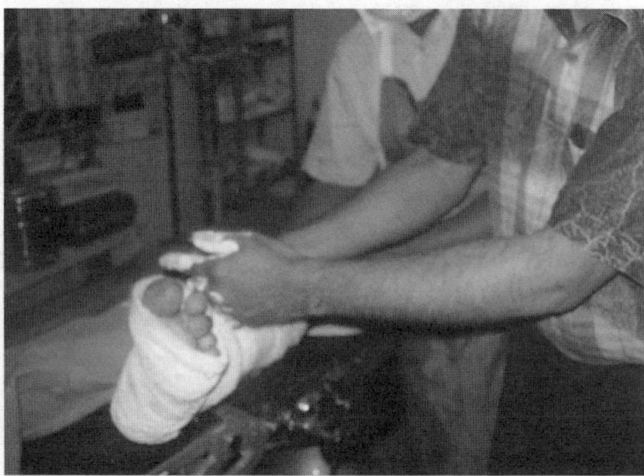

Fig. 41.5: Plaster application technique (1).

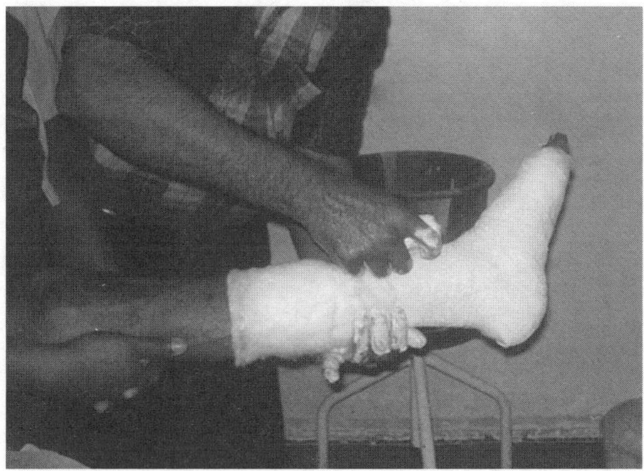

Fig. 41.6: Plaster application technique (2).

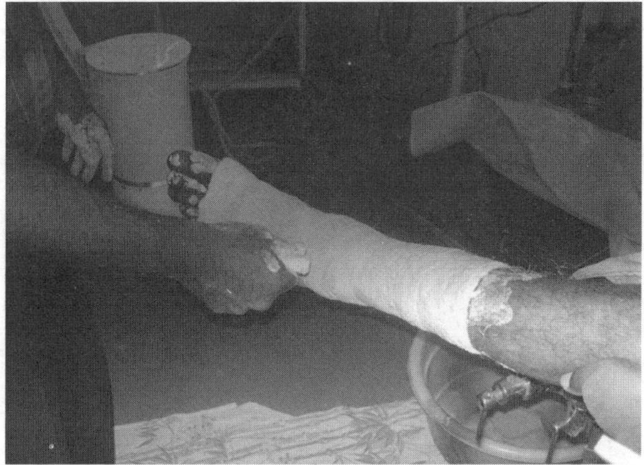

Fig. 41.7: Plaster application technique (3).

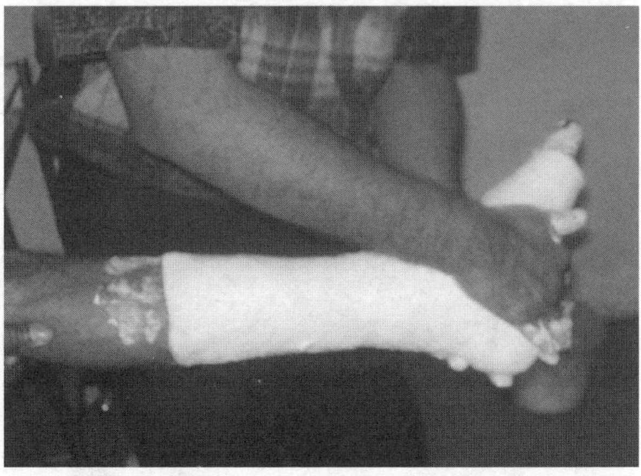

Fig. 41.8: Plaster application technique (4).

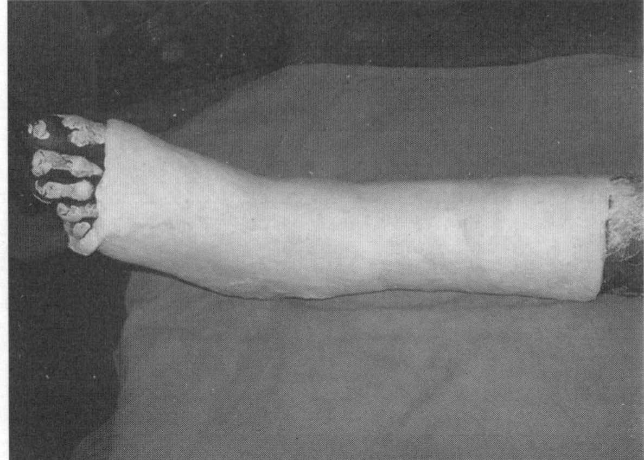

Fig. 41.9: Final appearance of the below knee plaster cast.

HEEL FRACTURE

Displaced Calcaneal Fracture

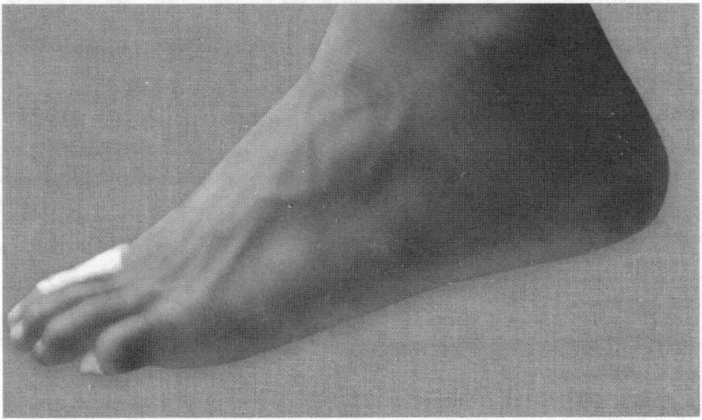

Fig. 41.10: Clinical deformity.

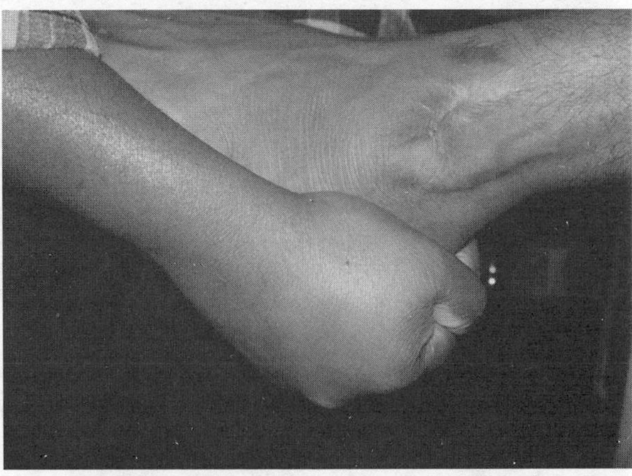

Fig. 41.11: Reduction of the deformity (1).

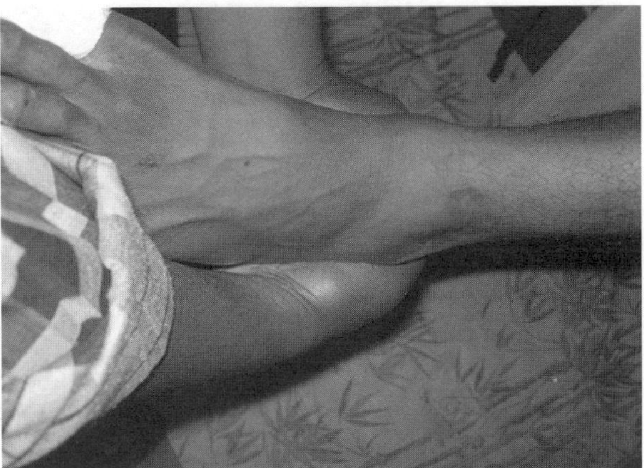

Fig. 41.12: Reduction of the deformity (2).

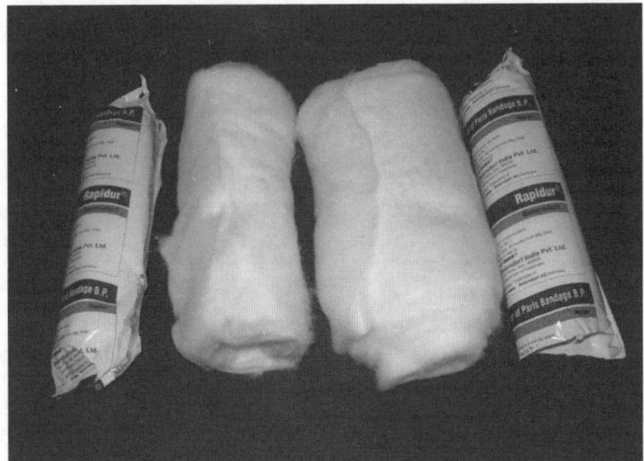

Fig. 41.13: Preparation for plaster application (1).

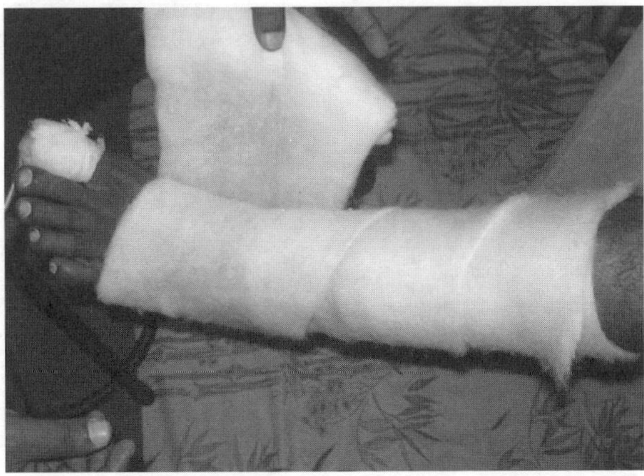

Fig. 41.14: Preparation for plaster application (2).

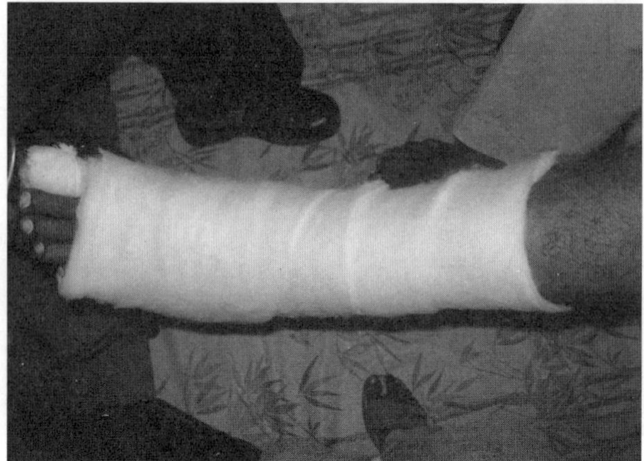

Fig. 41.15: Preparation for plaster application (3).

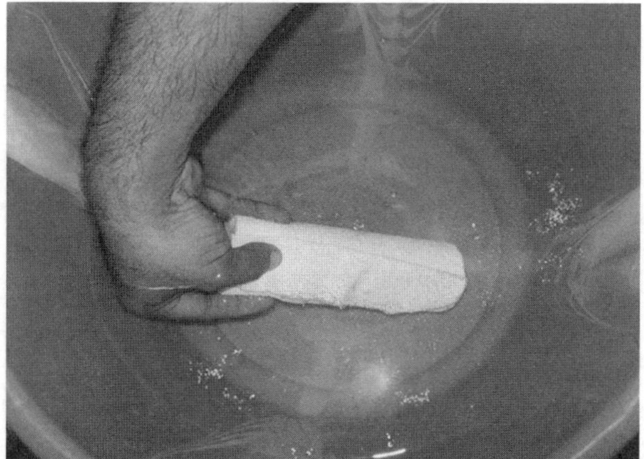

Fig. 41.16: Preparation for plaster application (4).

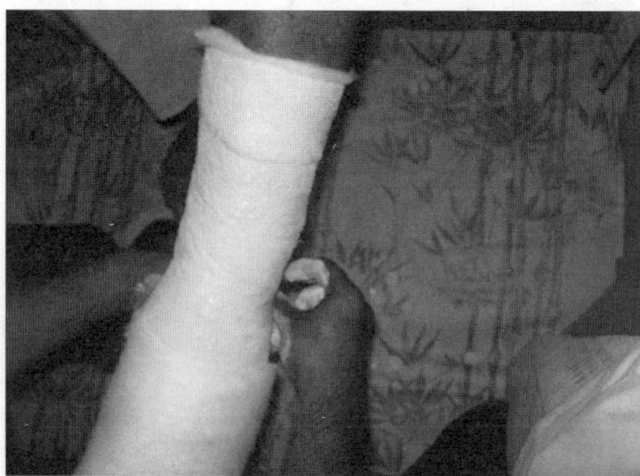

Fig. 41.17: Preparation for plaster application (5).

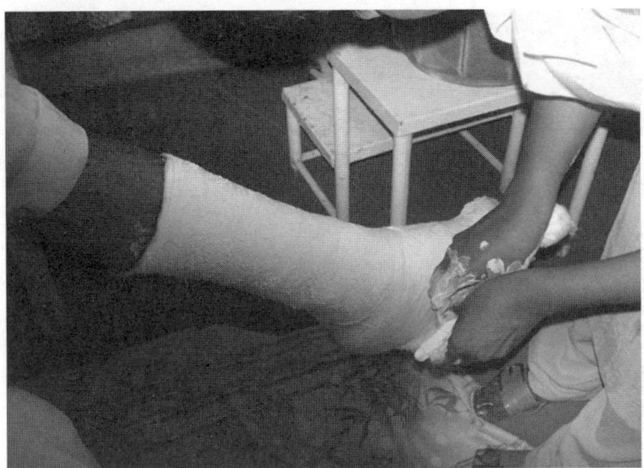

Fig. 41.18: Technique of plaster cast application (1).

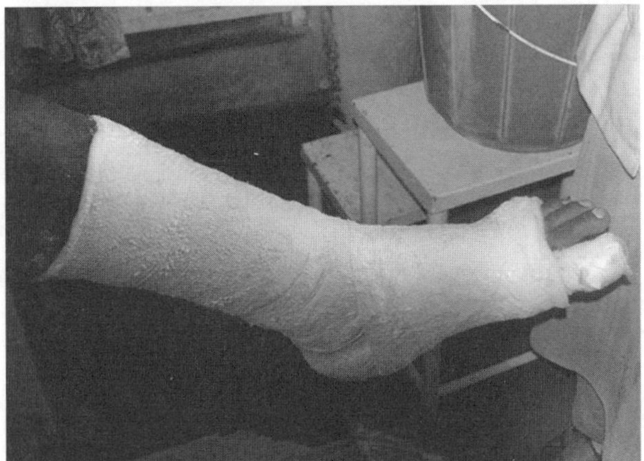

Fig. 41.19: Technique of plaster cast application (2).

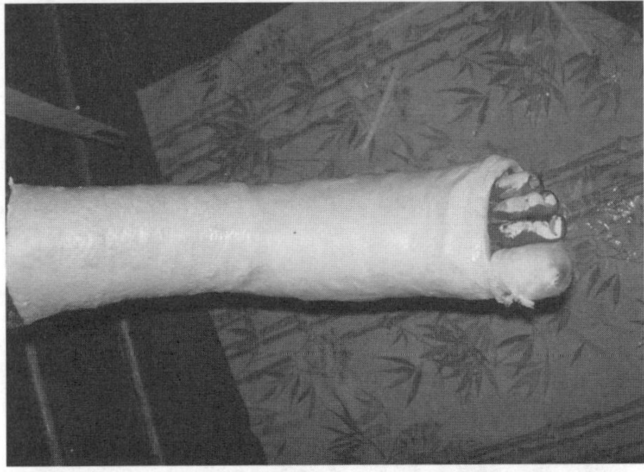

Fig. 41.20: Technique of plaster cast application (3).

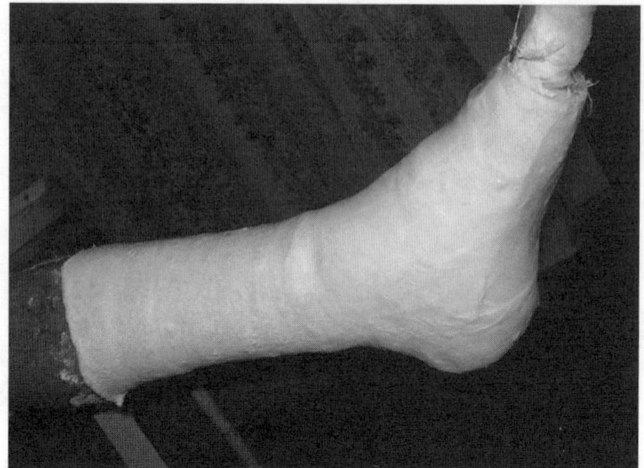

Fig. 41.21: Final look.

JONES FRACTURE

Fracture Base of V Metatarsal Bone

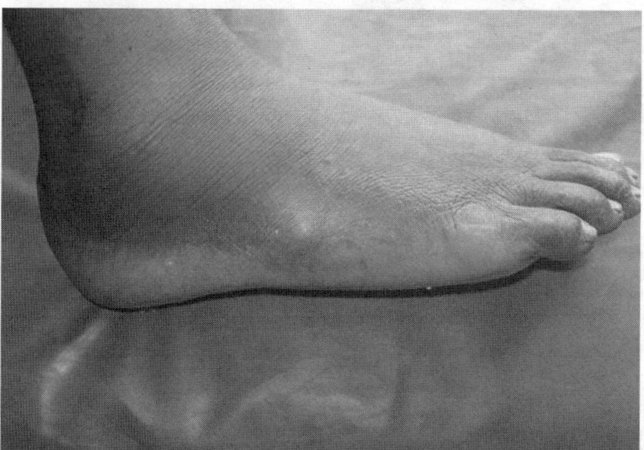

Fig. 41.22: Clinical deformity (1).

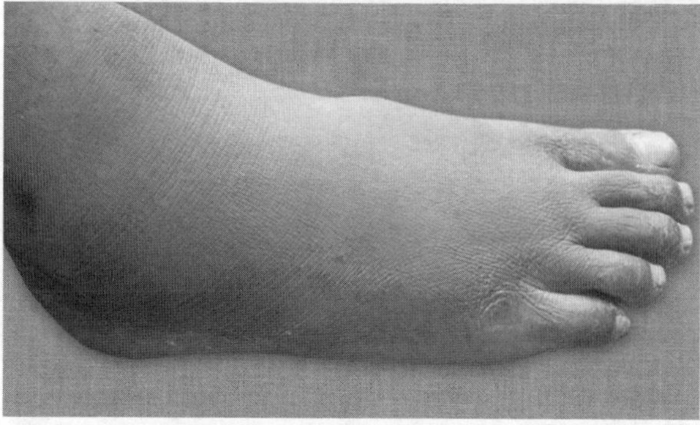

Fig. 41.23: Clinical deformity (2).

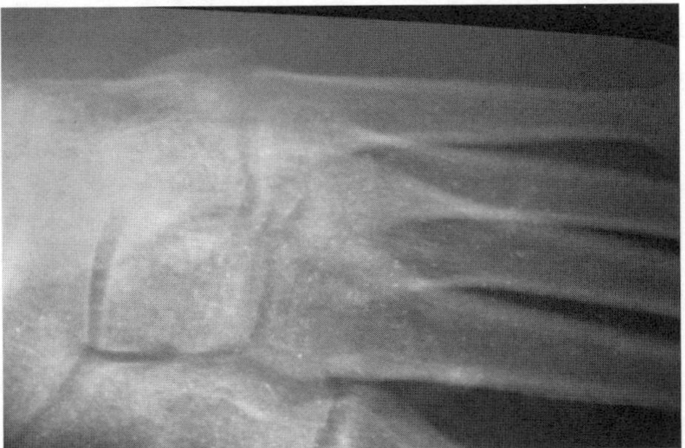

Fig. 41.24: Plain X-ray.

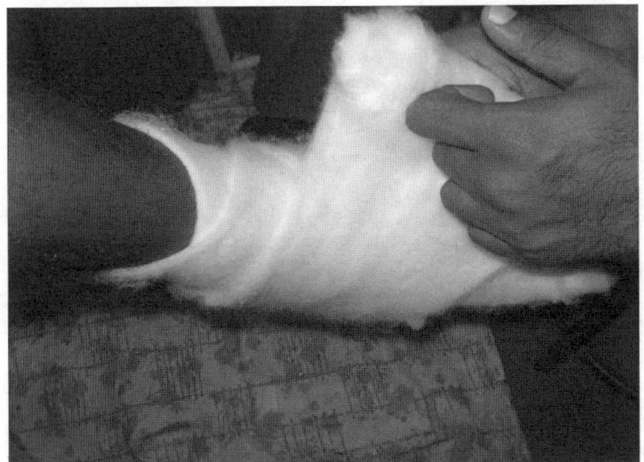

Fig. 41.25: Technique of plaster application (1).

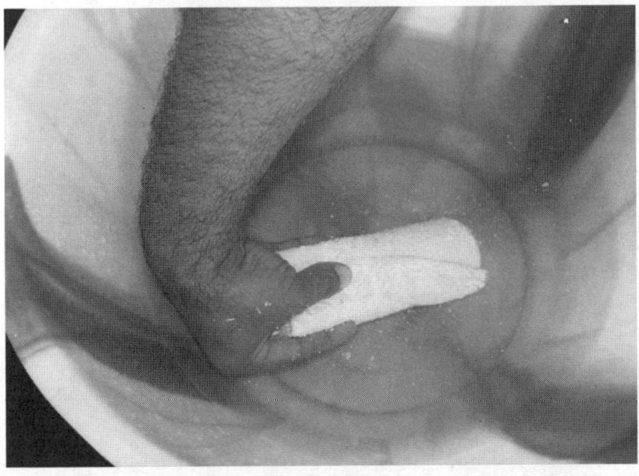

Fig. 41.26: Technique of plaster application (2).

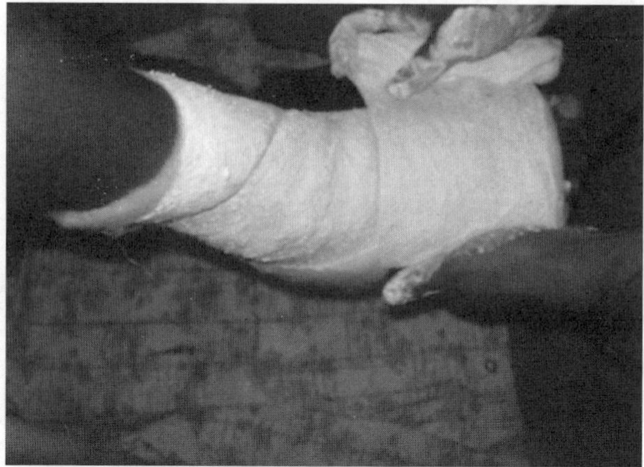

Fig. 41.27: Technique of plaster application (3).

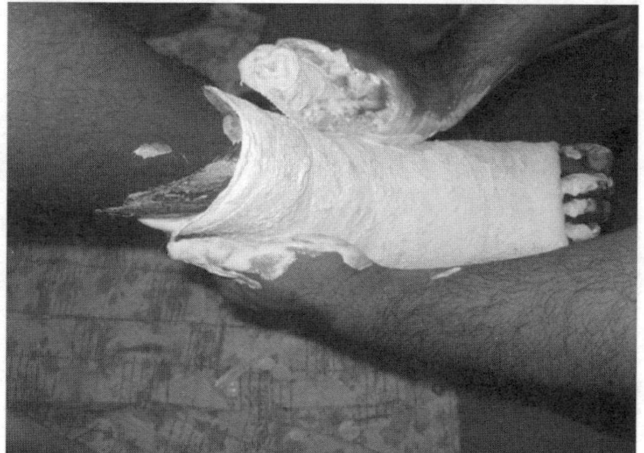

Fig. 41.28: Technique of plaster application (4).

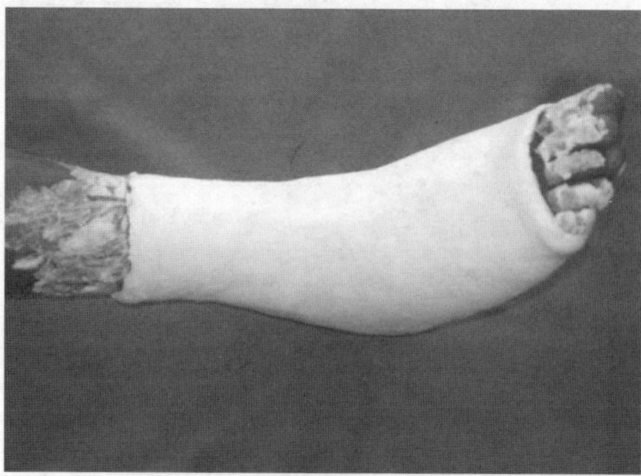

Fig. 41.29: Plaster applied.

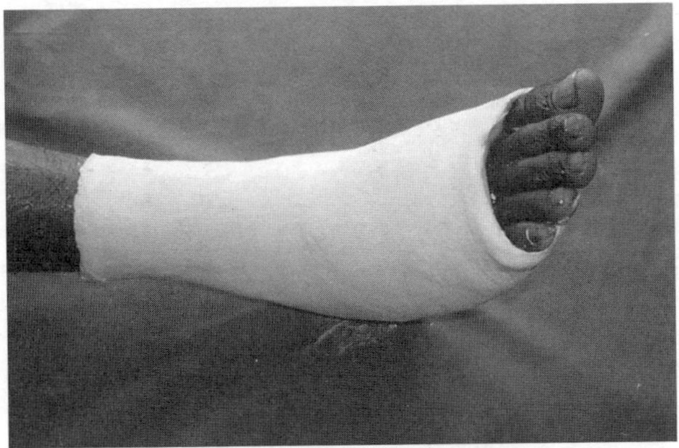

Fig. 41.30: Final look.

METATARSAL FRACTURES

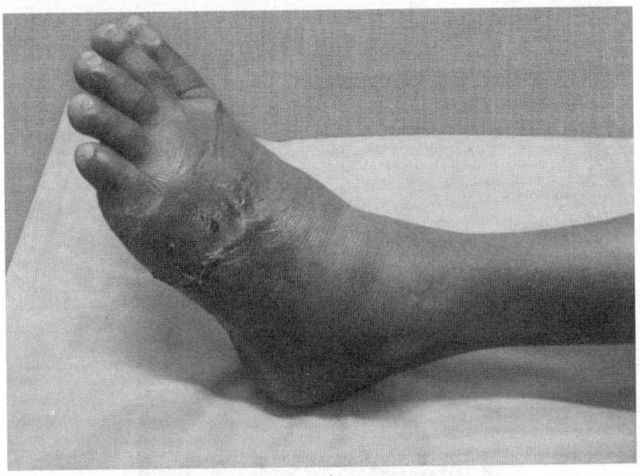

Fig. 41.31: Clinical deformity (1).

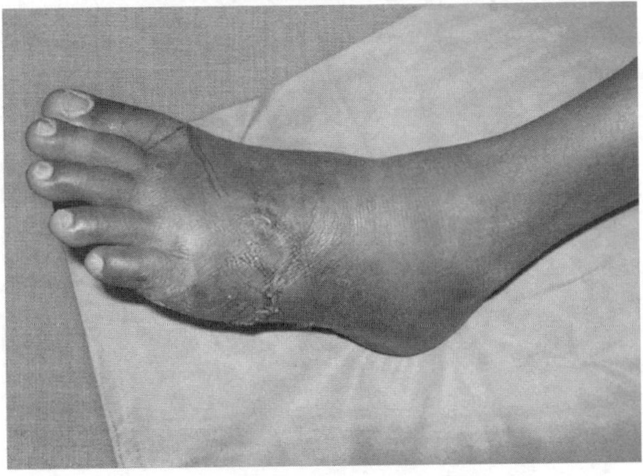

Fig. 41.32: Clinical deformity (2).

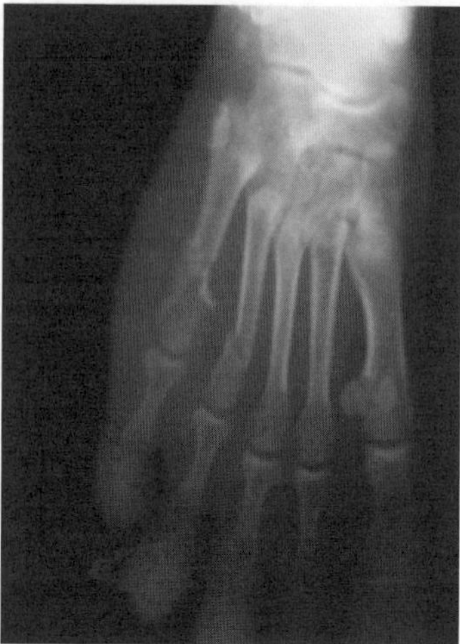

Fig. 41.33: Plain X-ray (1).

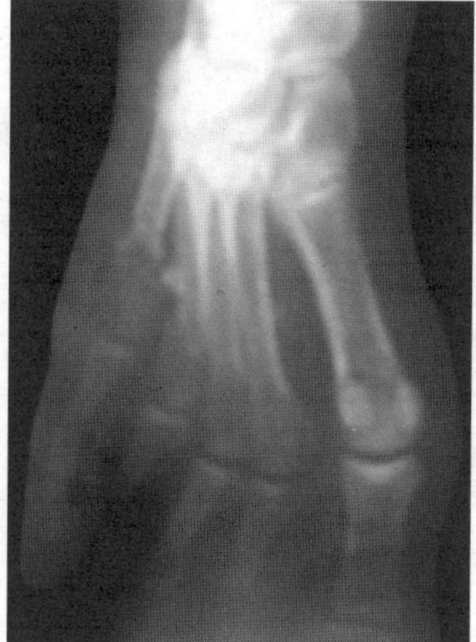

Fig. 41.34: Plain X-ray (2).

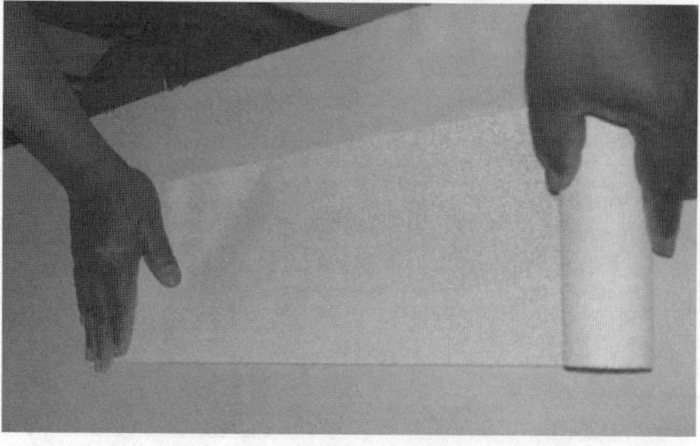

Fig. 41.35: Technique of plaster slab (1).

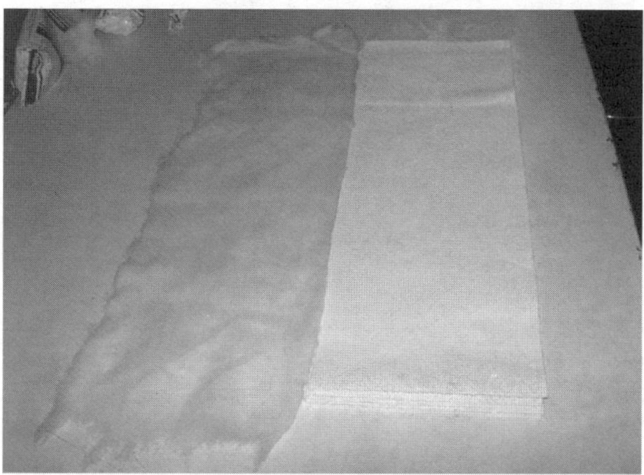

Fig. 41.36: Technique of plaster slab (2).

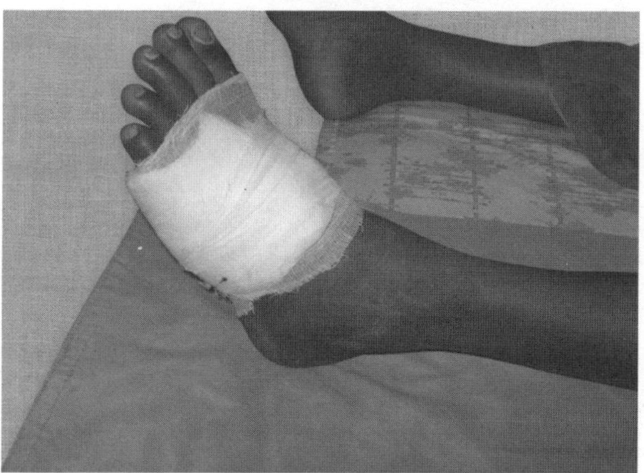

Fig. 41.37: Technique of plaster slab (3).

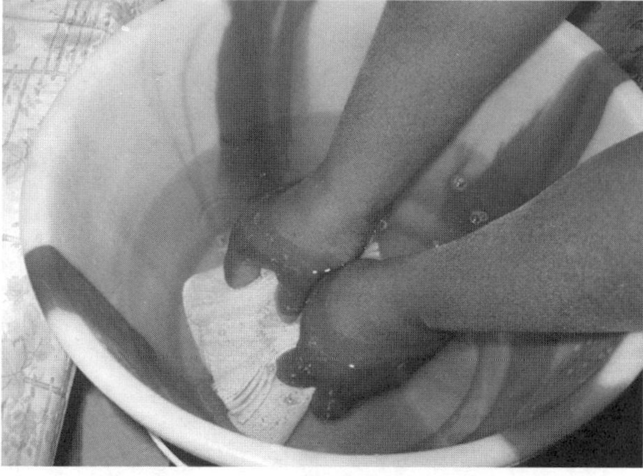

Fig. 41.38: Technique of plaster slab (4).

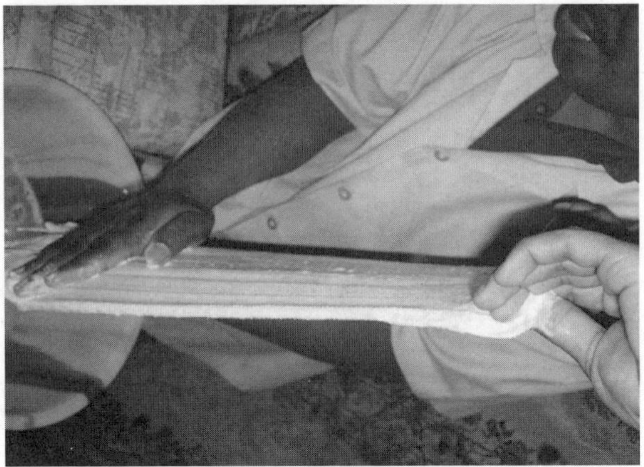

Fig. 41.39: Technique of plaster slab (5).

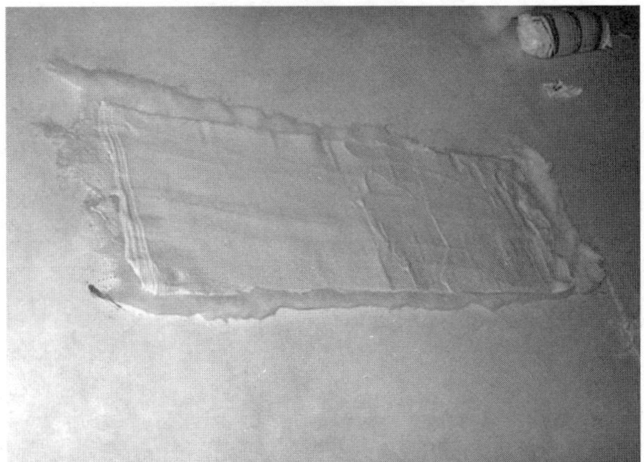

Fig. 41.40: Technique of plaster slab (6).

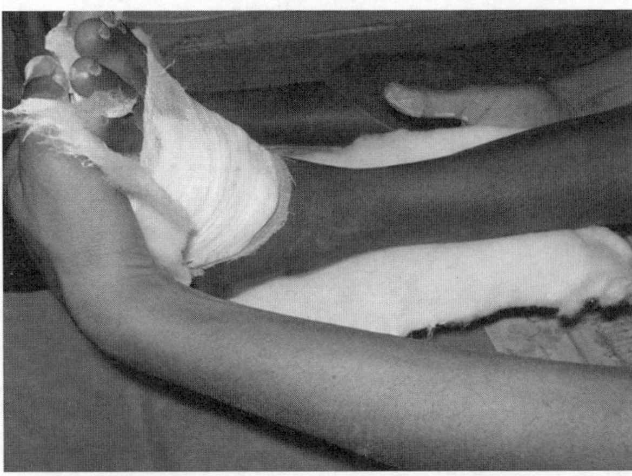

Fig. 41.41: Technique of plaster slab (7).

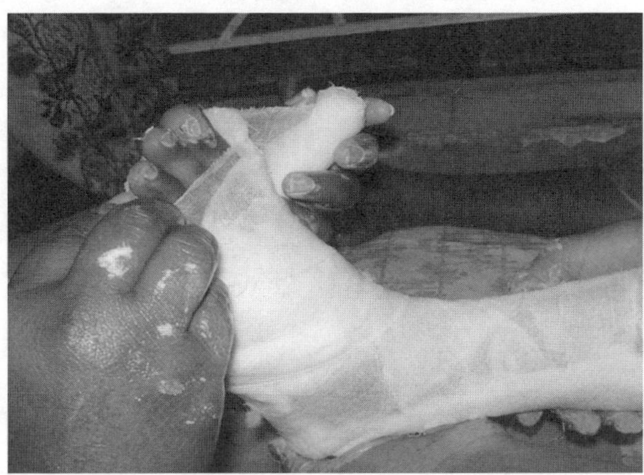

Fig. 41.42: Technique of plaster slab (8).

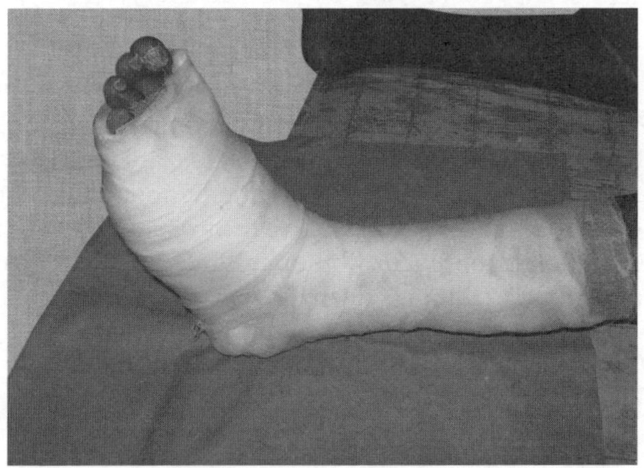

Fig. 41.43: Final look.

42
CHAPTER

Conventional Plaster Splints

PLASTER BANDAGES – BRIEF HISTORY

In Holland, in 1852 Antonius Mathijsen (1805–1878), a military surgeon, was on the look out of an immobilizing bandage that would permit the safe transport of patients with gunshot injuries to specialized treatment centers. He sought a bandage that could be used at once, would become hard in minutes and be adaptable to the extremity. Thus, he introduced plaster of Paris (POP) in 1876 at the centennial exhibition in Philadelphia. The use of POP bandages as cast and slabs became popular after his death.

GENERAL PRINCIPLES OF THE CONSERVATIVE METHODS OF FRACTURE TREATMENT

❖ **No treatment:** Some fractures needs no treatment. Nonsteroidal anti-inflammatory drugs (NSAIDs) and rest suffices, e.g., rib fractures (because of the efficient splinting action of the intercostal muscles).
❖ **Strapping:** Merely strapping certain fractures to the adjacent normal structures like in undisplaced phalanx fracture of fingers and toes is sufficient. Other fractures that are treated by strapping are fracture of clavicle, scapula, proximal humeral fractures, etc.
❖ **Slings:** These are used to treat undisplaced upper limb fractures or as first aid measures.
❖ **Plaster treatment methods:** Two modalities are described.
   a. *Merely support by plaster slabs or splints:* In undisplaced fractures, incomplete fractures, stress fractures, fatigue fractures, support by POP slab often suffices.
   b. *Reduction and support with plaster cast:* Displaced fractures need to be reduced under general anesthesia before splinting with plaster casts. Reduction can be brought about either by manipulative traction and counter traction methods or by skeletal or skin traction. Principles of closed reduction have already been discussed. Plaster of Paris plays a big role in the conservative management of fractures.
   c. *Spica cast:* This is a plaster cast, which encircles a part of the body other than the limb. For example, hip spica, thumb spica, etc.
   d. *Traction:* This comparatively plays a less important role and is discussed in detail in a separate section.

> **Remember**
>
> The cardinal rule of reducing any displaced fracture is to reverse the mechanism of injury preferably under general anesthesia and muscle relaxation.

All you Wanted to Know About Plaster of Paris Splint

History

The name plaster of Paris originated from an accident to a house built on deposit of gypsum near the city of Paris. The house was accidentally burnt down. When it rained on the next day, it was noted that the footprints of the people in the mud had set rock hard. Mathysen, a Dutch surgeon, first used plaster of Paris in orthopedics in 1852. It is made from gypsum, which is a naturally occurring mineral. It is commercially available since 1931.

Chemical Formula

It is a hemihydrated calcium sulphate. To make plaster of Paris, gypsum is heated to drive off water. When water is added to the resulting powder, original mineral reforms and is set hard.

$$2\,(CaSO_4 .\ 2\,H_2O) + Heat \leftrightarrow 2(CaSO_4 .\ \tfrac{1}{2}\,H_2O) + 3H_2O$$

POP Types

Indigenous prepared from ordinary cotton bandage role smeared with POP powder.

Commercial: Plaster of Paris rolls commercially prepared consists of rolls of muslin stiffened by starch, POP powder and an accelerator substance like alum. This commercial preparation sets very fast and gives a neat finish unlike the indigenous ones.

Why is plaster of Paris an ideal splint?

- It is cheap.
- It is easily available.
- It is comfortable.
- It is easy to mould.
- It is quick setting.
- It is strong and light.
- It is easy to remove.
- It is permeable to radiography.
- It is permeable to air and hence underlying skin can breathe.
- It is noninflammable.

Its Various Forms

Plaster of Paris is used in four forms as slab, cast, spica, and functional cast brace.

Slab

It is a temporary splint used in the initial stages of fracture treatment and during first aid. It is useful to immobilize the limbs postoperatively and in infections. It is made up of half by POP and half by bandage roll and hence can accommodate the swelling in the initial stages of fractures.

Slab is prepared according to the required length. There are three methods of applying a slab:

1. *Dry method:* Here the slab is prepared first and then dipped in water (commonly employed).
2. *Wet method:* Here the slab is prepared after dipping the POP roll in water. This is rare and requires experience.
3. *Pattern method:* Here the slabs are fashioned in the desired way before dipping it in water.

Casts

Here the POP roll completely encircles the limb **(Figs. 42.1 A to D)**. It is used as a definitive form of fracture treatment and to correct deformities. There are two methods of applying a POP cast:

1. *Traditional cast (Bologna cast):* Here generous amount of cotton padding is applied to the limb before putting the cast. This is the commonly employed method.
2. *Three-tier cast:* Here stockinette is used first over which cotton padding is done before applying the POP cast.

Spica

This encircles a part of the body, e.g., hip spica for fracture around the hip **(Fig. 42.1C)**, thumb spica for fracture scaphoid.

Functional Cast Brace

This is used for fracture tibia after initial immobilization **(Fig. 42.1D)**.

Rules of Application of POP Casts
1. Choose the correct size, 8 inches for the thigh, 6 inches for the leg, and 4 inches for the forearm.
2. A joint above and a joint below should be included. Accordingly, we have an above elbow **(Fig. 42.1A)** or below elbow, POP cast or slab and above knee **(Fig. 42.1B)** or below knee POP cast or slab. This is done to eliminate movements of the joints on either side of the fractures. However, this is not a hard and fast rule in certain fractures, like a below elbow cast in Colles' fracture, which often suffices.
3. It should be moulded with the palm and not the fingers for fear of indentation.
4. The joints should be immobilized in functional positions.
5. The plaster should just snugly fit and should not be too tight or too loose.
6. Uniform thickness of the plaster is preferred.

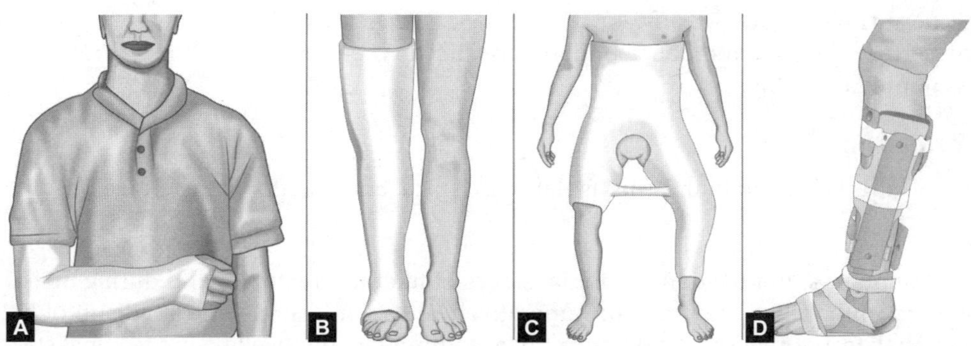

Figs. 42.1A to D: Types of plaster applications: (A) Above elbow cast; (B) Above knee cast; (C) Hip spica; (D) Functional cast brace.

Stages of Plastering

First stage: Involves application of POP slab or cast **(Fig. 42.2)**.

Second stage or cast setting stage: This is change of POP to gypsum and is defined as the time taken to form a rigid dressing after contact with water.

Third stage or green stage: This is the just set wet cast.

Fourth stage or cast drying: By evaporation of excess water when the cast dries. This results in a mature cast with multiple air pockets through which the skin breathes.

Complications of POP

Due to tight fit
- Pain
- Pressure sores
- Compartmental syndromes
- Peripheral nerve injuries
- Cast syndrome (Also called Cast disease).

Due to improper application
- Joint stiffness
- Plaster blisters and sores
- Breakage.

Due to plaster allergy
- Allergic dermatitis.

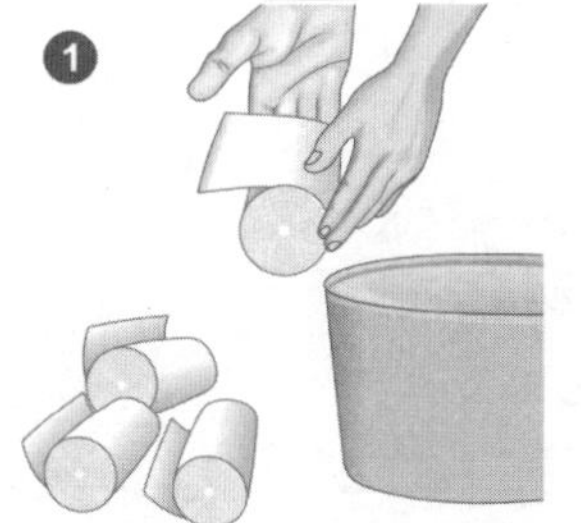

Unwrap the required number of bandages and keep ready for immersion. Wet only one bandage at a time

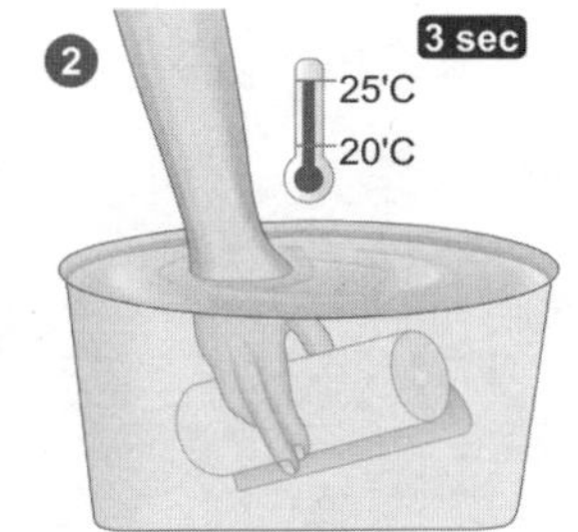

Immerse in a bowl of clean, tepid water diagonally until bubbles cease (approx. 3 seconds). Change water frequently

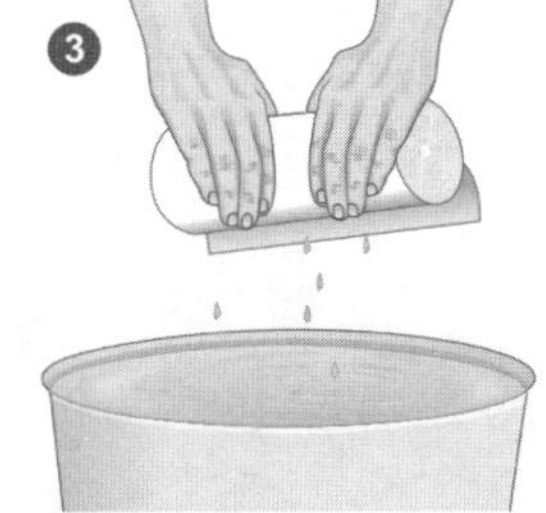

Remove bandage and gently squeeze it from edges to center to expel surplus water

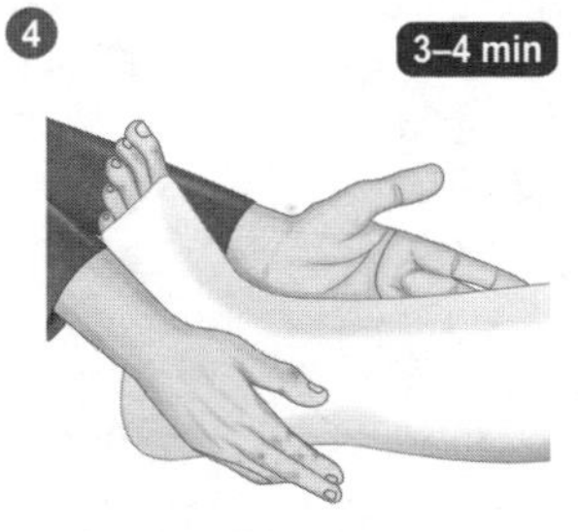

Normal setting time is 3–4 minutes. To retard, use common borax

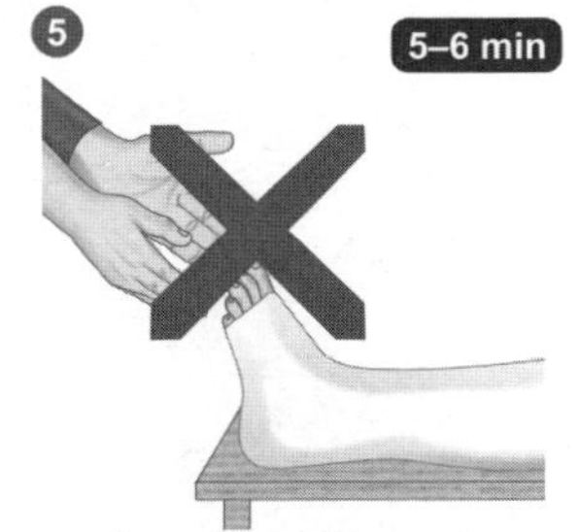

Do not mould the cast after 5–6 minutes

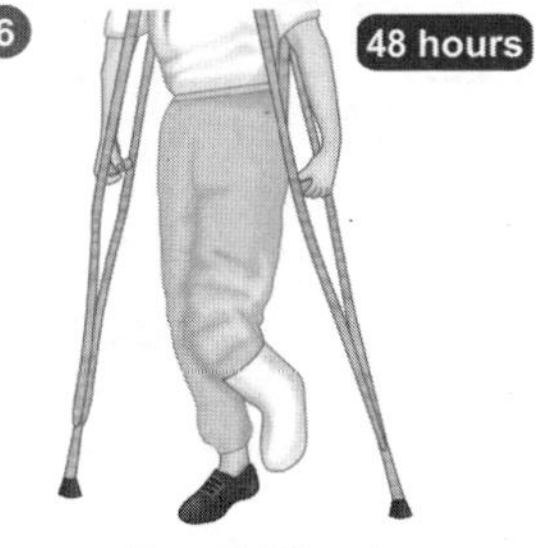

No weightbearing before 48 hours

Fig. 42.2: Steps of application of plaster cast.

Unpleasant Facts about Cast Disease

- ❖ Muscle atrophy.
- ❖ Osteoporosis.
- ❖ Joint stiffness.
- ❖ Muscle weakness.
- ❖ Skin breakdown.
- ❖ Compartmental syndrome.
- ❖ Blister formation.

Remember about POP

- ◂◂ Used first in the city of Paris
- ◂◂ The ideal splint
- ◂◂ Slab for temporary and initial treatment
- ◂◂ Casts for definitive treatment
- ◂◂ Spica for hip fracture, etc.
- ◂◂ Functional cast brace for early mobilization

Index

Page numbers followed by *f* refer to figure.